NATIONAL ACADEMIES

Sciences
Engineering
Medicine

NATIONAL
ACADEMIES
PRESS
Washington, DC

Measuring Meaningful Outcomes for Adult Hearing Health Interventions

Committee on Meaningful
Outcome Measures in Adult
Hearing Health Care

Board on Health Care Services

Health and Medicine Division

Consensus Study Report

NATIONAL ACADEMIES PRESS 500 Fifth Street, NW Washington, DC 20001

This activity was supported by contracts between the National Academy of Sciences and the Centers for Disease Control and Prevention, the Defense Health Agency (contract no. HT942524P0098), the Department of Veterans Affairs, the National Institute on Aging and the National Institute on Deafness and Other Communication Disorders under a contract with the National Institutes of Health (contract no. HHSN263201800029I and task order no. 75N98023F00011), and NAS Endowment.

International Standard Book Number-13: 978-0-309-99237-4
International Standard Book Number-10: 0-309-99237-0
Digital Object Identifier: https://doi.org/10.17226/29104
Library of Congress Control Number: 2025938400

This publication is available from the National Academies Press, 500 Fifth Street, NW, Keck 360, Washington, DC 20001; (800) 624-6242; http://www.nap.edu.

Suggested citation: National Academies of Sciences, Engineering, and Medicine. 2025. *Measuring meaningful outcomes for adult hearing health interventions.* Washington, DC: National Academies Press. https://doi.org/10.17226/29104.

The **National Academy of Sciences** was established in 1863 by an Act of Congress, signed by President Lincoln, as a private, nongovernmental institution to advise the nation on issues related to science and technology. Members are elected by their peers for outstanding contributions to research. Dr. Marcia McNutt is president.

The **National Academy of Engineering** was established in 1964 under the charter of the National Academy of Sciences to bring the practices of engineering to advising the nation. Members are elected by their peers for extraordinary contributions to engineering. Dr. Tsu-Jae Liu is president.

The **National Academy of Medicine** (formerly the Institute of Medicine) was established in 1970 under the charter of the National Academy of Sciences to advise the nation on medical and health issues. Members are elected by their peers for distinguished contributions to medicine and health. Dr. Victor J. Dzau is president.

The three Academies work together as the **National Academies of Sciences, Engineering, and Medicine** to provide independent, objective analysis and advice to the nation and conduct other activities to solve complex problems and inform public policy decisions. The National Academies also encourage education and research, recognize outstanding contributions to knowledge, and increase public understanding in matters of science, engineering, and medicine.

Learn more about the National Academies of Sciences, Engineering, and Medicine at **www.nationalacademies.org**.

Reviewers

This Consensus Study Report was reviewed in draft form by individuals chosen for their diverse perspectives and technical expertise. The purpose of this independent review is to provide candid and critical comments that will assist the National Academies of Sciences, Engineering, and Medicine in making each published report as sound as possible and to ensure that it meets the institutional standards for quality, objectivity, evidence, and responsiveness to the study charge. The review comments and draft manuscript remain confidential to protect the integrity of the deliberative process.

We thank the following individuals for their review of this report:

RICHARD ALBA, City University of New York
KATHERINE BOUTON, Hearing Loss Association of America
CHRIS GREAME, Health Care Executive
RONALD HAYS, University of California, Los Angeles
ROBERT KAPLAN, Stanford University
RYAN McCREERY, Boys Town National Research Hospital
TODD RICKETTS, Vanderbilt University Medical Center
HINRICH STAECKER, University of Kansas Medical Center
ANDREW VERMIGLIO, East Carolina University
BLAKE WILSON, Duke University
SARAH WINGFIELD, University of Texas Southwestern Medical Center
YU-HSIANG WU, The University of Iowa

Although the reviewers listed above provided many constructive comments and suggestions, they were not asked to endorse the conclusions or recommendations of this report nor did they see the final draft before its release. The review of this report was overseen by **DAVID B. REUBEN,** University of California, Los Angeles, and **DAN G. BLAZER, II,** Duke University. They were responsible for making certain that an independent examination of this report was carried out in accordance with the standards of the National Academies and that all review comments were carefully considered. Responsibility for the final content rests entirely with the authoring committee and the National Academies.

Acknowledgments

The study committee and the Health and Medicine Division project staff take this opportunity to recognize and thank the many individuals who shared their time and expertise to support the committee's work and to inform deliberations. The committee appreciates the sponsors of this study for their generous financial support: the Centers for Disease Control and Prevention, the Defense Health Agency, the Department of Veterans Affairs, the National Institute on Aging, the National Institute on Deafness and Other Communication Disorders, and NAS Endowment. The contents provided do not necessarily represent the official views of the sponsors.

Over the course of its meetings, the committee heard from many people who shared their stories about their hearing difficulties, particularly regarding what outcomes are most meaningful to them. The committee thanks the participants from its public sessions: Katherine Bouton, Chris Greame, Suzanne Johnston, Eric Matson, Russell Misheloff, Elizabeth Pentin, Kerry Sullivan, and Wynne Whyman. The committee is also grateful for the many submissions to this committee by adults with hearing difficulties as well as their clinicians and care partners.

Additionally, the committee benefited greatly from discussions with representatives of the project's sponsors, hearing health care clinicians, and representatives from professional groups who participated during the committee's open sessions:

Yulia Carroll, Centers for Disease Control and Prevention
Lee Cottrell, Balance and Hearing Institute at Farragut ENT & Allergy
Patricia Gaffney, American Academy of Audiologists

Kelly King, National Institute on Deafness and Other Communication
    Disorders, National Institutes of Health
Rachel McArdle, Veterans Health Administration
Erica Person, Flex Audiology
Sierra Sharpe, International Hearing Society
Donna Smiley, American Speech-Language-Hearing Association
Alicia Spoor, Academy of Doctors of Audiology
Tim Steele, Associated Audiologists, Inc.

The committee is grateful to Erin Giovannetti and Bryan Luce for their
early contributions to this project. Deep appreciation goes to the many
staff within the National Academies who provided support at various
times throughout this project, especially to Violet Bishop, Lori Brenig, Sam
Gerard, Megan Lowry, Amber McLaughlin, Rebecca Morgan, Leslie Sim,
and Taryn Young. The committee and project staff are grateful to Robert
Pool for his drafting and editorial assistance to prepare this report.

Contents

7   **DISSEMINATION AND IMPLEMENTATION**   195

APPENDIXES

Boxes, Figures, and Tables

BOXES

FIGURES

TABLES

Acronyms and Abbreviations

AAA	American Academy of Audiology
ABR	auditory brainstem response
ACT	Audible Contrast Threshold
ADA	Academy of Doctors of Audiology
APHAB	Abbreviated Profile of Hearing Aid Benefit
APHAP	Abbreviated Profile of Hearing Aid Performance
ASHA	American Speech-Language Hearing Association
AURONET	Auditory Rehabilitation Outcomes Network
BKB-SIN	Bamford-Kowal-Bench Speech in Noise
CESD-5	Center for Epidemiologic Studies Depression Scale 5
COM-B	capability, opportunity, motivation-behavior
COMET	Core Outcome Measures in Effectiveness Trials
COMiT'ID	Core Outcome Measures in Tinnitus International Delphi
COS	core outcome set
COSI	Client-Oriented Scale of Improvement
COSMIN	COnsensus-based Standards for the selection of health Measurement INstruments
COS-STAD	Core Outcome Set-STAndards for Development
CPHI	Communication Profile for the Hearing Impaired
CQMC	Core Quality Measures Collaborative

dB	decibel
dB HL	decibels hearing level
dB SPL	decibels sound pressure level
DIN	Digits-in-Noise
DSL v.5	Desired Sensation Level Version 5
EHIMA	European Hearing Instrument Manufacturers Association
EHR	electronic health record
ENT	ear, nose, and throat
EQ-5D	European Quality of Life 5-Dimension
ET-F	2022 EuroTrak in France
ET-G	2022 EuroTrak in Germany
FDA	U.S. Food and Drug Administration
FUEL	Framework for Understanding Effortful Listening
gEAR	gene Expression Analysis Resource
GHABP	Glasglow Hearing-Aid Benefit Profile
HALex	Health and Activities Limitation Index
HEAL	Helping to End Addiction Long-term
HHI	Hearing Handicap Inventory
HHIA	Hearing Handicap Inventory for Adults
HHIE	Hearing Handicap Inventory for the Elderly
HHIE-S	Hearing Handicap Inventory for the Elderly—Screening
HINT	Hearing in Noise Test
HLAA	Hearing Loss Association of America
HUI2	Health Utilities Index 2
HUI3	Health Utilities Index 3
ICF	International Classification of Functioning, Disability, and Health
IHS	International Hearing Society
ILD	interaural level difference
IOI	International Outcome Inventory
IOI-HA	International Outcome Inventory for Hearing Aids
IRT	item response theory
ITD	interaural timing difference
MCID	minimal clinically important difference
MDC	minimal detectable change
MT2022	MarkeTrak

NAL-NL2	National Acoustic Laboratories Non-Linear 2
NHANES	National Health and Nutrition Examination Survey
NHS	National Health Service
NIDCD	National Institute on Deafness and Other Communication Disorders
NIH	National Institutes of Health
NIHL	noise-induced hearing loss
NORA	National Occupational Research Agenda
NQF	National Quality Forum
OMERACT	Outcome Measures in Rheumatology
OMER-ED	Outcome Measures in Rheumatology Education
OTOF	otoferlin
PHAB	Profile of Hearing Aid Benefit
PHAP	Profile of Hearing Aid Performance
PHQ-9	patient health questionnaire
POD-Vis	Probing Outcomes Data with Visual Analytics
PQM	Partnership for Quality Measurement
PROM	patient-reported outcome measure
PROMIS	Patient-Reported Outcome Measurement Information System
PROMIS-29	Patient-Reported Outcomes Measurement Information System 29
QoL	quality of life
QuickSIN	Quick Speech-in-Noise
QWB-SA	Quality of Well-Being scale—self-administered
RE-AIM	reach, adoption, implementation, and maintenance
RHHI	Revised Hearing Handicap Inventory
RHHI-S	Revised Hearing Handicap Inventory—Screening
SEM	standard error of measurement
SF-6D	Short-Form 6-Dimension
SNR	signal-to-noise ratio
SPIRIT	Standard Protocol Items: Recommendations for Interventional Trials
SRM	standardized response mean
SRT	speech recognition threshold
SSQ	Speech, Spatial, and Qualities of Hearing Scale
TINNET	TINnitus research NETwork

VA   Department of Veterans Affairs

WHO   World Health Organization
WHODAS II   World Health Organization's Disability Assessment
              Scale II
WIN   Words-in-Noise

Summary

Hearing loss is the most common sensory disorder in the United States, and the prevalence and severity of hearing loss—and hearing difficulties—increase with age. While approximately one in five Americans experience hearing loss, most individuals with hearing loss (about 83 percent) are over the age of 50. The term *hearing loss* is generally used to reflect a diagnosis based on a clinical measurement of hearing ability, often using the pure-tone audiogram.[1] The term *hearing difficulties*, on the other hand, is more strongly associated with hearing trouble perceived by the individual and may or may not be reported by adults with measured hearing loss. Hearing difficulties may also be perceived by adults without measurable hearing loss. The value of interventions for hearing difficulties in adults depends, in part, on what aspects of an individual's lived experience matter the most to that person. Evaluations of the effectiveness of interventions that do not consider these important lived experiences may not accurately capture individuals' perceptions of their functional abilities or the effect their hearing difficulties have on their quality of life.

While diagnostic tests are used to determine the cause of signs and symptoms, outcome measures are used to evaluate an intervention's effect. When assessing the effect of an intervention, researchers and clinicians can consider a multitude of outcomes to measure. A core outcome set

---

[1] In this report, the committee favors the use of the term *adult with hearing difficulties*, which is more focused on perceived troubles with hearing. However, the term *hearing loss* is used when referring specifically to a measured impairment, diagnosis, or when citing an original source.

recommends the specific outcomes (i.e., areas of hearing, communication, and beyond) that should be measured and reported, at a minimum. The use of a core outcome set—and of specific corresponding measures (i.e., the tools or instruments used to assess those core outcomes)—can enhance the consistency and quality of research, facilitate the comparison of different interventions, support clinical decision making, and focus on the outcomes that matter the most to adults with hearing difficulties. However, although several groups have created core outcome sets for specific hearing loss etiologies or interventions, no core outcome set has been broadly accepted by the hearing health community.

STATEMENT OF TASK AND STUDY FOCUS

With support from a coalition of sponsors, the National Academies of Sciences, Engineering, and Medicine (the National Academies) formed the Committee on Meaningful Outcome Measures in Adult Hearing Health Care in late 2023. The committee comprised 13 members with a broad range of expertise, including hearing health care, etiology of and interventions for hearing loss (and hearing difficulties), outcome measurement, primary care, disability and rehabilitation, quality of life, health disparities, public health, and epidemiology. The sponsors charged the committee with examining the state of the science in outcomes research for hearing health interventions in adults and to recommend the outcomes (the core outcome set) and corresponding outcome measures that should be used across interventions and settings at this time, with an emphasis on the outcomes that are most meaningful to adults with hearing difficulties and the clinicians who treat them.[2] The committee also was charged with making recommendations on areas of needed research on meaningful outcome domains (including hearing, communication, and domains beyond hearing and communication)[3] and on the approaches needed to guide the development and refinement of standardized measures.

This report focuses on meaningful outcomes and the measures used to evaluate the efficacy and effectiveness of interventions rather than focusing on the types of assessments used to diagnose hearing loss or determine candidacy for various devices. While the committee contends that outcome measurement is an important part of clinical practice and research, this study does not focus on whether outcome measurement should be done. Rather, the committee starts with the assumption that outcome measurement is being performed and provides recommendations for the outcomes

---

[2] The complete statement of task is presented in Chapter 1 of this report.

[3] A health outcome reflects a change in health attributable to an intervention. Several related outcomes may be grouped into a category called an *outcome domain.*

that are most meaningful to measure and the measures that are most appropriate to use in order to create more consistency in outcome measurement for hearing health interventions.

BACKGROUND

The most common causes of hearing loss are age; exposures to noise, ototoxic drugs or chemicals; and genetics. Age-related hearing loss begins in early adulthood and progresses gradually. A range of risk factors exacerbate age-related hearing loss, including gender, ethnicity, environment, lifestyle, health comorbidities, and genetics. Some common characteristics of age-related and noise-induced hearing loss are progressive bilateral hearing loss, an inability to hear sounds at high frequencies, and challenges understanding speech, particularly in complex listening situations such as with background noise. Several approaches to treating hearing loss exist, and the choice of intervention may depend upon the etiology of the individual's hearing loss and their goals. However, hearing aids have been the most common treatment for several decades.

COMMITTEE PROCESS

The committee followed several general best practices that have been identified for developing core outcome sets, including specifying a clear scope, involving key partners, and using a consensus process.

For this study, the scope was largely specified by the statement of task, although with refinement from the committee. The committee considered a wide range of etiologies but primarily focused on acquired adult-onset hearing loss (and hearing difficulties), which is most often caused by aging, noise exposure, or both. While the committee considered all adults (age 18 and older), it focused primarily on older age groups. The committee considered its scope to include a wide range of interventions, including devices, rehabilitation and training strategies, and pharmaceuticals and biological therapies; per the statement of task, the committee did not consider surgically placed prosthetic devices. The committee approached its work broadly to be able to apply its recommendations to both current and emerging individual-level interventions as well as to a range of settings and purposes. The committee focused on outcomes related directly to the effectiveness of the intervention itself and excluded the assessment of outcomes that could be highly influenced by systems or practice patterns, such as cost-effectiveness or patient satisfaction. The accessibility and affordability of hearing health care, which were examined in the 2016 National Academies report *Hearing Health Care for Adults*, were beyond this committee's scope of work.

In any National Academies consensus study it is standard practice to include key partners and use a consensus process, although the particular approach to consensus will vary from study to study. The committee's review of best practices for core outcome set development found that there is currently wide variation in the specifics of how consensus is reached on the components of a core outcome set. In many cases a Delphi-type voting process is used, with multiple parties and multiple rounds of balloting determining the final core outcome set. This committee chose, by contrast, to rely on an evidence-based review and synthesis of the literature to identify a set of core outcomes as well as the best measures to assess those outcomes. While the committee recognizes that there may be some isolated situations where its recommendations will not apply, it sought to develop recommendations that would be as broadly applicable as possible. The committee further recognizes that the measurement of additional outcomes will likely be warranted in many contexts.

Figure S-1 provides an overview of the committee's overall process for determining a core outcome set and corresponding measures. While assembling an initial list of outcomes to consider for the core set, the committee simultaneously examined the hearing health outcome literature to begin an inventory of existing outcome measures for each of the candidate core outcomes.

Core Outcome Set

The committee's first step in determining a core outcome set was to consider an extensive list of potential outcome domains and individual outcomes based on literature reviews of outcomes typically reported in studies of hearing interventions. The committee also hosted public webinars to hear directly from adults with hearing difficulties as well as clinicians and professional groups, and the committee established an online platform to invite comments from members of the public. Working with the information gathered from these sources, the committee conducted multiple iterative discussions of the evidence identified to create a comprehensive and clearly defined set of outcomes to be considered for a core outcome set.

As shown in Figure S-2, the committee considered both proximal and distal outcomes. Proximal outcomes are evaluated at the time of intervention (i.e., verification that the intervention was applied successfully). Distal outcomes are the outcomes that are typically most meaningful to adults with hearing difficulties.

Next, the committee conducted a more in-depth exploration into which outcomes are the most meaningful to adults with hearing difficulties and their clinicians. In general, the meaningfulness of an outcome reflects the perceived importance of that outcome by adults with hearing difficulties and by clinicians.

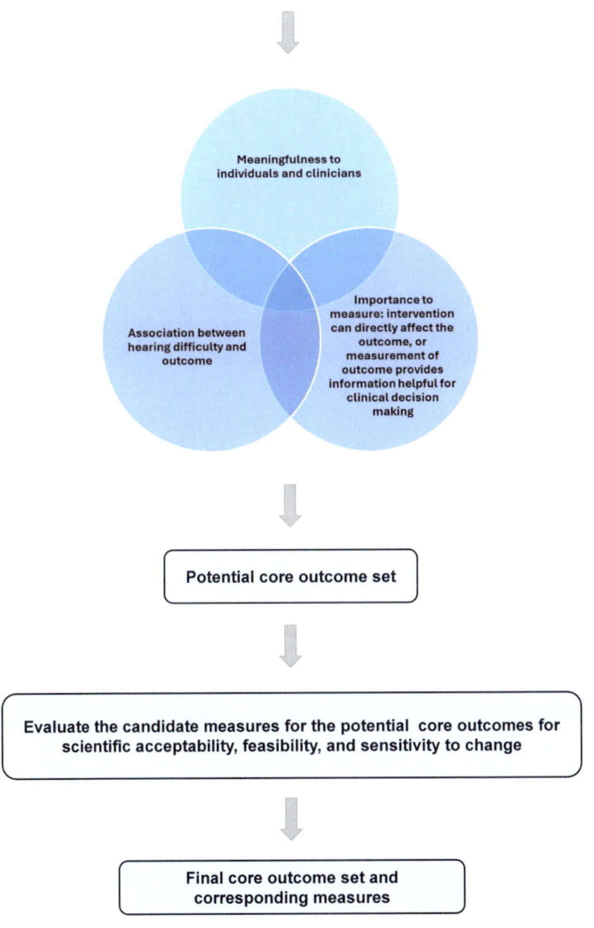

FIGURE S-1 Overview of the committee's process.

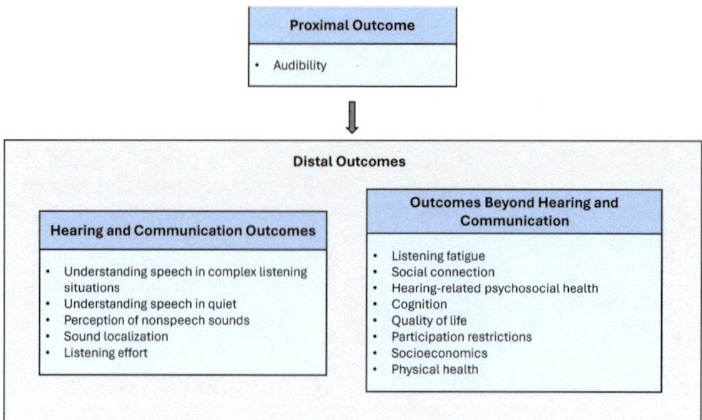

FIGURE S-2 Proximal and distal outcomes of hearing health interventions.

Recognizing that any single outcome will be meaningful to some individuals or populations, and may depend on context, the committee sought to determine which outcomes are meaningful across populations. Given the limited direct evidence regarding the most meaningful outcomes, the committee also considered evidence of the prevalence and severity of hearing-related complaints among those with hearing difficulties. A related concept, importance to measure, reflects whether an intervention can directly affect the outcome or whether measurement of the outcome provides information that would be helpful for clinical decision making.[4] Since the committee was charged with recommending a core outcome set that applies across settings, interventions, a range of severities, and multiple etiologies of hearing loss, the committee concluded that any outcome in the core outcome set needs to be universally meaningful and important to measure across all contexts. The broadness of the scope of applications of the core outcome set also means that it needs to be feasible to measure in all contexts.

Therefore, after amassing a list of outcomes to consider, the committee used three main criteria to narrow down the outcomes to be considered for the core set (see Figure S-1). First, the committee required that the outcome be consistently defined across the literature and have a strong, established association with hearing difficulties. Second, the committee asked that the outcome be meaningful for virtually all adults with hearing difficulties and clinicians. Finally, the committee considered the evidence for importance

---

[4] The availability of outcome measures to assess a particular outcome is implicit to this criterion, given that generating evidence of the effect of the intervention on the outcome requires the use of measures. The consideration of the quality of existing measures occurred after the committee determined candidate outcomes.

to measure. To be considered for the core set, the outcome would need to meet all these criteria.

Outcome Measures

After narrowing the candidate core outcomes under consideration, the committee consulted its list of potential measures to recommend. For outcomes with multiple possible measures, the committee initially narrowed the list of outcome measures to be examined primarily based on the amount and quality of available evidence regarding the development and psychometric assessment of that measure. Next, the committee developed a set of criteria for a full evaluation of the remaining candidate measures, which included scientific acceptability (including reliability, validity, and sensitivity to change) and feasibility. The committee carefully reviewed the literature on the psychometrics of each candidate measure, using value judgments regarding the amount and quality of the evidence for each criterion, noting that no single measure had robust evidence for all criteria. Through a series of iterative discussions regarding the available evidence for each measure, the committee determined the final core outcome set and the best existing measure for each core outcome.

RECOMMENDATIONS

Audibility is defined as the ability to detect sound across a broad frequency range and across a range of input levels. Improvement of audibility is expected to be accomplished at the time of the intervention. The particular approach to improving audibility is chosen according to the individual's type, configuration, and degree of hearing loss and the target of the treatment. Therefore, the measurement of this proximal outcome (to verify that the intervention has been applied successfully) cannot be achieved with a single approach for all contexts and so is not included in the committee's core set. However, the committee concluded that the improvement of audibility is fundamental to the success of the intervention and requires verification using appropriate methods. Even so, improved audibility alone does not guarantee that the intervention will have the anticipated effect on everyday function; such effects are distal outcomes, and their measurement captures essential aspects of a treatment's effectiveness. Therefore, the committee's recommendations relate to measurement of the more meaningful distal outcomes of hearing health interventions.

The following sections describe the committee's recommendations in five key areas:

1. Core outcome set,
2. Standardized outcome measures,

3. Future research on outcomes,
4. Measure development and refinement, and
5. Uptake of the core outcome set and measures.

Core Outcome Set

As noted earlier, the committee created a comprehensive and clearly defined set of outcomes to be considered for a core outcome set. Significant literature supports several outcomes as being meaningful to adults with hearing difficulties and clinicians, as being associated with hearing difficulties, and as being important to measure. These outcomes are well defined, and adequate measures of the outcomes exist that meet the committee's criteria to warrant their use in various contexts. In settling on a core outcome set, the committee also considered factors that influence the burden of assessing that set overall (e.g., number of outcomes, availability of measures, mode of administration, time of administration). Table S-1 outlines the committee's overall conclusion for each outcome considered for the core set.

The committee determined that two outcomes have the strongest evidence for inclusion in a core outcome set: understanding speech in complex listening situations and hearing-related psychosocial health.[5]

Recommendation 5-1:[6] Individuals and organizations engaged in hearing health interventions should adopt the following outcomes as a core outcome set in both research and clinical settings:

- **Understanding speech in complex listening situations**
- **Hearing-related psychosocial health**

The committee emphasizes that this core outcome set should be considered as a foundation for hearing-health outcome assessment following intervention—that is, this set represents the minimum that should be measured across settings and intervention types. This does not imply that other outcomes are not meaningful or should be unexamined.

---

[5] While the term *speech in noise* is typically used, the committee prefers the use of *speech in complex listening situations*, which includes understanding speech in a variety of contexts including noisy environments, accented language, multiple speakers, with music playing, and other situations that complicate an individual's ability to understand speech.

[6] The committee's recommendations are numbered according to the chapter of the main report in which they appear. Thus, Recommendation 5-1 is the first recommendation in Chapter 5.

TABLE S-1 Outcomes in Hearing, Communication, and Beyond Considered for the Core Set

Outcome	Conclusion
Hearing and Communication	
Understanding speech in complex listening situations	Meaningful and a key complaint. Important to measure (intervention can impact outcome), and existing measures have a sufficient amount of psychometric data supporting the quality of the measures.
Perception of nonspeech sounds (e.g., music, nature)	Meaningful to specific subpopulations but not a key complaint. Psychometric data for existing measures are limited. Interventions meeting needs for speech in complex listening situations often meet needs for this outcome.
Understanding speech in quiet	Meaningful, but not a key complaint. Interventions meeting needs for speech in complex listening situations typically meet needs for this outcome.
Sound localization	Meaningful, but less frequently raised as a significant difficulty compared with other outcomes. A lack of feasible measures with a sufficient amount of psychometric data supporting the quality of the measures for sound localization specifically. Measure development and refinement needed.
Listening effort	Meaningful, but the outcome is inconsistently defined and measured. Measure development and refinement needed.
Beyond Hearing and Communication	
Listening fatigue	Meaningful, but the outcome is inconsistently defined and measured. Measure development and refinement needed.
Social connection	Meaningful, but there is insufficient evidence that the intervention has a significant clinical effect on the outcome at the individual level.
Hearing-related psychosocial health	Meaningful, important to measure (intervention can affect outcome), and existing measures have a sufficient amount of psychometric data supporting the quality of the measures.
Cognition	Meaningful, but there is inconsistency in the cognitive construct being measured. Insufficient evidence exists that the intervention has a significant clinical effect on the outcome at the individual level.

continued

TABLE S-1 Continued

Outcome	Conclusion
Quality of life	Meaningful, but there is inconsistency in the definition of the outcome and in the underlying constructs being measured. Many hearing-related factors contribute to quality of life; however, outside the key constructs of psychological, social, and emotional health, which are covered by hearing-related psychosocial health, current studies offer mixed results on the effect of hearing interventions on quality of life.
Socioeconomic effects	Might be meaningful to specific subpopulations and types of research, but not a key complaint.
Participation restrictions	Outcome is inconsistently defined and measured.
Physical health	Not a key complaint. Insufficient evidence exists that interventions have a significant clinical effect on the outcome.

Standardized Outcome Measures[7]

Many outcome measures have been developed to assess the outcomes of understanding speech in complex listening situations and hearing-related psychosocial health. The committee focused on the measures with the most available information concerning their psychometric development and use. First, the committee documented the descriptive characteristics of the studies used in each measure's development, including the population studied, the number of participants, the setting, and how the measure is scored. Next the committee evaluated each measure according to a series of criteria including scientific acceptability and feasibility (by setting).[8]

For the assessment of the outcome of understanding speech in complex listening situations, the committee concluded that both behavioral measures and self-report measures are necessary. While behavioral measures have face validity, are considered by some to be more objective, and are readily available, these measures often lack data on their sensitivity to change and do not necessarily correlate with an individual's perception of their improvement.

For the self-report measure, the committee narrowed the candidates down to the Abbreviated Profile of Hearing Aid Benefit (APHAB) (and the APHAB-global score in particular) and the Speech, Spatial and Qualities

---

[7] The word *standardized* is used here in a broad sense to indicate that the same measures are being used for specific outcomes and that there are prescribed materials and procedures for the use of these measures. The committee does not imply that the measures are part of national or international standards.

[8] See Appendix C for the committee's detailed evaluation process.

of Hearing Scale (SSQ). While both measures have a sufficient amount of psychometric data regarding the quality of the measure and both are available in multiple languages, the APHAB (and the APHAB-global score in particular) has a greater focus on scenarios of complex listening situations, whereas the SSQ includes a mix of speech, spatial location, and sound qualities. Therefore, the committee concluded that the APHAB-global score currently is the best candidate for assessing an individual's experience with understanding speech in complex listening environments.

For the behavioral measure, the committee narrowed the candidates down to the Quick Speech-in-Noise (QuickSIN) test and the Words-in-Noise (WIN) test. The QuickSIN, which evaluates an individual's ability to understand sentences, may be more familiar to audiologists and somewhat shorter to administer. However, psychometric evaluation of the QuickSIN shows more limited evidence on the reliability and consistency of the measurement over time. The WIN, which evaluates an individual's ability to understand single words, has had a much more rigorous psychometric development and evaluation (including significant evidence for test–retest reliability), is currently used as part of the National Institutes of Health (NIH) toolbox, and is available in Spanish (although additional validation of the Spanish WIN is needed).

For hearing-related psychosocial health, the committee ultimately zeroed in on variations of the Hearing Handicap Inventory (HHI). The well-studied HHI for the Elderly (HHIE) was eliminated primarily because of its length and because psychometric analyses favor the 18-item Revised HHI (RHHI). The shorter screening version (RHHI-S) had less robust research on psychometric strength of the measure. The RHHI, a relatively new measure, has undergone rigorous item analysis but lacks explicit data regarding reliability and sensitivity to change following intervention. Given that 18 of the 25 items included in the HHIE are common to the RHHI, the committee relied on evidence regarding the reliability and sensitivity to change for the HHIE when considering the RHHI.

Overall, current outcome measures are imperfect, but there is adequate evidence to support the standard use of specific measures at this time.

Recommendation 6-1: When assessing outcomes in hearing health, clinicians, researchers, and individuals should use the following outcome measures for each of the outcomes in the core outcome set:

a. Understanding speech in complex listening situations
   i. Abbreviated Profile of Hearing Aid Benefit global score (APHAB-Global)
   ii. Words-in-Noise (WIN) test
b. Hearing-related psychosocial health
   i. Revised Hearing Handicap Inventory (RHHI)

The committee recognizes the potential burden of assessing outcomes with three different measures and emphasizes that it will be important to determine the timing and frequency of the outcome measurements that will deliver optimal information. Additionally, it will not necessarily be required to evaluate each measure at each encounter, and self-report measures could be completed by the adult with hearing difficulties in advance of a clinical or research encounter. Finally, the committee reemphasizes that supplemental measures will likely be needed, depending on the specific context of the outcome measurement, including verification of audibility as appropriate.

Future Research on Outcomes

For many of the outcomes of interest, the committee found limited evidence and determined that more research is needed—both to better understand which outcomes are most meaningful for adults with hearing difficulties and for clinicians and also to better define and build the evidence base for these outcomes as potential candidates for an updated core outcome set.

Limited *direct* research has been performed to determine which outcomes are most meaningful for adults with hearing difficulties and for clinicians. Existing evidence is mostly indirect, as it is usually derived from surveys of satisfaction with interventions or studies of the prevalence and severity of hearing difficulties, and these are typically based on (1) constrained surveys wherein the choices are developed by others (e.g., researchers and clinicians) and (2) varying degrees of direct input from those with hearing difficulties.

Recommendation 4-1: Sponsors of hearing health research should fund additional research to engage adults with hearing difficulties, their communication partners, and clinicians to determine the most meaningful outcomes based on direct evidence from adults with hearing difficulties.

Several meaningful outcomes need further research for various reasons. For example, some outcomes are inconsistently defined, and measurement is inconsistent in terms of the underlying constructs examined. Furthermore, many of the outcomes considered by the committee lack robust evidence on the importance to measure—that is, whether the intervention itself can result in significant clinical change in the outcome, particularly at the level of the individual.

Recommendation 5-2: Sponsors of hearing health research should fund research to build the evidence base on the clinical effect of hearing

health interventions on key outcomes that are meaningful to adults with hearing difficulties and clinicians.

Examples of the types of research needed by outcome are provided in Table S-2.

Additional research will help determine which outcomes might be appropriate for an updated core outcome set. The committee recognizes that while this research is warranted, some outcomes may never rise to the level of a core set to be used across hearing health interventions because the outcome may never be meaningful to all subpopulations. However, this type of research will be useful both for reconsidering outcomes for an overarching core set and also for understanding their use as supplemental outcomes to be measured for specific populations or contexts.

Measure Development and Refinement

The committee recognizes that the measurement of hearing health outcomes requires an improvement in psychometric rigor overall. Research on measure development and refinement is needed to improve the quality of existing measures, including the previously recommended measures. For example, statistical approaches such as item response theory and linking

TABLE S-2 Areas of Needed Research by Outcome

Outcome	Research Needed on Outcome
Perception of nonspeech sounds (e.g., music)	Determine which subpopulations consider this most meaningful.
Listening effort and listening fatigue	Research the separate constructs warranted. Currently, definitions and theoretical approaches are not consistent.
Social connection	Determine the intervention's effect on clinical outcomes.
Hearing-related psychosocial health	Determine the differences of effects on social versus emotional health (currently not distinctly measured).
Cognition	Determine the intervention's effect on clinical outcomes and mechanism for effect.
Quality of life	Determine a clear and consistent definition with common metrics across conditions.
Socioeconomic impacts	Determine the intervention's effect on the outcome.
Participation restrictions	Develop a consistent definition. Define the outcome independent of individual underlying constructs and overlapping outcomes.
Physical health	Determine the intervention's effect on clinical outcomes.

may help with the refinement of existing measures. Additionally, research on sensitivity to change, associations among core outcomes, and variations of existing measures may also help with measure refinement.

> **Recommendation 6-2: Sponsors of hearing health research should fund further psychometric evaluation of the measures recommended for the core outcome set. Specific areas of research include the following:**

a. Development of links and crosswalks
   i. Words-in-Noise (WIN) test versus Quick Speech-in-Noise (QuickSIN) test
   ii. Among different variations of the Hearing Handicap Inventory (HHI)
b. Establishment of the sensitivity to change relative to intervention (including minimal detectable change and minimal clinically important difference) for the WIN, the global score from the Abbreviated Profile of Hearing Aid Benefit (APHAB-global), the Revised HHI (RHHI), and the screening (RHHI-S)
c. Development of WIN (and QuickSIN) in other languages
d. Assessment of associations among the set of core outcomes to further establish the independence and uniqueness of each measure
e. Application of item response theory to further develop and refine the recommended outcome measures

Research beyond the currently recommended measures is needed to build evidence for the use of measures not recommended by this committee that might be reconsidered for an updated core outcome set.

> **Recommendation 6-3: Sponsors of hearing health research should fund research to develop and refine hearing health outcome measures beyond the currently recommended measures, including:**

a. Broader psychometric development of the Quick Speech-in-Noise (QuickSIN) test;
b. Exploration of the use of the digits-in-noise test as an outcome measure; and
c. Exploration of the usefulness of high-quality language agnostic tests for sound processing in complex listening situations.

Uptake of Core Outcome Set and Measures

Dissemination and implementation science develops approaches to increasing the uptake of research innovations and of the resulting evidence-based interventions. Dissemination refers to active efforts to spread information to targeted audiences, while implementation refers to the process of translating that knowledge into action. Both strategies seek to create a change in behavior that leads to the uptake of a new practice—in this case, the use of the core outcome set and corresponding measures when outcome measurement is being undertaken. Several facilitators and barriers have been identified that are specifically related to the uptake of core outcome sets. Facilitators include knowledge of the core outcome set (including its purpose), understanding how to use it and recognizing that its use does not preclude the use of other outcomes, and understanding the rigor of its development. Barriers include lack of awareness, costs, measurement burden, and a preference for continuing current practices.

The first step in encouraging the adoption of the core outcome set and corresponding measures includes engaging in a robust dissemination strategy to ensure that researchers, health care professionals, and adults with hearing difficulties have the necessary awareness and knowledge of the core outcome set and measures.

> **Recommendation 7-1: Health academic organizations and programs, professional organizations, researchers, and consumer groups should disseminate information about the importance of the core outcome set to clinicians of first contact (e.g., primary care clinicians), hearing health clinicians (e.g., students, audiologists, otolaryngologists), and adults with hearing difficulties.**

Strategies for dissemination include providing information and training on the core outcome set and corresponding measures through formal educational, clinical and research-focused training programs, websites, meetings, continuing education, and webinars. The committee notes that disseminating this information to different partners will likely require a multipronged approach. The committee purposefully includes primary care and other clinicians of first contact among the targets of dissemination because these partners will often be the first to evaluate the concerns of patients reporting hearing difficulties. Furthermore, adults with hearing difficulties themselves need to be included in the dissemination efforts to encourage a whole health approach to care.

Dissemination of information alone, however, is insufficient to ensure uptake. It will be important to develop strategies for creating incentives to use the core outcome set as well as strategies for alleviating burdens to its use. Such strategies can come from a variety of sources, including requirements for use in research, incorporation of the outcome measures into electronic health records (to both allow for ease of use by the clinician and to enable patients to answer self-report questionnaires in advance), and use in value-based care.

Recommendation 7-2: To create incentives for the use of the core outcome set and corresponding measures the following should occur:

a. Sponsors of research on hearing health interventions should require the use of the core outcome set and corresponding measures (at a minimum), unless scientifically justified for exclusion.
b. Electronic health record (EHR) vendors should incorporate the Abbreviated Profile of Hearing Aid Benefit and Revised Hearing Handicap Inventory into EHRs.
c. Insurers who require outcome measures should require the use of the recommended measures.

One of the main purposes of developing and using a core outcome set (and corresponding measures) is to allow for the pooling of data to compare the effectiveness of interventions and to develop a more robust evidence base that helps improve clinical care. The committee recognizes that NIH already has existing platforms for the centralized sharing of data.

Recommendation 7-3: To facilitate big data meta-analyses, the National Institutes of Health should develop a national database to allow clinicians and researchers to benchmark the use of the core outcome set and corresponding measures as well as their results.

One highly effective strategy for encouraging the uptake of core outcome sets in other fields is having a central entity take responsibility for developing and updating the core outcome set. The committee recognizes the importance of ensuring the consistency of what is measured and how it is measured over time. However, as new evidence emerges, the core outcome set will need to be revisited. The purpose will not be to just add more core outcomes, but to consider which ones should remain part of the core or which ones should be considered for supplemental measurement, as appropriate. The committee notes that several federal agencies provide substantial funding and work in hearing health research and hearing health care delivery and therefore are well positioned to collaborate to support ongoing evaluation and support for a core outcome set.

Recommendation 7-4: After an adequate level of new research has been gathered, the National Institutes of Health, the Department of Defense, and the Veterans Administration should collaborate to revisit the core outcome set.

Finally, while following the recommendations for dissemination and implementation of the core outcome set can help encourage uptake, there will still likely be gaps in understanding which approaches work best for specific target audiences in the hearing health field.

Recommendation 7-5: Sponsors of hearing health research should fund research on comprehensive implementation science approaches to identify additional key facilitators for and barriers to the uptake and use of the core outcome set and corresponding measures.

CONCLUSION

The development and use of a core outcome set and standardized outcome measures for hearing health interventions in adults will help better determine the effectiveness of various interventions and allow for comparison across interventions, sites, and time. Moving forward, significant investments in research to better define the most meaningful outcomes and improve the rigor of measure development and refinement will be needed to better understand the full functional effect of hearing interventions. Finally, robust and multicomponent approaches to dissemination and implementation that provide incentives for the use of the core outcome set will be key to its uptake. Overall, consistent approaches to outcome measurement that focus on the outcomes that matter the most to adults with hearing difficulties, as well as to clinicians who may be involved in their care, will ultimately improve those individuals' everyday hearing function.

1

Introduction

Hearing loss is "the most prevalent sensory disorder in the United States," with approximately 22 percent of the population (nearly 73 million individuals) experiencing hearing loss (Haile et al., 2024, p. 261). The prevalence and severity of hearing loss (as well as of hearing difficulties increase with age (Haile et al., 2024). Similar trends are seen when individuals are asked about their perceptions of their own hearing difficulties (Dillard et al., 2024; Humes, 2023a,b). The value of interventions for hearing loss in adults depends, in part, on what aspects of an individual's lived experience with hearing loss matter the most to that person. Evaluations of the effectiveness of interventions may not reflect an individual's perception of their functional abilities or the effect that their hearing difficulties have on their quality of life. That is, changes in various outcomes that might be statistically significant at the group level and used as evidence for the effectiveness of an intervention may have no bearing on an individual's assessment of their own improvement.

STUDY ORIGIN AND STATEMENT OF TASK

With support from a coalition of sponsors, including the National Institutes of Health (the National Institute on Deafness and Other Communication Disorders and the National Institute on Aging), the Centers for Disease Control and Prevention (CDC), the Defense Health Agency, and the Department of Veterans Affairs (VA), the National Academies of Sciences, Engineering, and Medicine (the National Academies) formed the Committee on Meaningful Outcome Measures in Adult Hearing Health Care in late 2023. The sponsors charged the committee with examining the state of the science in outcomes

---

BOX 1-1
Statement of Task

An ad hoc committee of the National Academies of Sciences, Engineering, and Medicine will examine the state of the science in outcomes research for interventions in adult hearing health care (excluding surgically placed prosthetic devices), with an emphasis on measures that are meaningful to the individual and the clinician. The committee will determine a core set of existing standard outcome measures, define the core outcome domains (including hearing, communication, and other domains) that should be measured, and develop strategies and a set of recommendations to guide the development of standardized and meaningful measures that are fit for use in different settings.

Specifically, the committee will:

- Identify and engage appropriate partners, including relevant federal agencies, the academic/professional community of researchers and clinicians, professional organizations, industry, and patient/consumer groups, to gain their perspectives as input to committee deliberations.
- Provide a brief contextual background describing the contribution of hearing to overall health and well-being, the etiology of hearing loss, the personal and societal costs of untreated hearing loss, the benefits of treatment for hearing loss, and disparities in treatment.

---

research for interventions in adult hearing health care with an emphasis on measures that are meaningful to adults with hearing difficulties and the clinicians who treat them (see the full statement of task in Box 1-1).

PREVIOUS WORK OF THE NATIONAL ACADEMIES

Previous reports from the National Academies relevant to this current study include the titles listed in the following paragraphs.

Hearing Loss: Determining Eligibility for Social Security Benefits critically evaluates the measures used to diagnose hearing loss and quantify hearing function for Social Security benefits. The report recommends a standard otolaryngological examination and an audiological examination. Additionally, for adults, the report recommends a pure-tone threshold test, a speech threshold test, a speech recognition test, and an objective physiological test (NRC, 2005).

Hearing Loss Research at NIOSH: Reviews of Research Programs of the National Institute for Occupational Safety and Health (2006) assesses the effect of the Hearing Loss Research Program on worker health and safety, and recommends effective leadership in program planning and implementation,

- Broadly describe the various interventions (e.g., hearing aids, rehabilitative strategies or training, pharmaceutical or biological therapies, etc.).
- Describe the outcome measures currently available to assess hearing function and communication in adults, available measures in outcome domains beyond communication (e.g., social connectivity, activity limitations, participation restrictions, economic productivity) that should be measured, and gaps where development of new outcome measures is urgently needed.
- Identify in which settings the metrics are most applicable (e.g., establishing efficacy in clinical trials, assessing patient response in clinical care and by type of intervention, conducting hearing health monitoring, assessing patient satisfaction).
- Provide recommendations on the standardized use of existing outcome measures for hearing health, including hearing, communication, and other domains ("core set of measures"), and the necessary qualities and strategies for adoption of new meaningful measures that could be implemented in the short term as well as longer timeframes with an eye toward large-scale adoption and standardization (e.g., national databases and repositories).

In the circumstance where robust evidence is lacking or absent, the committee is encouraged to make recommendations based on sound scientific reasoning in the context of the current health care environment.

improvements in evaluations, and incorporation of the expertise of epidemiologists and noise control engineers to improve surveillance data for occupational hearing loss and workplace noise exposure (IOM and NRC, 2006).

Noise and Military Service: Implications for Hearing Loss and Tinnitus recommends consistent use of hearing protection and required audiograms before exposure and after exposure to make it possible to better pinpoint the cause of hearing loss. The report notes that these audiogram records should include questions evaluating hearing loss and measuring hearing thresholds at 8000 Hz and that individuals with significant changes between audiograms should receive additional monitoring. The report also recommends improving the Defense Occupational and Environmental Health Readiness System to track reports of tinnitus and exposures to hazardous noise and allow Veterans Administration personnel to access these records for disability claims (IOM, 2006).

Hearing Loss and Healthy Aging: Workshop Summary examines how age-related hearing loss affects healthy aging and how public and private parties can collaborate to address this issue (IOM and NRC, 2014). Panels included consumer perspectives, the connection between hearing loss and healthy aging, current approaches to hearing health care delivery, innovative models of care, hearing technologies, contemporary issues in hearing health care, and collaborative strategies for the future.

Hearing Healthcare for Adults: Priorities for Improving Access and Affordability emphasizes that many adults with hearing loss do not seek or receive treatment. The report recommends increased efforts by relevant government agencies, advocacy groups, and nonprofit organizations to "collect, analyze, and disseminate prospective population-based data," to collaborate with each other and align best practices, to inform patients about their rights regarding their audiograms and hearing aid programming history, and to collaborate with providers incentivizing diversity and cultural competence in the field. The report also recommended that the Food and Drug Administration establish a new category of over-the-counter wearable hearing devices (NASEM, 2016).

The Promise of Assistive Technology to Enhance Activity and Work Participation evaluates products and technologies that assist adults with disabilities, including hearing impairments. The report summarizes the existing information, accommodations offered by employers, and associated costs (NASEM, 2017).

Functional Assessment for Adults with Disabilities discusses how to assess an adult's mental and physical abilities relative to their workplace demands and how to collect this information (NASEM, 2019). The report considers the measures of functional hearing. Overall, the report concluded that "determinations about a person's ability to sustain full-time work are more complicated than can be indicated by an assessment of individual body structures, functions, or impairments."

Transforming Human Health: Celebrating 50 Years of Discovery and Progress summarizes human health milestones (NASEM, 2022). The report briefly covers the history of newborn hearing screening, restoring hearing through cochlear implants, the first digital hearing aid, and efforts to remove background noise from hearing aids.

STUDY APPROACH

The Committee on Meaningful Outcome Measures in Adult Hearing Health Care consisted of 13 members with a broad range of expertise, including hearing health care (both clinical care and research), etiology of and interventions for hearing loss, outcome measurement (e.g., patient-reported outcome measures), primary care (e.g., family medicine, geriatrics, and nursing), disability and rehabilitation, quality of life, health disparities, public health, and epidemiology. Appendix E provides brief biographies of the committee members, fellows, and staff.

The committee deliberated during seven full committee meetings and many working group calls between December 2023 and March 2025. Additionally, the committee held three virtual public webinars and invited panelists to offer comments to inform the committee's deliberations. The panelists provided valuable input from a broad range of perspectives, including adults with hearing difficulties, clinicians, and hearing health professional groups. The committee also completed an extensive search of the peer-reviewed literature and the gray literature, including publications by private organizations, advocacy groups, and government entities. In addition, the committee established an online system for collecting narratives from clinicians and adults with hearing difficulties on measuring outcomes of hearing health intervention. Selected quotes from these narratives are included in Chapter 4.

Definitions and Terminology

The sections below present some definitions and distinctions in terminology developed by the committee that are important for the focus of this report. For a full list of definitions, see Appendix A.

Outcomes and Outcome Domains

An intervention's health outcome is the effect of the intervention on one's health. That is, health outcomes refer to changes in the health of an individual or population after an intervention. Several related outcomes may be grouped into a category called an outcome domain. For example, an outcome domain of speech communication includes many individual outcomes such as understanding speech in quiet, understanding speech in noise, and perception of nonspeech sounds.

Core Outcome Set

A core outcome set is an agreed-upon standardized minimum set of meaningful outcomes that are measured and reported across settings and interventions. When assessing the effect of an intervention, researchers and clinicians can consider a multitude of outcomes to measure. A core outcome set recommends, at a minimum, the specific outcomes to be measured and reported. The use of a core set of outcomes (and corresponding standardized measures) helps to enhance the consistency and quality of research, allows for the pooling of data, and facilitates the comparison of different interventions.

Outcome Measures

"Outcome measures reflect the impact of the health care service or intervention on the health status of patients" (AHRQ, 2015). While the terms *measure*, *measurement tool*, and *measurement instrument* are used interchangeably and are fairly synonymous, this report will use the term *measure*.

Diagnostic Assessment versus Outcome Assessment

A diagnostic test or assessment is used to identify a condition or disease, and the results from a diagnostic assessment can help determine a treatment plan or intervention, if needed (Deeks and Bossuyt, 2023). By contrast, outcome measures are used to evaluate an intervention's effect on an individual. This report focuses on meaningful outcomes and the measures used to evaluate the efficacy and effectiveness of interventions, rather than focusing on the types of assessments used to diagnose hearing loss or determine candidacy for various devices.

Meaningfulness versus Importance to Measure

In general, the meaningfulness of an outcome reflects the perceived importance of that outcome by adults with hearing difficulties and clinicians. For this study, given the limited direct evidence on which outcomes are perceived as most meaningful, the committee used evidence on the prevalence and severity of hearing-related complaints among adults with hearing difficulties as supplemental evidence of meaningfulness. A related concept, importance to measure, reflects whether an intervention has the ability to directly affect the outcome or whether measurement of the outcome provides information that would be helpful for clinical decision making.

Hearing Loss versus Hearing Difficulties

In this report, the committee elected to use the term *adult with hearing difficulties* rather than *adult with hearing loss* whenever possible. Hearing loss is generally used to reflect a clinical measurement of hearing ability, often using the pure-tone audiogram. Hearing difficulties, on the other hand, are more strongly associated with hearing trouble perceived by the individual and may or may not be reported by adults with audiometric hearing loss. Hearing difficulties may also be perceived by individuals who do not have audiometric hearing loss (Spankovich et al., 2018). Furthermore, hearing difficulties may be undiagnosed (especially when they are mild), whereas hearing loss is most often a clinical diagnosis. The term *hearing loss* is used in this report in cases of direct quotes or as defined in cited studies or when specifically appropriate to a discussion of diagnosis.

Study Focus

Outcome measurement is important in health care, as the resulting data can help clinicians, researchers, and individuals understand which interventions work best for which populations and thereby improve the patient experience (ICHOM, n.d). While the committee does believe that outcome measurement is an important part of clinical practice and research, this study does not focus on the question of whether outcome measurement should be done. Rather, it starts with the assumption that outcome measurement is being performed and, given that, presents the evidence on how outcome measurement should be carried out in the field of hearing health. In addition, this study focuses primarily on assessing the efficacy and effectiveness of interventions for hearing health rather than on ways to assess hearing health as a part of the diagnostic process or process for determining candidacy for various devices. Determination of the legitimacy of the target disorder as well as assessment of the diagnostic accuracy of measures was also outside of the committee's scope of work. Instead, the committee starts with the assumption that hearing loss has been properly diagnosed, and a treatment has been applied. The study and associated recommendations target the twin issues of what is most meaningful to measure (core outcome set) and which measures are most appropriate to use in order to create more consistency in outcome measurement for hearing health interventions.

Generally speaking, the first step in the development of a core outcome set is setting the scope of what the core outcome set will cover. While in this case the scope was largely determined by the statement of task, the committee set the following parameters for its examination of evidence. This study focuses on adults with hearing difficulties; while the committee considered all adults (age 18 and older), it focused primarily on older age groups, as the prevalence of hearing loss and hearing difficulties increases with age. The committee also considered a wide range of etiologies, but primarily focused on acquired, adult-onset hearing loss, which is most often caused by aging, noise exposure, or both. The committee considered its scope to apply to a wide range of interventions such as devices (including some assistive devices at the level of the individual), rehabilitation and training strategies, and pharmaceuticals and biological therapies. It approached its work broadly so as to apply its recommendations to both current and emerging interventions. The committee's focus was on interventions at the level of the individual rather than systemic approaches (e.g., hearing loops).[1] Furthermore, the committee also focused on improvement due to a single intervention (e.g., based on the comparison of aided versus unaided listeners) rather than comparing results among intervention types or different technologies or determining why people abandon the use of certain devices. Per the statement of task, the committee excluded consideration of

---

[1] A hearing loop is an assistive listening system placed in a public setting that helps transmit sound directly from a microphone into hearing aids (equipped with telecoils) and cochlear implants. This system "can make speech and music in public places more understandable" (HLAA, 2025).

surgically placed prosthetic devices (e.g., cochlear implants, bone-anchored hearing aids).

The committee focused on outcomes related directly to the efficacy and effectiveness of the intervention itself and excluded the assessment of outcomes that could be highly influenced by systems or practice patterns such as cost-effectiveness and patient satisfaction. The committee did not consider the effects of interventions on the family, friends, and care partners of adults with hearing difficulties. Additionally, the focus of the committee's work was not on the accessibility or affordability of hearing health care, which was the focus of a previous National Academies report *Hearing Health Care for Adults: Priorities for Improving Access and Affordability* (2016).

Committee Process

In its work, the committee followed several general best practices that have been identified for developing core outcome sets, including specifying a clear scope, involving key partners, and using a consensus process (see Chapter 3). For this study, as described above, the statement of task (with refinement from the committee) largely specified the scope. In any National Academies consensus study it is standard practice to include key partners and use a consensus process, although the particular approach to consensus will vary from study to study. However, the committee's review of best practices for core outcome set development found that there is currently wide variation in the specifics of how core outcome sets are developed. For example, in many cases a Delphi-type voting process is used, with multiple parties and multiple rounds of balloting determining the outcome set. Another valid approach, the one used by this committee, is an evidence-based review and synthesis of the literature, for defining a broadly applicable core outcome set in hearing health care as well as the best measures to assess those outcomes. While the committee recognizes that there may be some isolated situations where its recommendations will not apply, it sought to develop recommendations that would be as broadly applicable as possible. The committee further recognizes that the measurement of additional outcomes may be warranted in many contexts.

Figure 1-1 provides an overview of the committee's overall process for determining a core outcome set (i.e., which areas of hearing, communication, and beyond should be assessed for impact of the intervention) and corresponding measures (i.e., which tools or instruments to use to assess the core outcomes). Note that while assembling an initial list of outcomes to consider for the core set, the committee simultaneously examined the hearing health outcome literature to begin an inventory of existing outcome measures for each of the candidate core outcomes (see Appendix B).

Committee Process

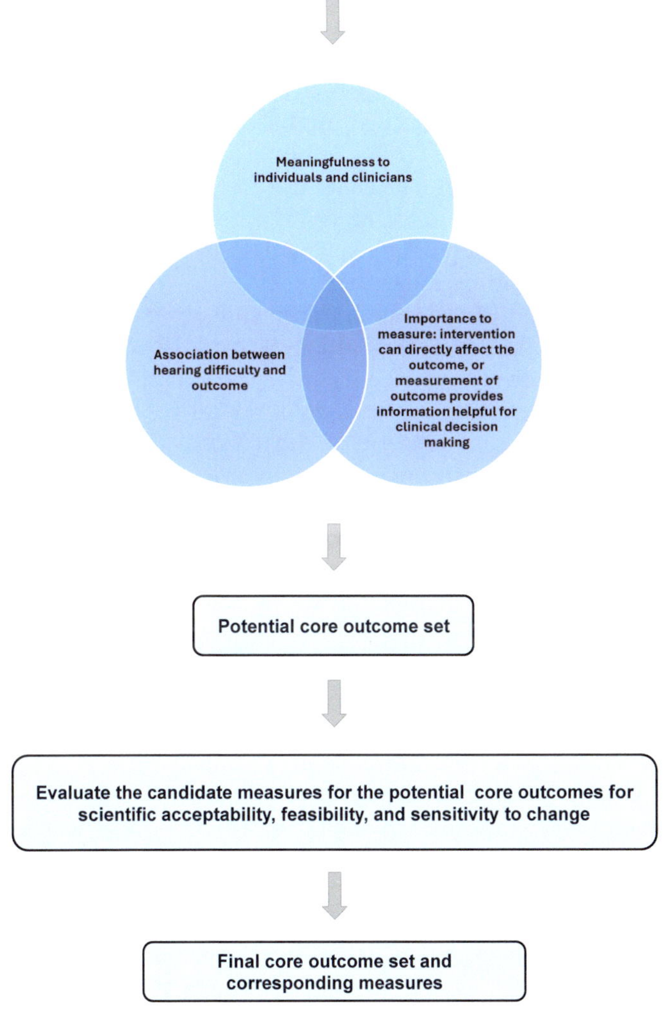

FIGURE 1-1 Overview of the committee's process.

Core Outcome Set

In determining the core outcome set, the committee first needed to identify which outcome domains and individual outcomes to consider. Although several other groups have created core outcome sets for specific hearing loss etiologies or interventions, there is a lack of consistency in which outcomes have been measured. Therefore, the committee first considered an extensive list of outcomes based on literature reviews of outcome domains and individual outcomes typically reported in studies of hearing interventions. The committee also hosted public webinars to hear directly from adults with hearing difficulties, clinicians, and hearing health professional organizations. An online platform that members of the public could use to submit their comments also was established. Based on the information collected from these sources, the committee conducted multiple iterative discussions to create a comprehensive and clearly defined set of outcomes to be considered for a core outcome set. Chapter 5 of this report defines the outcomes identified by the committee and describes the connection between each outcome and hearing difficulties.

Next, the committee conducted a more in-depth exploration into which of these outcomes are the most meaningful to adults with hearing difficulties and to their clinicians. As noted earlier, meaningfulness was defined as a combination of perceived importance of the outcome, prevalence of difficulty in that outcome, and severity of the difficulty. The committee looked to several evidence-based sources for determining the meaningfulness of the outcome. First, the committee reviewed the existing peer-reviewed literature as well as industry and consumer group surveys regarding which outcomes were most meaningful. Additionally, the committee considered information gathered through public webinars and the project's public call for comments. See Chapter 4 for evidence of meaningfulness.

Since the committee was charged with recommending a core outcome set that applies across interventions (excluding surgical implants), in multiple settings (e.g., clinic, research), for multiple purposes (e.g., efficacy, effectiveness), and a range of severities and etiologies of hearing loss, the committee concluded that any outcome in the core set needs to be universally meaningful and important to measure across all contexts. The broadness of the scope of applications of the core outcome set also means that the core set needs to be feasible to measure in all contexts. Therefore, after amassing a list of outcomes to consider (see Chapter 5), the committee used several criteria to narrow down the outcomes to be considered for the core set (see Figure 1-1).

First, the committee required that the outcome needed to be consistently defined across the literature and have a strong established association with hearing difficulties; several outcomes were excluded from consideration for the core outcome set because either the evidence on the connection between the outcome and hearing difficulties is inconclusive or because the outcome is poorly defined in the literature and follows no consistent definition. Second, the outcome needed to be meaningful for virtually all adults with hearing difficulties and clinicians. The committee recognizes that any single outcome will be meaningful to some individuals or populations, and depends on context, but the committee sought to determine which outcomes were meaningful across populations. Finally, the committee considered the evidence for "importance to measure"—that is, the extent to which hearing health interventions can significantly affect the outcome or whether measurement of the outcome helps inform treatment. The ability to measure the outcome is implicit to this criterion, given that the existence of evidence of the intervention's effect on the outcome requires the availability of measures to generate such evidence.

Outcome Measures

With an initial list of outcomes to consider for the core set, the committee next consulted its list of potential measures to recommend for each of the candidate core outcomes; see Appendix B for the committee's initial measure inventory. For some outcomes the committee found multiple possible measures and narrowed the list of outcome measures to be examined based on the amount of available evidence on the development and psychometric assessment of that measure. The committee developed a set of criteria for measure evaluation that included scientific acceptability (including reliability, validity, and sensitivity to change) and feasibility (see Chapter 6 and Appendix C). The committee carefully reviewed the literature on the psychometric properties of each candidate measure, using value judgments regarding the sufficiency of the amount and quality of the evidence for each criterion. Through iterative discussions, the committee determined the final core outcome set and the best existing measure for each core outcome.

Dissemination and Implementation

For the final part of its charge, the committee reviewed general evidence on best practices for dissemination and implementation as well as for best practices specifically for the uptake of core outcome sets. Chapter 7 provides further details of this evidence.

ORGANIZATION OF REPORT

This introductory chapter provides the study context, charge to the committee, and committee approach. Chapter 2 presents a contextual background of adult hearing health care, including an overview of etiologies of hearing loss and types of interventions. Chapter 3 describes general principles for the development of core outcome sets and the identification of appropriate measures. Chapter 4 describes the concepts of meaningfulness and importance to measure in hearing health care, providing evidence from various sources. Chapter 5 reviews outcomes for hearing health care, and Chapter 6 explores the measurement of those outcomes. Finally, Chapter 7 considers various strategies to encourage the uptake of core outcome sets and the use of standardized measures. The report has five appendixes: Appendix A is a glossary of terms, Appendix B contains a measure inventory (as part of the committee's early evidence-gathering phase), Appendix C includes the committee's measure evaluation worksheet, Appendix D provides a side-by-side comparison of two of the measures considered by the committee for a core outcome, and Appendix E presents the biosketches of the committee members and project staff.

REFERENCES

AHRQ (Agency for Healthcare Research and Quality). 2015. *Types of health care quality measures*. https://www.ahrq.gov/talkingquality/measures/types.html (accessed May 22, 2024).

Deeks, J. J., and P. M. Bossuyt. 2023. Evaluating medical tests. In *Cochrane handbook for systematic reviews of diagnostic test accuracy*. Version 2.0., Pp. 19–33. https://doi.org/10.1002/9781119756194.ch2

Dillard, L. K., L. J. Matthews, and J. R. Dubno. 2024. Prevalence of self-reported hearing difficulty on the Revised Hearing Handicap Inventory and associated factors. *BMC Geriatrics* 24(510). https://doi.org/10.1186/s12877-024-04901-w.

Haile, L. M., A. U. Orji, K. M. Reavis, P. S. Briant, K. M. Lucas, F. Alahdab, T. W. Bärnighausen, A. W. Bell, C. Cao, X. Dai, S. I. Hay, G. Heidari, I. M. Karaye, T. R. Miller, A. H. Mokdad, E. Mostafavi, Z. S. Natto, S. Pawar, J. Rana, A. Seylani, J. A. Singh, J. Wei, L. Yang, K. L. Ong, and J. D. Steinmetz. 2024. Hearing loss prevalence, years lived with disability, and hearing aid use in the United States from 1990 to 2019: Findings from the Global Burden of Disease Study. *Ear and Hearing* 45(1).

HLAA (Hearing Loss Association of America). 2025. *Hearing loop technology*. https://www.hearingloss.org/find-help/hearing-assistive-technology/hearing-loop-technology (accessed March 11, 2025).

Humes, L. E. 2023a. U.S. population data on hearing loss, trouble hearing, and hearing-device use in adults: National Health and Nutrition Examination Survey, 2011-12, 2015-16, and 2017-20. *Trends in Hearing* 27. https//doi.org/10.1177/23312165231160978.

Humes, L. E. 2023b. U.S. population data on self-reported trouble hearing and hearing-aid use in adults: National Health Interview Survey, 2017-2018. *Trends in Hearing* 27. https://doi.org/10.1177/23312165231160967.

ICHOM (International Consortium for Health Outcomes Measurement). n.d. *Why measure outcomes?* https://www.ichom.org/why-measure-outcomes/ (accessed November 12, 2024).

IOM (Institute of Medicine). 2006. *Noise and military service: Implications for hearing loss and tinnitus*. Washington, DC: The National Academies Press.

IOM and NRC (National Research Council). 2006. *Hearing loss research at NIOSH: Reviews of research programs of the National Institute for Occupational Safety and Health*. Washington, DC: The National Academies Press.

IOM and NRC. 2014. *Hearing loss and healthy aging: Workshop summary.* Washington, DC: The National Academies Press.

NASEM (National Academies of Sciences, Engineering, and Medicine). 2016. *Hearing health care for adults: Priorities for improving access and affordability.* Washington, DC: The National Academies Press.

NASEM. 2017. *The promise of assistive technology to enhance activity and work participation.* Washington, DC: The National Academies Press.

NASEM. 2019. *Functional assessment for adults with disabilities.* Washington, DC: The National Academies Press.

NASEM. 2022. *Transforming human health: Celebrating 50 years of discovery and progress.* Washington, DC: The National Academies Press.

NRC (National Research Council). 2005. *Hearing loss: Determining eligibility for Social Security benefits.* Washington, DC: The National Academies Press.

Spankovich, C., V. B. Gonzalez, D. Su, and C. E. Bishop. 2018. Self reported hearing difficulty, tinnitus, and normal audiometric thresholds, the National Health and Nutrition Examination Survey 1999-2002. *Hearing Research* 358:30–36.

2

Contextual Background of Adult Hearing Health Care

As noted in Chapter 1, hearing loss is "the most prevalent sensory disorder in the United States" (Haile et al., 2024, p. 261). Many adults remain unaware of mild hearing loss because it occurs slowly over the course of years and it often remains unnoticed by the individual and undiagnosed (Contrera et al., 2016). Another reason for delays in hearing health care is the psychological resistance to admitting difficulty with hearing (Gates and Mills, 2005). Family members and friends often are the first to notice a hearing loss. Alternatively, older adults may view hearing difficulties as an inevitable rite of passage associated with aging, which deemphasizes the importance of seeking care. On the other hand, adults who seek interventions may have challenges accessing care (e.g., physical health, cost, access) (NASEM, 2016). Today, hearing cannot be fully restored, but a variety of interventions can improve communication, social engagement, and the ability to carry out daily activities. This chapter provides an overview of the prevalence and severity of hearing loss and hearing difficulties, the different etiologies of hearing loss, a variety of disparities in both the prevalence and severity of hearing loss, the different types of interventions, and the settings for evaluating the effectiveness of these interventions.

PREVALENCE AND SEVERITY OF HEARING LOSS AND HEARING DIFFICULTIES

As shown in Figure 2-1, both the prevalence and severity of hearing loss increase with age (Haile et al., 2024). Similarly, as shown in Figure 2-2, the prevalence of self-reported trouble hearing also increases with age (Dillard et al., 2024; Humes, 2023a,b, 2024).

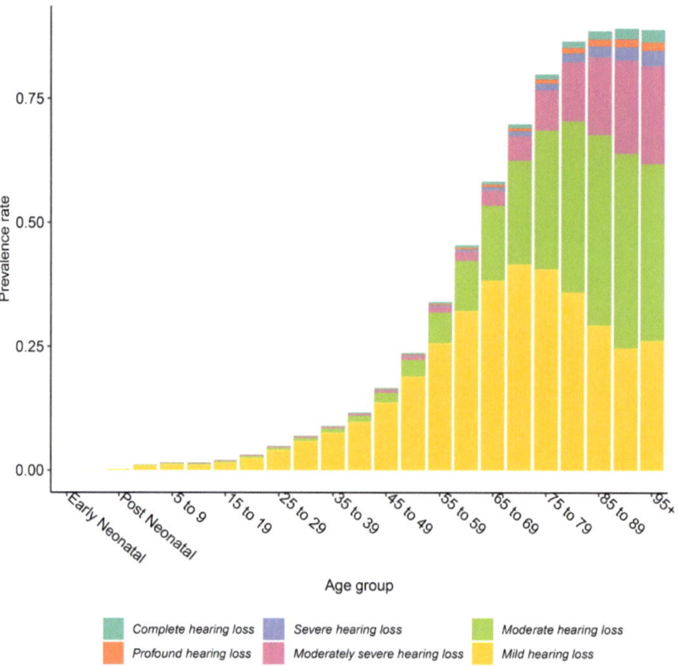

FIGURE 2-1 Prevalence and severity of hearing loss by age.
SOURCE: Haile et al., 2024. CC BY.

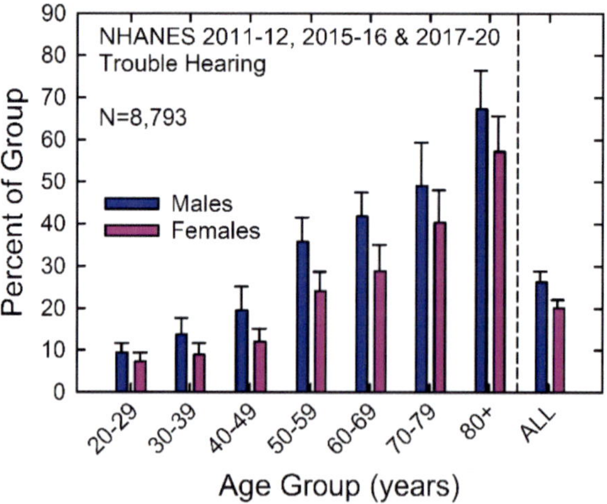

FIGURE 2-2 Prevalence of self-reported trouble hearing among U.S. adults aged 20 and older.
NOTE: NHANES = National Health and Nutrition Examination Survey.
SOURCE: Humes, 2023a. CC-BY-NC.

While approximately 22 percent of the U.S. population overall has hearing loss (Haile et al., 2024), 83 percent of individuals with hearing loss are over age 50 (Haile et al., 2024), and about 65 percent of adults over age 70 experience hearing loss (Reed et al., 2023). About one-quarter of adults report trouble hearing (Humes, 2023a). Additionally, some adults experiencing hearing difficulties do not demonstrate measurable hearing loss when tested. For example, as noted by Grant and colleagues (2021) in their examination of functional hearing and communication deficits, "recent studies suggest that some blast-exposed patients with normal to near-normal-hearing thresholds not only have an awareness of increased hearing difficulties, but also poor performance on various auditory tasks (sound source localization, speech recognition in noise, binaural integration, gap detection in noise, etc.)" (p. 1615). Estimates of the number of individuals who experience hearing difficulties in the absence of measurable hearing loss vary widely in the literature, in part due to differences in the definition of "normal audiometric threshold" as well as differences in the study population (Grant et al., 2021; Parthasarathy et al., 2020; Spankovich, et al., 2018; Tremblay et al., 2015).

ETIOLOGY OF HEARING LOSS

Hearing loss can be classified as mild, moderate, severe, profound, or complete (Haile et al., 2024). Approximately 64 percent of all cases of hearing loss are mild (where one has difficulty understanding speech in noise), and about 25 percent are moderate (where one has difficulty hearing and understanding in noise and sometimes in quiet or on the phone) (Haile et al., 2024). Furthermore, the National Health and Nutrition Examination Survey asks adults (aged 20 and older) about their perceived hearing condition; data from recent surveys show that about 76 percent of respondents described their hearing as excellent or good, and 21 percent said they had "a little" to "moderate" trouble (Humes, 2024).

The three basic types of hearing loss are conductive, sensorineural, and mixed hearing loss, a combination of conductive and sensorineural hearing loss in the same ear (see Figure 2-3; ASHA, n.d. a,b,c; CDC, 2024). Conductive hearing loss is when sound energy is decreased when passing through the outer and/or middle ear on its way to the inner ear (Anastasiadou and Al Khalili, 2023; CDC, 2024). Causes of conductive hearing loss include fluid in the middle ear (due to colds or allergies), infection, earwax, tumors, foreign bodies, or congenital deformities (ASHA, n.d. a). Sensorineural hearing loss, the most prevalent type of permanent hearing loss, reflects difficulty in transforming the sound energy into neural electrical energy at the cochlea or cochlear nerve, owing to deterioration of the cochlear hair cells or nerve. Sensorineural hearing loss both diminishes and distorts the

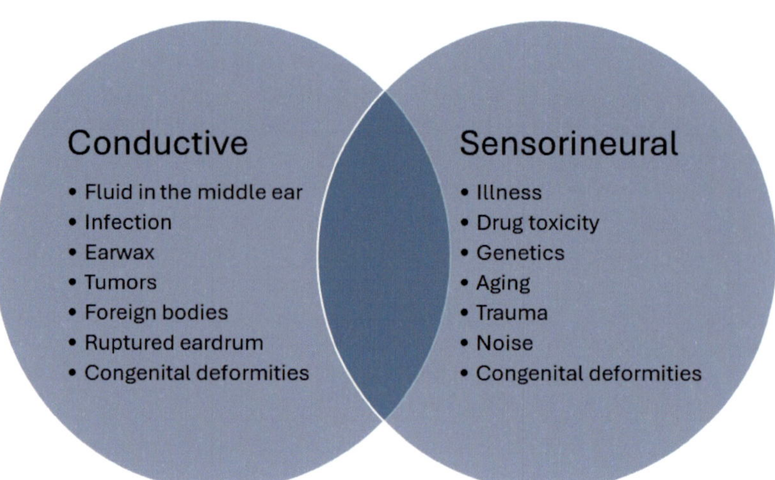

FIGURE 2-3 Basic types of hearing loss.
SOURCES: ASHA, n.d. a,b,c; Cleveland Clinic, 2023.

sensory encoding of sound (Anastasiadou and Al Khalili, 2023). Causes of sensorineural hearing loss include illness (e.g., viral infections, high blood pressure, stroke, diabetes), drug toxicity, genetics, aging, trauma, noise, and congenital deformities (ASHA, n.d. c; Cleveland Clinic, 2023). Mixed hearing loss is a combination of both conductive and sensorineural hearing loss occurring simultaneously in the same ear (ASHA, n.d. b). Hearing loss can occur unilaterally, meaning it is only in one ear, or bilaterally (i.e., in both ears) (CDC, 2024). Hearing loss can also be symmetrical (same degree and configuration of hearing loss in both ears), or asymmetrical (the amount of loss is different between ears).

The most common causes of hearing loss are age; exposures to noise, ototoxic drugs, or chemicals; and genetics (Cunningham and Tucci, 2017, p. 3). The etiologies of hearing loss are explained in more detail below.

Age-Related Hearing Loss

Adult-onset hearing loss is primarily attributable to "the effects of aging on the auditory system," which include "not only the degenerative effects of aging on the cochlea but also by the accumulated effects of exposure to noise and ototoxic drugs" (Cunningham and Tucci, 2017, p. 3). Age-related hearing loss begins in early adulthood and progresses gradually (Gates and Mills, 2005). A range of risk factors exacerbate age-related hearing loss including "biological age, gender, ethnicity, environment, lifestyle health comorbidities, and genetic predisposition" (Bowl and Dawson, 2019, p. 2).

The effects of aging (and other exposures) affect the cochlea, particularly the hair cells and the stria vascularis, and frequently result in significant and irreversible hearing loss (Cunningham and Tucci, 2017).

Some common characteristics of age-related hearing loss include progressive bilateral hearing loss, inability to hear sounds at high frequencies, and challenges understanding speech, especially in noise (Cunningham and Tucci, 2017). In addition to hair cell pathology resulting in sensorineural hearing loss, age-related pathology of synapses and the ascending neural pathway has been shown in mouse models (Sergeyenko et al., 2013) and human temporal bones (Viana et al., 2015; Wu et al., 2021). While synaptic and afferent loss are difficult to distinguish in humans, some evidence suggests potential associations between age-related damage to the afferent neural pathway and speech-in-noise declines (Johannesen et al., 2019). Listening difficulties in complex listening situations (particularly in a noisy environment) are a common patient complaint and can occur with or without audiometric hearing loss.

Noise-Induced Hearing Loss

Medicine has long been aware of noise-induced hearing loss (Hawkins and Schacht, 2005). The Centers for Disease Control and Prevention estimates that the prevalence of noise-induced hearing loss among adults in the United States is 24 percent (Carroll et al., 2017). Noise-induced hearing loss can be unilateral or bilateral (Natarajan et al., 2023). Transient or moderate exposure can cause temporary hearing loss that will return to baseline thresholds in hours or several days at most (Ding et al., 2019). Long-term and or high-dose noise exposure causes permanent irreparable hearing loss (Ding et al., 2019). Continual exposure to intense noise destroys the hair cells in the inner ear, which detect vibrations and amplify sounds (Ding et al., 2019). Hair cells are not able to regenerate; this damage is permanent. Noise exposure occurs in everyday life such as loud music, movie theaters, vehicles, and power tools and in occupational environments such as factories, utilities (e.g., power generation, natural gas distribution, sewer treatment systems), forestry, bars and nightclubs, and sporting events (Cunningham and Tucci, 2017; Masterson and Themann, 2024; NIOSH, 2024; Themann and Masterson, 2019).

In addition to hair cell pathology resulting in sensorineural hearing loss, noise-induced pathology of synapses and the ascending neural pathway has been shown in mouse models (Kujawa and Liberman, 2009). There is significant interest in where the risk of noise-induced synaptic pathology begins in humans (Bramhall et al., 2019; Dobie and Humes, 2017) and the National Occupational Research Agenda (NORA) for Hearing Loss Prevention includes a call for research investigating suprathreshold deficits as a consequence of noise exposure and possible noise-induced pathology including both noise-induced synaptic pathology and outer hair cell loss (NORA, 2019). Recent noise exposure can cause deficits in the understanding of speech in noise in the absence of changes in the audiogram (Grinn et al., 2017), and a history of noise exposure is associated with poorer performance on speech-in-noise tests (for review see Le Prell and Clavier, 2017). Figure 2-4 demonstrates examples of safe and unsafe levels of noise in occupational and nonoccupational settings (Natarajan et al., 2023).

Drug-Induced Hearing Loss

Ototoxic medications that treat cancer, serious infections, and heart disease can damage the ear and cause hearing loss (Campo et al., 2013; Cone

Breathing	10 dB	
Ticking watch	20 dB	
Average room noise	30-50 dB	**Safe sound level**
Normal conversation/ background music	60 dB	
Average office noise	70 dB	
Landscaping equipment (inside house)	75 dB	
Vacuum / inside an airplane	80 dB	
City traffic (inside a car) / noisy restaurant	85 dB	
Subway, shouted conversation	90-95 dB	**Repeated or prolonged exposure could lead to NIHL over time**
Pro sports events/ car horn at 16 ft	95-100 dB	
Motorcycle, stereo	100 dB	
Chainsaw, leafblower, snowmobile	106-115 dB	
Music concert, ambulance siren	120 dB	**Can result in immediate and permanent hearing loss after a single close-range exposure**
Jet engine taking off	140 dB	
Gun shot	140-60 dB	

FIGURE 2-4 Noise exposure levels.
NOTE: NIHL = noise-induced hearing loss.
SOURCE: Natarajan et al., 2023. CC BY 4.0.

et al., n.d.; Schacht et al., 2012). Approximately one million individuals are exposed to platinum-based cancer treatments annually resulting in a global burden of about 500,000 cases of hearing loss every year (Dillard et al., 2022). For example, cisplatin, which is used commonly to treat many types of cancer, is held in the inner ear for months to years after administration where it kills certain types of cells essential for hearing (Lee et al., 2024). Another class of ototoxic drugs are aminoglycoside antibiotics used for the treatment of gram-negative bacterial infections killing cochlear hair cells impairing high-frequency hearing (Lee et al., 2024). Loop diuretics used to treat high blood pressure and congestive heart failure (e.g., ethacrynic acid, furosemide, and bumetanide) can cause temporary hearing loss during treatment (Ding et al., 2002; Forge, 1982; Martínez-Rodríguez et al., 2007). When diuretics are prescribed with other ototoxic drugs, the damage to the ear is multiplied and results in worsening the degree of hearing loss (Ding et al., 2002; Komune and Snow, 1981; Li et al., 2011).

Hearing Loss Attributable to Chemical Exposures

In addition to noise exposure, workers in some industries also are exposed to ototoxic chemicals that can cause hearing loss (Campo et al., 2013). Industries that may have workers at risk of environmental exposure to such chemicals include "printing, painting, boat building, construction, glue manufacturing, metal products, chemicals, petroleum, leather products, furniture making, agriculture, and mining" (Campo et al., 2013, p. 5). The risk for workers in these industries comes primarily from exposure to aromatic solvents, which are vital ingredients in "adhesives, paints, lacquers, varnishes, printing inks, degreasers, fuel additives, glues, and thinners. . .plastics, rubber articles, and glass fibers" (Campo et al., 2013, p. 5). Firefighters also are at high risk of exposure because of the inhalation of smoke from burning toxic items like lead paint, batteries, and pressure-treated wood (Campo et al., 2013). Ototoxic chemicals primarily poison the hair cells or may damage other elements of the organ of Corti, which is essential for transmitting auditory signals (Campo et al., 2013). Growing evidence suggests that noise exposure compounds these chemicals' toxic effects, furthering the damage, which is a significant concern since both exposures are often present in the same environment.

Genetic Hearing Loss

In addition to age and environmental exposures, genetics also influence age-related hearing loss (WHO, 2021). About half of the cases of early-onset hearing loss have a genetic etiology, but the extent to which genetics influence adult hearing loss is under researched (Penn Medicine, n.d.). Current research estimates that adult-onset hearing loss is 25 to 55 percent hereditary resulting from mutation of genes that are required for hearing (Cunningham and Tucci, 2017). Preliminary research has been done on what genes may predispose someone to noise-induced or age-related hearing loss, but additional research is needed to fully understand to what extent one's genetics predisposes hearing loss (Penn Medicine, n.d.).

Idiopathic Sudden Sensorineural Hearing Loss

Idiopathic sudden sensorineural hearing loss is typically a unilateral, sensorineural hearing loss that occurs within a 72-hour period (Rauch, 2008). Recovery correlates to the severity of the hearing loss. People with mild hearing loss are likely to recover fully. People with moderate hearing loss often recover some but will not fully recover. People with severe hearing loss rarely recover fully (Rauch, 2008). Sudden sensorineural hearing loss may be attributable to an array of causes including Meniere's disease, trauma, autoimmune disease, syphilis, Lyme disease, and perilymphatic fistula (Rauch, 2008). It also can occur because of a spinal tap or an intracranial surgery. In most cases, the sudden sensorineural hearing loss is termed idiopathic as the cause is not known. Steroid treatment is generally considered to be the standard of care even though the scientific evidence for its efficacy is insufficient (Chandrasekhar et al., 2019; Marx et al., 2018).

DISPARITIES IN HEARING LOSS

A variety of factors contribute to disparities in hearing loss demographics as well as access to hearing health care. Several of these factors are described below.

Demographics

The prevalence of age-related hearing loss varies by race and sex. After adjusting for all demographic variables, White individuals report the highest rates of hearing loss (Lin et al., 2012; Humes 2023a, 2024). Generally, the factors identified for hearing loss also have emerged from analyses of national data on perceived hearing difficulties (Humes, 2023a,b). One explanation for the racial disparity in hearing loss is that higher levels of melanin may exist in the cochlea of Black individuals and melanin may decrease the risk of hearing loss (Lin et al., 2012). Both the rates of self-reported hearing difficulties (see Figure 2-2) and prevalence of hearing impairment are higher for men than women (Hoffman et al., 2017; Humes, 2023a,b, 2024). This is likely at least partially because of differences in noise exposure (Daniel, 2007; Helzner et al., 2005). Additionally, the hormone estrogen is protective against hearing loss, reducing risk, which can be a protective factor for women (Delhez et al., 2020; Reavis et al., 2023).

Access to Hearing Health Care

In addition to disparities in the prevalence of hearing loss itself, access to diagnostics and treatment for hearing loss is unequal among older adults in the United States. Disparities exist in both cost and insurance coverage. Prescription hearing aids cost about $2,700 per ear (Currie, 2025). Standard Medicaid programs are not required to cover hearing aids; therefore, coverage varies by state. In 2017, 28 states offered Medicaid coverage for "hearing aid assessment and associated services for adult beneficiaries meeting the inclusion criteria" (Arnold et al., 2017, p. 1479). The inclusion criteria also vary by state. Medicare Part B covers diagnostic evaluations only if the assessment is ordered by a physician and will not cover "hearing aids or examination for the purpose of prescribing, fitting, or changing hearing aids" (Center for Medicare Advocacy, 2024). If coverage is offered, it will be through Medicare Part C (also referred to as Medicare Advantage); this coverage is optional supplementary insurance that comes at additional costs (Malcolm et al., 2022). Hearing aids may be covered to some extent by a Medicare Advantage plan, but again this is not a requirement (Currie, 2025). In 2024, the European Federation of Hard of Hearing People (EFHOH), the European Association of Hearing Aid Professionals (AEA), and the European Hearing Instrument Manufacturers Association (EHIMA) collaborated publishing *Getting the Numbers Right on Hearing Loss Hearing Care and Hearing Aid Use in Europe* (Laureyns et al., 2024). The report found that "in countries where reimbursement is around 20 percent of the total cost, the uptake is 19 percent, but when reimbursement is around 50 percent, the uptake is 27 percent. When reimbursement is around 80 percent, the uptake increases to 41 percent, and when hearing aids are free of charge, uptake is 49 percent" (p. 8). These data show that when hearing aids are partially or even fully covered by insurance the uptake is still low.

As noted in the 2014 Institute of Medicine (IOM) and National Research Council (NRC) workshop summary *Hearing Loss and Healthy Aging:*

> Among nonadopters, cost is cited as the primary reason for not getting a hearing aid. Two-thirds of these people said that they would get a hearing aid if insurance or other programs provided 100 percent coverage, and 47 percent said they were likely to get a hearing aid if the price did not exceed $500. "Beyond the purchase of a home or a car, hearing aids and services can be the third most expensive purchase for many Americans with hearing loss over time." (pp. 78–79)

Beyond expenses, adults living in rural areas are more likely to experience delays in accessing hearing care (including hearing aids) because of the distance and availability of specialists (Chan et al., 2017). Chan and colleagues (2017) found that rural residents reported an average of 10.9 years between hearing loss onset and receiving a hearing aid compared to urban/suburban residents who reported an average of 7.9 years. A qualitative study of adults ages 50 to 78 living in Appalachian Kentucky reported that participants were frequently exposed to loud sounds like lawn mowers, hunting guns, and heavy power tools putting them at high risk of developing hearing difficulties (Powell et al., 2019). The participants in this study voiced concerns about the consequences of hearing loss like not being able to hear a fire alarm, not being able to speak on the phone, not hearing grandchildren, and impaired job performance (Powell et al., 2019).

Not only is the access to both primary care and hearing health care services more limited in remote settings, but more people in rural communities rely on Medicaid coverage making the cost of hearing aids unaffordable (Powell et al., 2019). One of the challenges for hearing health care access is awareness of hearing health and hearing health literacy among primary care providers who are often the first point of contact and source of referrals for hearing health care (Sydlowski et al., 2022).

CLASSES OF NONSURGICAL INTERVENTIONS

Several approaches to treating hearing loss exist, and the choice of intervention may depend on the etiology of the individual's hearing loss and their goals. The main categories of interventions include devices, rehabilitation and training strategies, and investigative pharmaceuticals and biological therapies. As delineated in the statement of task for this study, surgically implanted devices (e.g., cochlear implants, bone-anchored hearing aids) are not considered here.

Devices

Several devices have been developed for adults with hearing difficulties including assistive listening devices, prescription hearing aids, and over-the-counter hearing aids.

Assistive Listening Devices

Assistive listening devices are electroacoustic devices that are alternative or supplemental to the use of hearing aids. These devices may be used at the level of the individual (e.g., personal sound amplification devices and software) or at the systems level (e.g., hearing loops).[1] A systematic review of the effectiveness of these devices in adults identified 11 studies, but the overall conclusion was that high-quality evidence regarding the effectiveness of assistive listening devices was not available (Maidment et al., 2018). None of these studies included any of the outcome measures recommended in this study (see Chapter 6).

Prescription Hearing Aids

Prescription hearing aids are small electronic devices worn in or behind the ear that deliver amplified sound, tailored to the level of severity of the hearing loss (NIH, 2022). Although hearing aids cannot restore hearing fully, they improve hearing and speech comprehension for individuals with hearing loss. An audiologist or hearing instrument specialist fits and programs the device for the individual with hearing difficulties. They can program the hearing aid to provide amplification differentially based on frequency and input level to customize the device to an individual's hearing profile. The hearing aid wearer may be able to switch between different settings set by the provider for different listening environments.

Over-the-Counter Hearing Aids

In addition to prescription hearing aids, the Food and Drug Administration (FDA) has approved a new category for over-the-counter hearing aids (NIDCD, 2022). The passage of the *Over-the-Counter Hearing Aid Act of 2017* sought to improve access to hearing aids for individuals with perceived mild to moderate hearing loss.[2] Over-the-counter hearing aids are not suitable for individuals with severe hearing loss or for children (NIDCD, 2022). Although over-the-counter hearing aids may offer a more affordable intervention for treating hearing difficulties in adults who perceive mild to moderate challenges, these hearing aids still may remain unaffordable for many individuals with low socioeconomic status (Malcolm et al., 2022). Notably, as of 2024, software that renders existing amplification hardware (e.g., earbuds) as meeting the criteria for over-the-counter hearing aids has been approved by the FDA (FDA, 2024).

---

[1] A hearing loop is an assistive listening system placed in a public setting that helps transmit sound directly from a microphone into hearing aids (equipped with telecoils) and cochlear implants. This system "can make speech and music in public places more understandable" (HLAA, 2025).

[2] Congress.gov. Over-the-Counter Hearing Aid Act of 2017, S. 670, 115th Cong., 1st sess., https://www.congress.gov/bill/115th-congress/senate-bill/670.

Perceived Benefit and Potential Adverse Effects of Hearing Aids

Research on hearing interventions typically focuses on their efficacy (measured in carefully controlled conditions) or effectiveness (measured in real-world settings). While most hearing aid wearers receive some benefit from hearing aids, the nonuse of hearing aids (among those with hearing aids) is primarily attributable to limited perceived benefit or dissatisfaction with the device (such as discomfort) (Franks and Timmer, 2023; Kochkin, 2000; McCormack and Fortnum, 2013). There is some limited evidence that the use of hearing aids that fit poorly may have adverse effects such as blisters, headaches, dizziness, and problems with chewing and swallowing (Kochkin, 2000; Manchaiah et al., 2019; McCormack and Fortnum, 2013).

Rehabilitation and Education

Other forms of hearing intervention may not involve a device. Specifically, aural rehabilitation is a common intervention that is most often used in addition to fitted devices to help individuals explore treatment options and learn how to communicate better and supports them through the adjustment to their device (Boothroyd, 2007; Pratt, 2005). Boothroyd (2007) defined aural rehabilitation as "the reduction of hearing-loss-induced deficits of function, activity, participation, and quality of life through sensory management, instruction, perceptual training, and counseling" (p. 63). Aural rehabilitation includes a wide range of activities including auditory training, assistive listening devices, communication strategies, relaxation techniques, and support groups (Hearing Speech + Deaf Center, n.d.). A systematic review of auditory training found a general lack of strong evidence supporting its effectiveness in adults with mild to moderate hearing loss (Henshaw and Ferguson, 2013). Three active-control randomized controlled trials conducted since that systematic review also failed to establish the effectiveness of this intervention, especially in the context of generalizing task-specific learning to improvements in everyday hearing function (Henshaw et al., 2022; Humes et al., 2019; Saunders et al., 2016).

Interventions based on education involving information about their hearing aids and the use of communication strategies, as well as general hearing-related counseling, have also been studied frequently. However, these studies typically involve instructional intervention included as a supplement to hearing aid use (i.e., not as a stand-alone intervention). Some studies show statistically significant benefits of the instructional intervention, but the effects are generally small compared to the effects of hearing-aids alone (Abrams et al., 1992; Brännström et al., 2016; Kricos and Holmes,

1996; Malmberg et al., 2017, 2023; Molander et al., 2018; Preminger, 2003; Preminger and Ziegler, 2008; Preminger and Yoo, 2010; Sweetow and Sabes, 2006; Thorén et al., 2014). Other studies have not demonstrated statistically significant effects of the instructional intervention (Ferguson et al., 2016; Kricos et al., 1992 Saunders et al., 2016).

Pharmaceutical and Biological Therapies

Currently the FDA has not approved any pharmaceutical or biological therapies to treat hearing loss, but regenerative strategies for improving hearing loss are being investigated (Ajay et al., 2022; Lewis, 2021). In addition to treatment of hearing loss, there is significant interest in therapies for hearing loss prevention, tinnitus, and balance disorders. As of 2019, there were 43 biotechnology and pharmaceutical companies working on therapeutics for inner ear and central ear disorders including drug, cell, and gene-based treatments (Schilder et al., 2019). As of 2021, there were 23 assets in clinical trials and 56 in preclinical development (Isherwood et al., 2022). One of the major challenges is that preclinical study designs lack standardization, which limits the ability to assess the comparative efficacy of potential treatments (Le Prell, 2023). Clinical trials evaluating pharmaceutical interventions in human participants similarly lack standardization (Le Prell, 2021). In 2022, the FDA approved a proprietary sodium thiosulfate formulation (Pedmark) administered intravenously to reduce the risk of cisplatin ototoxicity in pediatric patients with localized non-metastatic solid tumors (Dhillon, 2023). As the first approved medicine for hearing loss prevention, it is a promising step forward.

Only three peer-reviewed papers from two companies are available on gene therapy for hereditary hearing loss in human patients (Lv et al., 2024; Qi et al., 2024; Wang et al., 2024). So far, all participants have been children with otoferlin (OTOF) mutations. At present, they all reported proximal outcomes like pure-tone audiograms, otoacoustic emissions, and auditory brainstem responses of various types in assessing the degree of restoration of hearing in these patients. Another report evaluating small-molecule therapy (CHIR99021+valproic acid) described improved speech intelligibility in a subset of the participants receiving the investigational agents with no improvements in any participants who received placebo (McLean et al., 2021). Like hearing aids and cochlear implants, gene-therapy approaches to treating hearing loss will and should follow a similar progression from proximal outcomes demonstrating the restoration of audibility to more distal outcome measures like speech understanding in quiet and in complex listening situations (see Chapter 5).

SETTINGS FOR OUTCOME MEASUREMENT

Evaluation of the effectiveness of hearing health interventions is done for various purposes and can take place in multiple settings including research and clinical care.

Research Settings

In addition to studies of the effect of interventions at the level of the individual, two specific settings for research include establishing efficacy and effectiveness in clinical trials and population-based research.

Establishing Efficacy and Effectiveness in Clinical Trials

A major research context for outcome measurement is in the establishment of efficacy and effectiveness of the intervention in clinical trials (Munro et al., 2021). Phase I trials are exploratory and aim to assess the safety and dosage of an intervention, including only a small number of healthy participants. Phase II trials estimate the efficacy of an intervention, including a small number of participants with the relevant health condition preliminarily. Efficacy is how well an intervention works in the ideal and controlled environment (Singal et al., 2014). Phase III trials measure efficacy with a larger study population (Munro et al., 2021). Study designs vary, but these trials compare people who receive the intervention to a control group who receive the current standard of care, or placebo when there is no standard of care. Then, Phase IV trials, which occur after drug approval, monitor for effectiveness and side effects in a large population over a long period.

Population Health Research

Outcome measurement for population-level research reflects "a population's dynamic state of physical, mental, and social well-being" (Parrish, 2010, p. 1). Outcome measures in population health can be used to create summary statistics, assess the distribution of an outcome in a population, and measure a population's overall health or well-being (Parrish, 2010). Summary statistics of health outcomes on a population level inform where additional research or policy changes may be necessary (Murray et al., 2002). Outcome measures in population health are also used to understand the distribution of health issues and shed light on health disparities (Murray et al., 2002). Understanding which subgroups are most affected by a particular health condition is necessary to appropriately target resources, interventions, and the potential harms and consequences of untreated hearing loss.

Population-level research is essential for suggesting a possible causal relationship (Cox and Wermuth, 2004; Hays and Peipert, 2021; Ling et al., 2023) and finding disease risk factors or predictors of treatment response. However, an inherent limitation of population-level research is transporting observational study risk estimates and clinical trial intervention effects to the individual level. Moreover, limited research exists on significant individual-level change associated with intervention in the hearing science and broader academic literature. An essential consideration in making recommendations for outcome measurement in clinical settings will be balancing the potential for individual-level change based off population-level evidence with other variables (e.g., patient-reported areas of concern, concordance of literature, proximal/distal outcome, characteristics of the intervention).

Clinical Settings

Clinical settings for outcome assessment include assessing patient response (in person), via telemedicine, and self-care.

Assessing Patient Response in Person

In the clinical setting, outcome measurement helps to assess the effect of an intervention on health and functioning and thereby inform the treatment plan. Behavioral measures may be used to objectively assess improvement in hearing difficulties, such as through various tests that assess an individual's ability to understand speech in a noisy environment (Billings et al., 2023). Additionally, the effects of an intervention may be assessed through the perspective of patient experience (i.e., through the use of patient-reported measures). Technological advancements have made the implementation of patient-reported outcome measures efficient by administering the measure (typically a questionnaire) online in advance of an appointment or on tablets in the clinician's office (Dobrozsi and Panepinto, 2015). By incorporating the patient's perspective into clinical care, clinicians can better understand what is meaningful to the patient and tailor interventions and treatment plans (Dobrozsi and Panepinto, 2015).

Telemedicine

Telemedicine, the delivery of health care services from a distance, has been used for decades but drastically increased in popularity during and after the COVID-19 pandemic (Hyder and Razzak, 2020). One of the main benefits of telemedicine is that it increases access and reduces the cost of traveling to a clinic, particularly for individuals in rural areas (D'Onofrio and Zeng, 2022). There is growing interest in tablet, computer, and smartphone-based audiometry, but the results may be compromised by the lack of a soundproof booth, which has been used to control background noise. Recent advances in both passive attenuation and active cancellation of noise as well as machine learning have alleviated this background noise issue to make tele-audiometry a reliable and accurate alternative to traditional audiometry for "air conduction, bone conduction, and contralateral masking" (D'Onofrio and Zeng, 2022, p. 4). Additionally, satisfaction with hearing aids with remote fitting and verification is comparable to traditional practices. Alternatives to remote or in-situ pure-tone audiometry include such tests as the digits-in-noise test (De Sousa et al., 2020; Smits et al., 2004) that use stimuli less vulnerable to the presence of background noise during testing yet are strongly correlated to the pure-tone test results. Patient-reported outcome measures are essential for measuring the effects of an intervention in the telemedicine setting (Mercadal-Orfila et al., 2024).

The availability of electronic versions of self-report outcome measurements means that patients can complete the questionnaire at home or anywhere with internet (Gibson and Pincus, 2021). A noninferiority trial of Veterans Administration patients evaluating hearing health outcomes (measured by the International Outcome Inventory for Hearing Aids) found that both teleaudiology and in-person audiology care were highly effective and found no clinically meaningful difference between the care delivery models (Pross et al., 2016). A single-blinded randomized controlled trial of 56 adults found that teleaudiology follow-up appointments "were of similar effectiveness" to in-person appointments (Teleaudiology Today, 2021). Telehealth has significant usefulness in a variety of hearing health care contexts, including not only use in noise and ototoxic exposure monitoring, but also expansion of access for patients and participants in rural and low-resource settings, and facilitating the evaluation of auditory outcomes in large-scale clinical trials (Robler et al., 2022). Ecological momentary assessment (EMA) is an alternative measurement technique that samples "subjects' current behaviors and experiences in real time, in subjects' natural environments" (Shiffman et al., 2008, p.1). EMA reduces recall bias and improves ecological validity, but they are time intensive for clinicians, researchers, and patients.

Self-Care

Over-the-counter hearing aids created a new setting in the hearing health world, which is self-care. The World Health Organization defines self-care as "the ability of individuals, families, and communities to promote and maintain their health, prevent disease, and cope with illness with or without the support of a health or care worker" (WHO, 2024). For hearing, this has been framed recently in the concept of "auditory wellness" (Humes, 2021; Humes et al., 2024). This care can range from administering medicines and diagnostics to intervening with devices and using digital tools. Consumers who purchase hearing aids over the counter will typically fit the devices themselves without the assistance of a hearing health professional. Instead of audiologists or hearing aid specialists, some consumers will rely on support and information from primary care clinicians and pharmacists (Berenbrok et al., 2021; Davis et al., 2025).

Adults with hearing difficulties who pursue over-the-counter hearing aids will usually not receive a traditional audiogram and will also not likely undergo formal outcome assessment. However, adults with hearing loss may be able to accurately administer some self-report outcome measures themselves. A framework for self-assessment of hearing difficulties, self-assessment of outcomes, and self-management of auditory wellness has been described recently (Humes et al., 2024). Such self-management has the potential to broaden the accessibility to hearing health care considerably.

FINDINGS

Finding 2-1: The prevalence and severity of both audiometric hearing loss and self-reported hearing difficulties increase with age.

Finding 2-2: Hearing loss and self-reported hearing difficulties affect approximately 1 in every 5 adults and about two-thirds of adults aged 70 and older.

Finding 2-3: Two-thirds of hearing loss cases are in adults over the age of 50.

Finding 2-4: The most common etiology of hearing loss is from the degenerative effects of aging, followed by noise exposure.

Finding 2-5: Currently, there are no cures for age-related or noise-induced hearing loss, but there are treatments that improve communication and mitigate many of the social and emotional consequences of hearing difficulties. Few people experience adverse side effects of treatment.

Finding 2-6: Outcomes of hearing health interventions may be assessed in a variety of settings and for a range of purposes.

REFERENCES

Abrams, H. B., T. Hnath-Chisolm, S. M. Guerreiro, and S. I. Ritterman. 1992. The effects of intervention strategy on self-perception of hearing handicap. *Ear and Hearing* 13(5):371–377.
Ajay, E., N. Gunewardene, and R. Richardson. 2022. Emerging therapies for human hearing loss. *Expert Opinion on Biological Therapy* 22(6):689–705.

Anastasiadou, S., and Y. Al Khalili. 2023. Hearing loss. In *Statpearls*. Treasure Island, FL: StatPearls Publishing

Arnold, M. L., K. Hyer, and T. Chisolm. 2017. Medicaid hearing aid coverage for older adult beneficiaries: A state-by-state comparison. *Health Affairs* 36(8):1476–1484.

ASHA (American Speech-Language-Hearing Association). n.d., a. *Conductive hearing loss.* https://www.asha.org/public/hearing/conductive-hearing-loss (accessed November 26, 2024).

ASHA. n.d., b. *Mixed hearing loss.* https://www.asha.org/public/hearing/mixed-hearing-loss (accessed November 26, 2024).

ASHA. n.d., c. *Sensorineural hearing loss.* https://www.asha.org/public/hearing/sensorineural-hearing-loss (accessed November 26, 2024).

Berenbrok, L. A., L. Ciemniecki, A. A. Cremeans, R. Albright, and E. Mormer. 2021. Pharmacist competencies for over-the-counter hearing aids: A Delphi study. *Journal of the American Pharmacists Association* 61(4):e255–e262.

Billings, C. J., T. M. Olsen, L. Charney, B. M. Madsen, and C. E. Holmes. 2023. Speech-in-noise testing: An introduction for audiologists. *Seminars in Hearing* 45(1). https://doi.org/10.1055/s-0043-1770155.

Boothroyd, A. 2007. Adult aural rehabilitation: What is it and does it work? *Trends in Amplification* 11(2):63–71.

Bowl, M. R., and S. J. Dawson. 2019. Age-related hearing loss. *Cold Spring Harbor Perspectives in Medicine* 9(8):1–14.

Bramhall, N., E. F. Beach, B. Epp, C. G. Le Prell, E. A. Lopez-Poveda, C. J. Plack, R. Schaette, S. Verhulst, and B. Canlon. 2019. The search for noise-induced cochlear synaptopathy in humans: Mission impossible? *Hearing Research* 377:88–103.

Brännström, K. J., M. Öberg, E. Ingo, K. N. T. Månsson, G. Andersson, T. Lunner, and A. Laplante-Lévesque. 2016. The initial evaluation of an internet-based support system for audiologists and first-time hearing aid clients. *Internet Interventions* 4:82–91.

Campo, P., T. C. Morata, and O. Hong. 2013. Chemical exposure and hearing loss. *Disease-a-Month* 59(4):119–138.

Carroll, Y. I., J. Eichwald, F. Scinicariello, H. J. Hoffman, S. Deitchman, M. S. Radke, C. L. Themann, and P. Breysse. 2017. Vital signs: Noise-induced hearing loss among adults—United States 2011–2012. *Morbidity and Mortality Weekly Report* 66(5):139–144.

CDC (Centers for Disease Control and Prevention). 2024. *Types of hearing loss.* https://www.cdc.gov/hearing-loss-children/about/types-of-hearing-loss.html (accessed September 18, 2024).

Center for Medicare Advocacy. 2024. *Medicare coverage of hearing care and audiology services.* https://medicareadvocacy.org/medicare-info/medicare-coverage-of-hearing-care-and-audiology-services (accessed October 4, 2024).

Chan, S., B. Hixon, M. Adkins, J. B. Shinn, and M. L. Bush. 2017. Rurality and determinants of hearing healthcare in adult hearing aid recipients. *Laryngoscope* 127(10):2362–2367.

Chandrasekhar, S. S., B. S. Tsai Do, S. R. Schwartz, L. J. Bontempo, E. A. Faucett, S. A. Finestone, D. B. Hollingsworth, D. M. Kelley, S. T. Kmucha, G. Moonis, G. L. Poling, J. K. Roberts, R. J. Stachler, D. M. Zeitler, M. D. Corrigan, L. C. Nnacheta, and L. Satterfield. 2019. Clinical practice guideline: Sudden hearing loss (update). *Otolaryngology-Head and Neck Surgery* 161(1_suppl):S1–S45.

Cleveland Clinic. 2023. *Hearing loss.* https://my.clevelandclinic.org/health/diseases/17673-hearing-loss (accessed January 3, 2025).

Cone, B., P. Dorn, D. Konrad-Martin, J. Lister, C. Ortiz, and K. Schairer. n.d. *Ototoxic medications (medication effects).* https://www.asha.org/public/hearing/ototoxic-medications (accessed November 16, 2023).

Contrera, K. J., M. I. Wallhagen, S. K. Mamo, E. S. Oh, and F. R. Lin. 2016. Hearing loss health care for older adults. *Journal of the American Board of Family Medicine* 29(3):394–403.

Cox, D. R., and N. Wermuth. 2004. Causality: A statistical view. *International Statistical Review* 72(3):285–305.

Cunningham, L. L., and D. L. Tucci. 2017. Hearing loss in adults. *New England Journal of Medicine* 377(25):2465–2473.

Currie, D. 2025. *Does Medicare & insurance cover hearing aids in 2025?* https://www.ncoa.org/adviser/hearing-aids/does-medicare-cover-hearing-aids (accessed January 11, 2025).

D'Onofrio, K. L., and F.-G. Zeng. 2022. Tele-audiology: Current state and future directions. *Frontiers in Digital Health* 3:788103.

Daniel, E. 2007. Noise and hearing loss: A review. *Journal of School Health* 77(5):225–231.

Davis, R. J., M. Lin, O. Ayo-Ajibola, D. D. Ahn, P. A. Brown, J. Parsons, T. F. Ho, and J. S. Choi. 2025. Over-the-counter hearing aids: A nationwide survey study to understand perspectives in primary care. *Laryngoscope* 135(1):299–307.

Delhez, A., P. Lefebvre, C. Péqueux, B. Malgrange, and L. Delacroix. 2020. Auditory function and dysfunction: Estrogen makes a difference. *Cellular and Molecular Life Sciences* 77(4):619–635.

De Sousa, K. C., D. W. Swanepoel, D. R. Moore, H. C. Myburgh, and C. Smits. 2020. Improving sensitivity of the digits-in-noise test using antiphasic stimuli. *Ear and Hearing* 41(2):442–450.

Dhillon, S. 2023. Sodium thiosulfate: Pediatric first approval. *Paediatric Drugs* 25(2):239–244.

Dillard, L. K., L. Lopez-Perez, R. X. Martinez, A. M. Fullerton, S. Chadha, and C. M. McMahon. 2022. Global burden of ototoxic hearing loss associated with platinum-based cancer treatment: A systematic review and meta-analysis. *Cancer Epidemiology* 79:102203.

Dillard, L. K., L. J. Matthews, and J. R. Dubno. 2024. Prevalence of self-reported hearing difficulty on the Revised Hearing Handicap Inventory and associated factors. *BMC Geriatrics* 24(510). https://doi.org/10.1186/s12877-024-04901-w.

Ding, D., S. L. McFadden, J. M. Woo, and R. J. Salvi. 2002. Ethacrynic acid rapidly and selectively abolishes blood flow in vessels supplying the lateral wall of the cochlea. *Hearing Research* 173(1–2):1–9.

Ding, T., A. Yan, and K. Liu. 2019. What is noise-induced hearing loss? *British Journal of Hospital Medicine* 80(9):525–529.

Dobie, R. A., and L. E. Humes. 2017. Commentary on the regulatory implications of noise-induced cochlear neuropathy. *International Journal of Audiology* 56(Supl 1):74–78.

Dobrozsi, S., and J. Panepinto. 2015. Patient-reported outcomes in clinical practice. *Hematology* 2015(1):501–506.

Ferguson, M., M. Brandreth, W. Brassington, P. Leighton, and H. Wharrad. 2016. A randomized controlled trial to evaluate the benefits of a multimedia educational program for first-time hearing aid users. *Ear and Hearing* 37(2):123–136.

FDA (Food and Drug Administration). 2024. FDA authorizes first over-the-counter hearing aid software. https://www.fda.gov/news-events/press-announcements/fda-authorizes-first-over-counter-hearing-aid-software (accessed Febuary 18, 2025).

Forge, A. 1982. A tubulo-cisternal endoplasmic reticulum system in the potassium transporting marginal cells of the stria vascularis and effects of the ototoxic diuretic ethacrynic acid. *Cell and Tissue Research* 226(2):375–387.

Franks, I., and B. H. B. Timmer. 2023. Reasons for the non-use of hearing aids: Perspectives of non-users, past users, and family members. *International Journal of Audiology* 63(10):794–801.

Gates, G. A., and J. H. Mills. 2005. Presbycusis. *Lancet* 366(9491):1111–1120.

Gibson, K. A., and T. Pincus. 2021. A self-report multidimensional health assessment questionnaire (MDHAQ) for face-to-face or telemedicine encounters to assess clinical severity (RAPID3) and screen for fibromyalgia (FAST) and depression (DEP). *Current Treatment Options in Rheumatology* 7(3):161–181.

Grinn, S. K., K. B. Wiseman, J. A. Baker, and C. G. Le Prell. 2017. Hidden hearing loss? No effect of common recreational noise exposure on cochlear nerve response amplitude in humans. *Frontiers in Neuroscience* 11:465.

Grant, K. W., L. R., Kubli, S. A. Phatak, H. Galloza, and D. S. Brungart. 2021. Estimated prevalence of functional hearing difficulties in blast-exposed service members with normal to near-normal-hearing thresholds. *Ear and Hearing* 42(6):1615–1626.

Haile, L. M., A. U. Orji, K. M. Reavis, P. S. Briant, K. M. Lucas, F. Alahdab, T. W. Bärnighausen, A. W. Bell, C. Cao, X. Dai, S. I. Hay, G. Heidari, I. M. Karaye, T. R. Miller, A. H. Mokdad, E. Mostafavi, Z. S. Natto, S. Pawar, J. Rana, A. Seylani, J. A. Singh, J. Wei, L. Yang, K. L. Ong, and J. D. Steinmetz. 2024. Hearing loss prevalence, years lived with disability, and hearing aid use in the United States from 1990 to 2019: Findings from the Global Burden of Disease study. *Ear and Hearing* 45(1):257–267.

Hawkins, J. E., and J. Schacht. 2005. Sketches of otohistory part 10: Noise-induced hearing loss. *Audiology and Neurotology* 10(6):305–309.

Hays, R. D., and J. D. Peipert. 2021. Between-group minimally important change versus individual treatment responders. *Quality of Life Research* 30(10):2765–2772.

Hearing Speech + Deaf Center. n.d. *What is aural rehabiliation.* https://hearingspeechdeaf.org/what-is-aural-rehabilitation/#:~:text=How%20Does%20Aural%20Rehabilitation%20Work,can%20reduce%20feelings%20of%20isolation (accessed January 5, 2025).

Helzner, E. P., J. A. Cauley, S. R. Pratt, S. R. Wisniewski, J. M. Zmuda, E. O. Talbott, N. De Rekeneire, T. B. Harris, S. M. Rubin, and E. M. Simonsick. 2005. Race and sex differences in age-related hearing loss: The health, aging and body composition study. *Journal of the American Geriatrics Society* 53(12):2119–2127.

Henshaw, H., and M. A. Ferguson. 2013. Efficacy of individual computer-based auditory training for people with hearing loss: A systematic review of the evidence. *PLoS One* 8(5):e62836.

Henshaw, H., A. Heinrich, A. Tittle, and M. Ferguson. 2022. Cogmed training does not generalize to real-world benefits for adult hearing aid users: Results of a blinded, active-controlled randomized trial. *Ear and Hearing* 43(3):741–763.

HLAA (Hearing Loss Association of America). 2025. *Hearing loop technology* https://www.hearingloss.org/find-help/hearing-assistive-technology/hearing-loop-technology (accessed March 11, 2025).

Hoffman, H. J., R. A. Dobie, K. G. Losonczy, C. L. Themann, and G. A. Flamme. 2017. Declining prevalence of hearing loss in US adults aged 20 to 69 years. *JAMA Otolaryngology – Head & Neck Surgery* 143(3):274–285.

Humes, L. E. 2021. An approach to self-assessed auditory wellness in older adults. *Ear and Hearing* 42(4):745–761.

Humes, L. E. 2023a. U.S. population data on hearing loss, trouble hearing, and hearing-device use in adults: National Health and Nutrition Examination Survey, 2011-12, 2015-16, and 2017-20. *Trends in Hearing* 27. https://doi.org/10.1177/23312165231160978.

Humes, L. E. 2023b. U.S. population data on self-reported trouble hearing and hearing-aid use in adults: National Health Interview Survey, 2017-2018. *Trends in Hearing* 27. https://doi.org/10.1177/23312165231160967.

Humes, L. E. 2024. Demographic and audiological characteristics of candidates for over-the-counter hearing aids in the United States. *Ear and Hearing* 45(5):1296–1312.

Humes, L. E., K. G. Skinner, D. L. Kinney, S. E. Rogers, A. K. Main, and T. M. Quigley. 2019. Clinical effectiveness of an at-home auditory training program: A randomized controlled trial. *Ear and Hearing* 40(5):1043–1060.

Humes L. E., S. Dhar, V. Manchaiah, A. Sharma, T. H. Chisolm, M. L. Arnold, and V. A. Sanchez. 2024. A perspective on auditory wellness: What it is, why it is important, and how it can be managed. *Trends in Hearing* 28. https://doi.org/10.1177/23312165241273342.

Hyder, M. A., and J. Razzak. 2020. Telemedicine in the United States: An introduction for students and residents. *Journal of Medical Internet Research* 22(11):e20839.

IOM (Institute of Medicine) and NRC (National Research Council). 2014. *Hearing loss and healthy aging: Workshop summary.* Washington, DC: The National Academies Press.

Isherwood, B., A. C. Gonçalves, R. Cousins, and R. Holme. 2022. The global hearing therapeutic pipeline: 2021. *Drug Discovery Today* 27(3):912–922.

Johannesen, P. T., B. C. Buzo, and E. A. Lopez-Poveda. 2019. Evidence for age-related cochlear synaptopathy in humans unconnected to speech-in-noise intelligibility deficits. *Hearing Research* 374:35–48.

Kochkin, S. 2000. MarkeTrakV: "Why my hearing aids are in the drawer": The consumers' perspective. *Hearing Journal* 53(2):34–41.

Komune, S., and J. B. Snow, Jr. 1981. Potentiating effects of cisplatin and ethacrynic acid in ototoxicity. *Archives of Otolaryngology* 107(10):594–597.

Kricos, P. B., and A. E. Holmes. 1996. Efficacy of audiologic rehabilitation for older adults. *Journal of the American Academy of Audiology* 7(4):219–229.

Kricos, P. B., A. E. Holmes, and D. A. Doyle. 1992. Efficacy of a communication training program for hearing-impaired elderly adults. *Journal of the Aural Rehabilitation Association* 24:69–80.

Kujawa, S. G., and M. C. Liberman. 2009. Adding insult to injury: Cochlear nerve degeneration after "temporary" noise-induced hearing loss. *Journal of Neuroscience* 29(45):14077–14085.

Laureyns, M., N. Bisgaard, L. Best, and S. Zimmer. 2024. *Getting the numbers right on hearing loss hearing care and hearing aid use in Europe.* https://www.ehima.com/wp-content/uploads/2024/03/Getting-the-numbers-right-on-Hearing-Loss-Hearing-Care-and-Hearing-Aid-Use-in-Europe-2024.pdf (accessed March 11, 2025).

Lee, J., K. Fernandez, and L. L. Cunningham. 2024. Hear and now: Ongoing clinical trials to prevent drug-induced hearing loss. *Annual Review of Pharmacology and Toxicology* 64(1):211–230.

Le Prell, C. G. 2023. Preclinical prospects of investigational agents for hearing loss treatment. *Expert Opinion on Investigational Drugs* 32(8):685–692.

Le Prell, C. G. 2021. Investigational medicinal products for the inner ear: Review of clinical trial characteristics in clinicaltrials.gov. *Journal of the American Academy of Audiology* 32(10):670–694.

Le Prell, C. G., and O. H. Clavier. 2017. Effects of noise on speech recognition: Challenges for communication by service members. *Hearing Research* 349:76–89.

Lewis, R. M. 2021. From bench to booth: Examining hair cell regeneration through an audiologist's scope. *Journal of the American Academy of Audiology* 32(10):654–660.

Li, Y., D. Ding, H. Jiang, Y. Fu, and R. Salvi. 2011. Co-administration of cisplatin and furosemide causes rapid and massive loss of cochlear hair cells in mice. *Neurotoxicity Research* 20:307–319.

Lin, F. R., P. Maas, W. Chien, J. P. Carey, L. Ferrucci, and R. Thorpe. 2012. Association of skin color, race/ethnicity, and hearing loss among adults in the USA. *Journal of the Association for Research in Otolaryngology* 13(1):109–117.

Ling, A. Y., M. E. Montez-Rath, P. Carita, K. J. Chandross, L. Lucats, Z. Meng, B. Sebastien, K. Kapphahn, and M. Desai. 2023. An overview of current methods for real-world applications to generalize or transport clinical trial findings to target populations of interest. *Epidemiology* 34(5):627–636.

Lv, J. H., X. Wang, Y. Cheng, D. Chen, L. Wang, Q. Zhang, Q. Cao, H. Tang, S. Hu, K. Gao, M. Xun, J. Wang, Z. Wang, B. Zhu, C. Cui, Z. Gao, L. Guo, S. Yu, L. Jiang, Y. Yin, J. Zhang, B. Chen, W. Wang, R. Chai, Z. Chen, H. Li, and Y. Shu. 2024. AAV1-hOTOF gene therapy for autosomal recessive deafness 9: A single-arm trial. *Lancet* 403(10441):2317–2325.

Maidment, D. W., A. B. Barker, J. Xia, and M. A. Ferguson. 2018. A systematic review and meta-analysis assessing the effectiveness of alternative listening devices to conventional hearing aids in adults with hearing loss. *International Journal of Audiology* 57(10):721–729.

Malcolm, K. A., J. J. Suen, and C. L. Nieman. 2022. Socioeconomic position and hearing loss: Current understanding and recent advances. *Current Opinion in Otolaryngology & Head and Neck Surgery* 30(5):351–357.

Malmberg, M., T. Lunner, K. Kähäri, and G. Andersson. 2017. Evaluating the short-term and long-term effects of an internet-based aural rehabilitation programme for hearing aid users in general clinical practice: A randomised controlled trial. *BMJ Open* 7(5):e013047.

Malmberg, M., K. Anióse, J. Skans, and M. Öberg. 2023. A randomised, controlled trial of clinically implementing online hearing support. *International Journal of Audiology* 62(5):472–480.

Manchaiah, V., H. Abrams, A. Bailey, and G. Andersson. 2019. Negative side effects associated with hearing aid use in adults with hearing loss. *Journal of the American Academy of Audiology* 30(6):472–481.

Martínez-Rodríguez, R., J. García Lorenzo, J. Bellido Peti, J. Palou Redorta, J. J. Gómez Ruiz, and H. Villavicencio Mavrich. 2007. [loop diuretics and ototoxicity]. *Actas Urologicas Espanolas* 31(10):1189–1192.

Marx, M., E. Younes, S. S. Chandrasekhar, J. Ito, S. Plontke, S. O'Leary, and O. Sterkers. 2018. International consensus (icon) on treatment of sudden sensorineural hearing loss. *European Annals of Otorhinolaryngology, Head and Neck Diseases* 135(1s):S23–S28.

Masterson, E. A., and C. L. Themann. 2024. Prevalence of hearing loss among noise-exposed US workers within the utilities sector, 2010-2019. *Journal of Occupational and Environmental Medicine* 66(8):648–653.

McCormack, A., and H. Fortnum. 2013. Why do people fitted with hearing aids not wear them? *International Journal of Audiology* 52(5):360–368.

McLean, W. J., A. S. Hinton, J. T. J. Herby, A. N. Salt, J. J. Hartsock, S. Wilson, D. L. Lucchino, T. Lenarz, A. Warnecke, N. Prenzler, H. Schmitt, S. King, L. E. Jackson, J. Rosenbloom, G. Atiee, M. Bear, C. L. Runge, R. H. Gifford, S. D. Rauch, D. J. Lee, R. Langer, J. M. Karp, C. Loose, and C. LeBel. 2021. Improved speech intelligibility in subjects with stable sensorineural hearing loss following intratympanic dosing of FX-322 in a phase 1b study. *Otology and Neurotology* 42(7):e849–e857.

Mercadal-Orfila, G., S. Herrera-Pérez, N. Piqué, F. Mateu-Amengual, P. Ventayol-Bosch, M. A. Maestre-Fullana, F. Fernández-Cortés, F. Barceló-Sansó, and S. Rios. 2024. Implementing systematic patient-reported measures for chronic conditions through the Naveta value-based telemedicine initiative: Observational retrospective multicenter study. *JMIR mHealth and uHealth* 12(1):e56196.

Molander, P., H. Hesser, S. Weineland, K. Bergwall, S. Buck, J. Jäder Malmlöf, H. Lantz, T. Lunner, and G. Andersson. 2018. Internet-based acceptance and commitment therapy for psychological distress experienced by people with hearing problems: A pilot randomized controlled trial. *Cognitive Behaviour Therapy* 47(2):169–184.

Munro, K. J., W. M. Whitmer, and A. Heinrich. 2021. Clinical trials and outcome measures in adults with hearing loss. *Frontiers in Psychology* 12:733060.

Murray, C. J., J. A. Salomon, C. D. Mathers, and A. D. Lopez. 2002. *Summary measures of population health: Concepts, ethics, measurement and applications*. Geneva, Switzerland: World Health Organization.

NASEM (National Academies of Sciences, Engineering, and Medicine). 2016. *Hearing health care for adults: Priorities for improving access and affordability*. Washington, DC: The National Academies Press.

Natarajan, N., S. Batts, and K. M. Stankovic. 2023. Noise-induced hearing loss. *Journal of Clinical Medicine* 12(6):2347.

NIDCD (National Institute on Deafness and Other Communication Disorders). 2022. *Over-the-counter hearing aids*. https://www.nidcd.nih.gov/sites/default/files/Documents/order/over-the-counter-hearing-aids-2024.pdf (accessed September 18, 2024).

NIH (National Institutes of Health). 2022. *Hearing aids*. https://www.nidcd.nih.gov/health/hearing-aids#hearingaid_01 (accessed November 16, 2023).

NIOSH (National Institute for Occupational Safety and Health). 2024. *Noise and hearing loss*. https://www.cdc.gov/niosh/noise/about/noise.html (accessed September 18, 2024).

NORA (National Occupational Research Agenda) Hearing Loss Prevention Cross-Sector Council. 2019. *National Occupational Research Agenda for hearing loss prevention.* https://www.cdc.gov/nora/councils/hlp/pdfs/National_Occupational_Research_Agenda_for_HLP_July_2019-508.pdf (accessed January 8, 2025).

Parthasarathy, A., K. E. Hancock, K. Bennett, V. DeGruttola, and D. B. Polley. 2020. Bottom-up and top-down neural signatures of disordered multi-talker speech perception in adults with normal hearing. *eLife* 9. https://doi.org/10.7554/eLife.51419.

Parrish, R. G. 2010. Measuring population health outcomes. *Preventing Chronic Disease* 7(4):A71.

Penn Medicine. n.d. *Genetic analysis at the new Penn Center for Adult-Onset Hearing Loss.* https://www.pennmedicine.org/departments-and-centers/otorhinolaryngology/about-us/newsletters/archive/2020-newsletters/genetic-analysis-for-adult-onset-hearing-loss#:~:text=In%20early%2Donset%20hearing%20loss,is%20the%20only%20diagnostic%20feature (accessed November 16, 2023).

Powell, W., J. A. Jacobs, W. Noble, M. L. Bush, and C. Snell-Rood. 2019. Rural adult perspectives on impact of hearing loss and barriers to care. *Journal of Community Health* 44(4):668–674.

Pratt, S. 2005. *Adult audiologic rehabilitation.* https://www.asha.org/articles/adult-audiologic-rehabilitation/#:~:text=According%20to%20Raymond%20Hull%2C%20aural,include%20a%20program%20of%20auditory (accessed May 22, 2024).

Preminger, J. E. 2003. Should significant others be encouraged to join adult group audiologic rehabilitation classes? *Journal of the American Academy of Audiology* 14(10):545–555.

Preminger, J. E., and J. K. Yoo. 2010. Do group audiologic rehabilitation activities influence psychosocial outcomes? *American Journal of Audiology* 19(2):109–125.

Preminger, J. E., and C. H. Ziegler. 2008. Can auditory and visual speech perception be trained within a group setting? *American Journal of Audiology* 17(1):80–97.

Pross, S. E., A. L. Bourne, and S. W. Cheung. 2016. Teleaudiology in the Veterans Health Administration. *Otology & Neurotology* 37(7):847–850.

Qi, J., F. Tan, L. Zhang, L. Lu, S. Zhang, Y. Zhai, Y. Lu, X. Qian, W. Dong, Y. Zhou, Z. Zhang, X. Yang, L. Jiang, C. Yu, J. Liu, T. Chen, L. Qu, C. Tan, S. Sun, H. Song, Y. Shu, L. Xu, X. Gao, H. Li, and R. Chai. 2024. AAV-mediated gene therapy restores hearing in patients with DFNB9 deafness. *Advanced Science* 11(11):2306788.

Rauch, S. D. 2008. Idiopathic sudden sensorineural hearing loss. *New England Journal of Medicine* 359(8):833–840.

Reavis, K. M., N. Bisgaard, B. Canlon, J. R. Dubno, R. D. Frisina, R. Hertzano, L. E. Humes, P. Mick, N. A. Phillips, M. K. Pichora-Fuller, B. Shuster, and G. Singh. 2023. Sex-linked biology and gender-related research is essential to advancing hearing health. *Ear and Hearing* 44(1):10–27.

Reed, N. S., E. E. Garcia-Morales, C. Myers, A. R. Huang, J. R. Ehrlich, O. J. Killeen, J. E. Hoover-Fong, F. R. Lin, M. L. Arnold, E. S. Oh, J. A. Schrack, and J. A. Deal. 2023. Prevalence of hearing loss and hearing aid use among US Medicare beneficiaries aged 71 years and older. *JAMA Network Open* 6(7):e2326320–e2326320.

Robler, S. K., L. Coco, and M. Krumm. 2022. Telehealth solutions for assessing auditory outcomes related to noise and ototoxic exposures in clinic and research. *Journal of the Acoustical Society of America* 152(3):1737–1754.

Saunders, G. H., S. L Smith, T. H. Chisolm, M. T. Frederick, R. A. McArdle, and R. H. Wilson. 2016. A randomized control trial: Supplementing hearing aid use with Listening and Communication Enhancement (LACE) auditory training. *Ear and Hearing* 37(4):381–396.

Schacht, J., A. E. Talaska, and L. P. Rybak. 2012. Cisplatin and aminoglycoside antibiotics: Hearing loss and its prevention. *Anatomical Record* 295:1837–1850.

Schilder, A. G. M., M. P. Su, H. Blackshaw, L. Lustig, H. Staecker, T. Lenarz, S. Safieddine, C. S. Gomes-Santos, R. Holme, and A. Warnecke. 2019. Hearing protection, restoration, and regeneration: An overview of emerging therapeutics for inner ear and central hearing disorders. *Otology and Neurotology* 40(5):559–570.

Sergeyenko, Y., K. Lall, M. C. Liberman, and S. G. Kujawa. 2013. Age-related cochlear synaptopathy: An early-onset contributor to auditory functional decline. *Journal of Neuroscience* 33(34):13686–13694.

Shiffman, S., A. A. Stone, and M. R. Hufford. 2008. Ecological momentary assessment. *Annual Review of Clinical Psychology* 4(1):1–32.

Singal, A. G., P. D. Higgins, and A. K. Waljee. 2014. A primer on effectiveness and efficacy trials. *Clinical and Translational Gastroenterology* 5(1):e45.

Smits, C., T. S. Kapteyn, and T. Houtgast. 2004. Development and validation of an automatic speech-in-noise screening test by telephone. *International Journal of Audiology* 43(1):15–28.

Spankovich, C., V. B. Gonzalez, D. Su, and C. E. Bishop. 2018. Self reported hearing difficulty, tinnitus, and normal audiometric thresholds, the National Health and Nutrition Examination Survey 1999–2002. *Hearing Research* 358:30–36.

Sweetow, R. W., and J. H. Sabes. 2006. The need for and development of an adaptive Listening and Communication Enhancement (LACE) program. *Journal of the American Academy of Audiology* 17(8):538–558.

Sydlowski, S. A., J. P. Marinelli, C. M. Lohse, and M. L. Carlson. 2022. Hearing health perceptions and literacy among primary healthcare providers in the United States: A national cross-sectional survey. *Otology and Neurotology* 43(8):894–899.

Teleaudiology Today. 2021. Measuring teleaudiology quality, effectiveness for hearing aid follow-ups. *Hearing Journal* 74(1):22.

Themann, C. L., and E. A Masterson. 2019. Occupational noise exposure: A review of its effects, epidemiology, and impact with recommendations for reducing its burden. *Journal of the Acoustical Society of America* 146(5):3879.

Thorén, E. S., M. Oberg, G. Wänström, G. Andersson, and T. Lunner. 2014. A randomized controlled trial evaluating the effects of online rehabilitative intervention for adult hearing-aid users. *International Journal of Audiology* 53(7):452–461.

Tremblay, K. L., A. Pinto, M. E. Fischer, B. E. Klein, R. Klein, S. Levy, T. S. Tweed, and K. J. Cruickshanks. 2015. Self-reported hearing difficulties among adults with normal audiograms: The Beaver Dam Offspring Study. *Ear and Hearing* 36(6):e290–e299.

Viana, L. M., J. T. O'Malley, B. J. Burgess, D. D. Jones, C. A. Oliveira, F. Santos, S. N. Merchant, L. D. Liberman, and M. C. Liberman. 2015. Cochlear neuropathy in human presbycusis: Confocal analysis of hidden hearing loss in post-mortem tissue. *Hearing Research* 327:78–88.

WHO (World Health Organization). 2021. *World report on hearing*. Geneva, Switzerland: World Health Organization.

WHO. 2024. *Self-care for health and well-being*. https://www.who.int/news-room/factsheets/detail/self-care-health-interventions#:~:text=Self%2Dcare%20is%20the%20ability,devices%2C%20diagnostics%20and%20digital%20tools (accessed December 3, 2024).

Wang, H., Y. Chen, J. Lv, X. Cheng, Q. Cao, D. Wang, L. Zhang, B. Zhu, M. Shen, C. Xu, M. Xun, Z. Wang, H. Tang, S. Hu, C. Cui, L. Jiang, Y. Yin, L. Guo, Y. Zhou, L. Han, Z. Gao, J. Zhang, S. Yu, K. Gao, J. Wang, B. Chen, W. Wang, Z. Chen, H. Li, and Y. Shu. 2024. Bilateral gene therapy in children with autosomal recessive deafness 9: Single-arm trial results. *Nature Medicine* 30:1898–1904.

Wu, P. Z., J. T. O'Malley, V. de Gruttola, and M. C. Liberman. 2021. Primary neural degeneration in noise-exposed human cochleas: Correlations with outer hair cell loss and word-discrimination scores. *Journal of Neuroscience* 41(20):4439–4447.

3

General Principles for Core Outcome Sets and Outcome Measurement

As noted in Chapter 1, outcome measurement is important in health care, as the resulting data can help clinicians, researchers, and individuals understand which interventions work best for which populations and thereby improve the patient experience (ICHOM, n.d.). Understanding which outcomes are most important to measure, as well as how to measure those outcomes, is the key to assessing the efficacy and effectiveness of various interventions. Furthermore, creating consistency in a field of health care through the use of a core outcome set (and corresponding standardized measures)[1] contributes to strengthening the evidence base and allowing for comparison across time, samples, and interventions. This chapter provides an overview of best practices for the development of core outcome sets, the assessment of outcome measures (in general), and the state of core outcome set development (and corresponding measurement) for hearing health interventions. The meaningfulness of specific outcomes are discussed in Chapter 4 and then more fully described and assessed in Chapter 5. Chapter 6 evaluates current measures for core outcomes.

---

[1] The word *standardized* is used here in a broad sense to indicate that the same measures are being used for specific outcomes, and that there are prescribed materials and procedures for the use of these measures. The committee does not imply that the measures are part of national or international standards.

OVERVIEW OF OUTCOMES AND
OUTCOME MEASURES

The Institute of Medicine proposed a framework where health care quality is described by the six aims of health care (i.e., safe, timely, effective, equitable, efficient, and patient-centered) (IOM, 2001). Quality of health care is assessed by structural, process, and outcome measures. Structural measures generally consider the provider's capacity and infrastructure while process measures generally consider whether the clinician or provider follows clinical practice guidelines (AHRQ, 2015). Outcome measures, the focus of this study, seek to quantify the effect of an intervention or treatment on health status in specific outcomes (Williamson et al., 2017).

Patient-reported outcome measures gather data directly from patients about their perceived health status and outcomes. Patient-reported outcomes have been defined as "any report of the status of a patient's health condition that comes directly from the patient, without interpretation of the patient's response by a clinician or anyone else" (NQF, 2013). Typical patient-reported outcomes in health care include health-related quality of life, symptoms and symptom burden, experience with care, functional status, and health behaviors (Churruca et al., 2021; NQF, 2013). As noted by Tysome and colleagues:

> Outcome measures are often clinician-[centered], measuring aspects that are deemed important primarily to health care professionals. However, it is our patients' well-being and the impact of our interventions on their lives that are most important in our practice. It follows that patient-[centered] outcomes should be [prioritized] in assessing both individual practice and reporting results of clinical trials. (Tysome et al., 2015, p. 512)

Patient-reported outcome measures are ideally standardized, psychometrically validated questionnaires that collect data directly from patients about their health-related priorities and outcomes (Churruca et al., 2021).

CORE OUTCOME SETS

When assessing the effect of an intervention on an individual's health, researchers and clinicians can consider measuring a multitude of outcomes. A core outcome set recommends what specific outcomes, at a minimum, researchers and clinicians should measure and report when assessing an intervention's effectiveness (Clarke and Williamson, 2016). Failure to report consistently defined outcomes, failure to use a common set of measures to evaluate those outcomes, or failure to evaluate outcomes prioritized by key partners (such as patients and clinicians) leads to research waste (Chalmers and Glasziou, 2009; Kirkham and Williamson, 2022; O'Connor and Brinker, 2013).[2]

The failure to measure a common set of outcomes has been noted across many areas in health care research. For example:

- An examination of 8,942 oncology clinical trials on ClinicalTrials. gov led to the identification of "more than 25,000 outcomes across oncology trials that occurred only once or twice" (Hirsch et al., 2013, p. 977).
- A review of 99 studies of bariatric surgery outcomes found that 85 percent of the 1,088 outcomes reported were only reported in one study (Hopkins et al., 2015).
- A review of 278 papers on the treatment of conductive and mixed hearing loss found 837 different outcomes were reported (Hill-Feltham et al., 2021).

Furthermore, researchers may define or measure commonly used outcomes differently (Williamson et al., 2017). For example, in the review of 99 studies of bariatric surgery outcomes, even common outcomes such as *weight loss* were either not defined or had contradictory definitions (Hopkins et al., 2015).

Core outcome sets and their corresponding measures have typically been defined for use in research (and clinical trials in particular) to enhance the consistency and quality of research, allow for meta-analysis of multiple smaller studies, and facilitate comparison of effectiveness among different interventions (to inform health care decision making) (Chiarotto et al., 2017; Clarke and Williamson, 2016; Kirkham et al., 2017; Kirkham and Williamson, 2022; Tysome et al., 2015; Williamson et al., 2017). As noted by Clarke and Williamson (2016):

> [T]he [standardization] which is achieved with a core outcome set is not intended to stifle innovation. The outcomes in the set should represent the minimum to be collected in all trials, and researchers should continue to measure and report additional outcomes of particular relevance to their topic. (p. 2)

Creating a comprehensive yet feasible core outcome set is challenging but not new to health care. Over the last few decades, hundreds of

---

[2] "Research waste refers to poor-quality research output that is often perceived as of minimal use to health policy makers and clinicians" (Sogi, 2023, p. 179).

core outcome sets have been developed for specific health conditions or specific populations in either research or clinical settings (or both) (Gargon et al., 2021; Kirkham et al., 2017; Prinsen et al., 2016a). The number of core outcome sets has been increasing, as has the number of sets intended for use in both research and clinical settings. However, Gargon et al. (2021) note that "further research is needed to understand and optimize the methods used to develop [core outcome sets] for multiple settings" (p. 9).

Best Practices for Developing a Core Outcome Set

The Core Outcome Measures in Effectiveness Trials (COMET) Initiative strives to raise awareness of problems with outcome measurement, encourage the development and implementation of evidence-based core outcome sets, promote patient engagement in the process, provide resources, and reduce duplication of efforts (Williamson et al., 2017). The *COMET Handbook* notes that developing a core outcome set requires engaging multiple partners to achieve consensus. This is typically done through an iterative Delphi process. However, "research to identify optimal methods of developing [core outcome sets] is ongoing and there is currently wide variation in the approaches used" to build consensus (Williamson et al., 2017, p. 6).

The Core Outcome Set-STAndards for Development (COS-STAD) project used a consensus-based process to identify methodological guidelines for the development of core outcome sets, noting that "no gold standard method for the development of a [core outcome set] currently exists" (Kirkham et al., 2017, p. 2). The COS-STAD project identified 11 minimum standards for the development of core outcome sets, "regardless of the specific consensus method chosen," but it did not address how to define or measure those outcomes (Kirkham et al., 2017). These standards fall into three main areas: scope specification, involvement of key partners, and consensus process.

Overall, core outcome set developers first need to determine *what* to measure (known as the scope) (Kirkham et al., 2017; Williamson et al., 2017). This includes specifying the health condition, the target population, specific interventions, and specific settings (i.e., research, routine care, or both). Next, the developers need to review the current evidence base in order to identify all potential core outcomes as well as to determine which outcomes are most important to measure (Williamson et al., 2017). Evidence may come from sources such as systematic reviews, published individual qualitative and quantitative studies, national datasets, and importantly, through direct input from key partners (including researchers, affected individuals, care partners, and clinicians) on what outcomes are the most meaningful to them. As noted by Clarke and Williamson (2016):

> If core outcome sets are to contribute to improvements in health and social care, by helping patients and the public, practitioners and policy makers to make better decisions about interventions, they need to contain the outcomes that really matter to these stakeholders. (p. 2)

Once the range of potential core outcomes has been identified, developers need to define outcomes with agreed-upon, unambiguous definitions of the outcome (Williamson et al., 2017). The process for coming to consensus on the set needs to be transparent. Criteria for determining the individual outcomes to be included in the core set need to be defined in advance, as well as how outcomes will be dropped or added during the process (Kirkham et al., 2017).

MEASUREMENT OF CORE OUTCOMES

A variety of outcome measures often exist that could be used to evaluate a specific outcome; this complicates the ability to compare interventions (Williamson et al., 2017). Once a core outcome set is established, the next challenge is to determine how to measure the individual outcomes (Clarke and Williamson, 2016). Two examples of published principles and methods to inform the process of identifying a core set of outcomes and their corresponding measures are described below.

Core Quality Measures Collaborative

The Core Quality Measures Collaborative (CQMC) published a series of principles for core set measure selection (CQMC, 2021). For creating core measure sets, it emphasizes that the set must be comprehensive and holistic to assess if care meets the full definition of high-quality care as defined by the Institute of Medicine (IOM, 2001). According to CQMC, measures should produce meaningful and useful information for patients, consumers, and clinicians. A core measure set needs to have a balance between specialty-specific measures and measures that are relevant across specialties and settings. The set should be as concise and efficient as possible to reduce the burden and include a mix of types of measures. CQMC recommends including patient-reported measures and standardized digital measures. It encourages the innovation of novel measures, particularly ones addressing the social determinants of health.

Additionally, CQMC has outlined a series of necessary measure characteristics, including that the measures should promote health and health care improvement, not have harmful unintended consequences, measure social needs, be scientifically sound, and balance innovation with burden.

COnsensus-based Standards for the selection of health Measurement INstruments

COnsensus-based Standards for the selection of health Measurement INstruments (COSMIN) is an international initiative focused on developing best practices for selecting appropriate outcome measures for both research and clinical practice (COSMIN, n.d.). COMET and COSMIN partnered to develop guidelines for the selection of measures for a core outcome set (Prinsen et al., 2016a,b). These guidelines were developed through a consensus-based Delphi process.

The best practices identified by COSMIN for selecting core measures mirrors the process for determining a core outcome set (see Figure 3-1). First, the outcome, domain, target population, and context of use need to be identified. The guideline further notes that separate measures may be needed for subgroups of the target population or by setting. Next, all existing measures need to be identified through the examination of systematic reviews, literature reviews, and other sources. Many different outcome measures need to be considered including "assessments by health professionals, biomarkers, clinical rating scales, imaging tests, laboratory tests, patient questionnaires, and performance-based tests" (Prinsen et al., 2016b, p. 2). Third, the outcome measures need to be evaluated for their quality. (See later in this section for a discussion of quality assessment of outcome measures.)

Finally, one measure needs to be selected for each core outcome, with recognition, as noted earlier, that a different or additional measure may be needed based on specific target population subgroups or settings. The COSMIN guideline notes:

> Ideally, an [outcome measure] included in a [core outcome set] has high-quality evidence for all measurement properties. However, in practice, there is often unknown or (very) low evidence for some measurement properties. (Prinsen et al., 2016a, p. 17)

The guideline suggests that some measures may be recommended based on a baseline of evidence for its quality, but that for others, further validation studies or the development of a new measure may be needed. Similar to the identification of the initial core outcome set, the guideline suggests using a consensus process to select the final outcome measures.

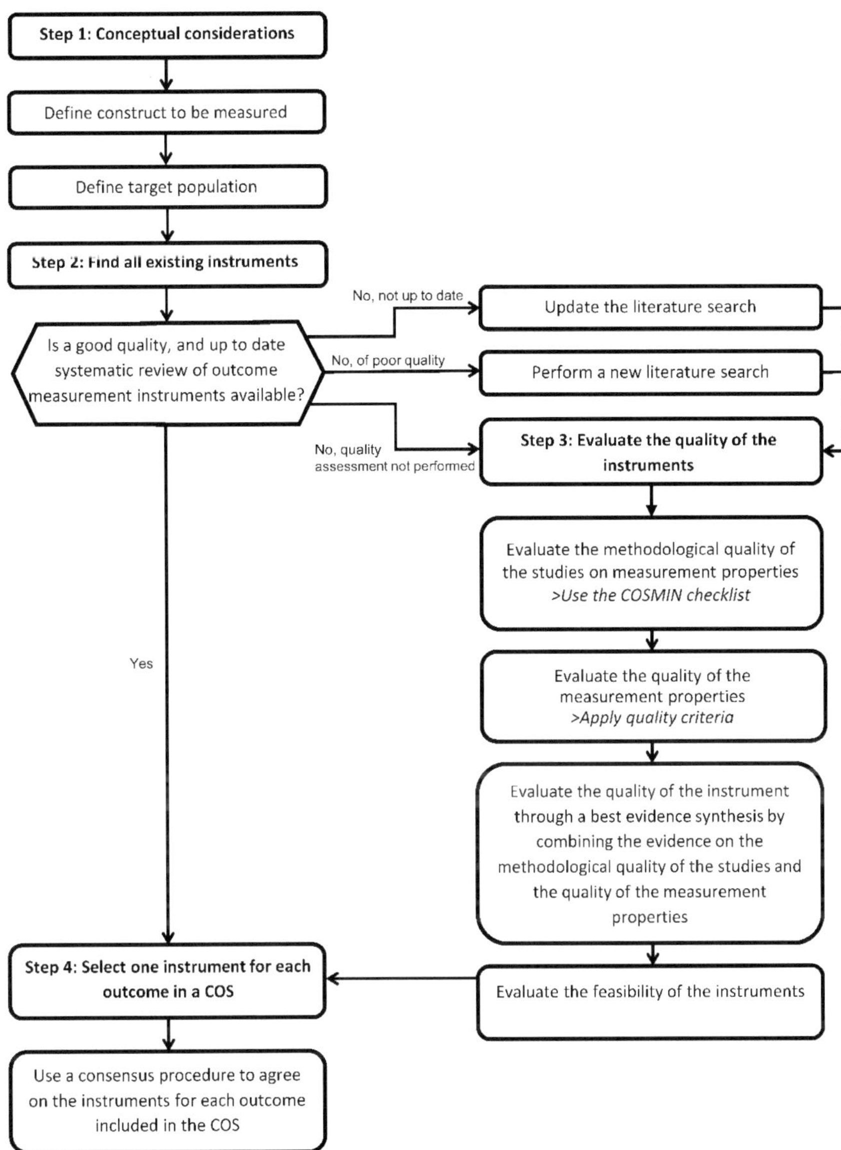

FIGURE 3-1 COSMIN guideline for selection of outcome measures for core outcome sets.
NOTE: COS = core outcome set; COSMIN = COnsensus-based Standards for the selection of health Measurement INstruments.
SOURCE: COSMIN, 2024b. CC BY 4.0.

ASSESSMENT OF OUTCOME MEASURES

Different groups use slightly different methodologies for assessing the quality of individual outcome measures. Some key initiatives are highlighted below.

Partnership for Quality Measurement

In 1999, the National Quality Forum (NQF) was established to promote consensus-based practices for quality measurement and public reporting (NQF, n.d. a). NQF, with support from the Centers for Medicare & Medicaid Services (CMS), developed a process for evaluating and endorsing measures, which also included the consideration of measure harmonization (consideration of other related or competing measures). As of March 2023, CMS now contracts with Battelle (under its Partnership for Quality Measurement [PQM]) as the consensus-based entity to review and endorse quality measures (NQF, n.d. b).[3]

Criteria for Endorsement

PQM uses five criteria to determine endorsement: importance, feasibility, scientific acceptability, use and usability, and equity (PQM, 2023). Importance reflects whether use of the measure can lead to improved outcomes and whether the outcome is meaningful to target populations. Feasibility considers the "people, tools, tasks, and technologies necessary to implement [the] measure" (PQM, 2024a). Scientific acceptability comprises the measure's reliability (whether the measure can be implemented consistently and the results are repeatable) and validity (whether the measure has been risk adjusted, and the score can identify good versus poor quality). Use and usability reflects whether the information gathered from the measure can be used by various partners (e.g., consumers, clinicians, policy makers) to improve care. Finally, the optional domain of equity reflects "the extent to which the measure can identify differences in care for certain patient populations" (PQM, 2024b).

COSMIN Guideline

As noted previously, COSMIN provides guidance on suggested methods for assessing both the quality of the studies of an outcome measure as well as the quality of the measure itself (Prinsen et al., 2016a). Similar to the PQM approach, COSMIN's criteria for high-quality measurement

---

[3] This responsibility was previously held by the National Quality Forum.

properties consider reliability (including internal consistency and measurement error), validity (including content validity, structural validity, and cross-cultural validity), and responsiveness (i.e., the ability of the measure to detect change over time). COSMIN specifically suggests first evaluating the measure for its content validity (i.e., does the content of the measure adequately reflect the outcome), including face validity. COSMIN suggests examining internal structure of the measure next, focusing on structural validity (i.e., can the scores of the measure adequately reflect the dimensionality of the outcome) and internal consistency (i.e., the interrelatedness of the measure items). Finally, it suggests other criteria be used as appropriate to the specific measure and context. The COSMIN guideline (Prinsen et al., 2016b) also recognizes the importance of considering various aspects of the feasibility of implementing each measure:

- Patient's comprehensibility
- Interpretability
- Ease of administration
- Length of the outcome measure
- Completion time
- Patient's mental ability level
- Ease of standardization
- Clinician's comprehensibility
- Type of outcome measure
- Cost of an outcome measure
- Required equipment
- Type of administration
- Availability in different settings
- Copyright
- Patient's physical ability level
- Regulatory agency's requirement for approval
- Ease of score calculation

CORE OUTCOME SETS AND MEASUREMENT FOR HEARING HEALTH INTERVENTIONS

No core outcome set has been broadly accepted by the hearing health community (Allen et al., 2022; Barker et al., 2015; Cox et al., 2000; Danermark et al., 2013; Granberg et al., 2014; Gurgel et al., 2012). In addition to the lack of consensus for the most meaningful outcomes, a variety of measures are being used to assess the same outcomes. For example, Granberg and colleagues (2014) performed a systematic review of outcome measures for hearing health interventions among studies separated into two pools. Pool 1 contained articles from large databases (i.e., MEDLINE,

CINAHL, EMBASE, and PsycInfo) and pool 2 contained articles from smaller databases (i.e., AMED, ERIC, Sociological Abstracts, PsycArticles, and CENTRAL). A total of 246 different outcome measures were identified among the 87 studies in pool 1, and 122 measures were identified among the 35 studies included in pool 2. Thirty-five percent of the outcome measures in pool 1 and 20 percent of the outcome measures in pool 2 involved audiometric measures of speech understanding under controlled test conditions. Furthermore, a study of the outcome measures used in the use of telehealth for both cochlear implant and hearing aid users showed that its "systematic literature review of 49 articles revealed over 250 discrete outcomes" (Laird et al., 2024, p. 1).

The use of multiple different measures further contributes to the inability to compare studies or pool data. As noted by Barker and colleagues, "A recommended core outcome set would not preclude researchers from including other measures relevant to an individual study but would at least provide a central dataset for meta-analysis" (Barker et al., 2015, p. 571). Moreover, the outcomes and corresponding measures currently being used may not adequately reflect the "real-world experiences and needs" of individuals with hearing difficulties (Moberly et al., 2023). The following sections highlight several distinct efforts to develop core outcome sets or define baseline outcome measures for hearing health interventions. These encompass both broad and more narrow aspects of hearing health.

International Outcome Inventory

In 1999, the Eriksholm Workshop on Measuring Outcomes in Audiological Rehabilitation Using Hearing Aids convened 15 experts to determine the state-of-the-art in self-report outcome measurement, to identify areas of disagreement or controversy, to outline approaches to resolving problems, and, in general, to work toward a coherent framework for outcome measurement that will encompass all of the goals and requirements for these kinds of data (Cox, 2000).

The group noted that outcome measurement serves different purposes, including to assess rehabilitative outcomes for an individual with hearing difficulties (in the clinical setting), to assess the effectiveness of a particular provider, to assess the effectiveness of a new intervention (e.g., clinical trials), and to evaluate the effect of the intervention on quality of life (Cox et al., 2000). The group agreed that "the characteristics of an optimal outcome measure vary as a function of the purpose of the measurement," and it endorsed "the concept of generating a brief universally applicable outcome measure" (Cox et al., 2000). The work of this group led to the development of the International Outcome Inventory for Hearing Aids (IOI-HA)—a seven-item questionnaire to evaluate the effectiveness of hearing aids (Cox and

Alexander, 2002). The group envisioned this measure as a supplement to outcome measures used for specific settings, interventions, or other narrower purposes as a means to pool research data across studies (Cox et al., 2000).

A version of the questionnaire exists both for hearing aids (IOI-HA) (Cox et al., 2000; Cox and Alexander, 2002) and for alternative interventions (IOI-AI), such as auditory training (Noble, 2002). The International Outcome Inventory measures are composed of seven separate items, each assessing one of the following areas:

1. hours of use,
2. benefit,
3. residual activity limitations,
4. satisfaction,
5. residual participation restrictions,
6. impact on others, and
7. quality of life.

The International Outcome Inventory measures assume that each of the seven domains assessed is important and independent from the others such that results are typically displayed as an array of seven scores compared to norms for each of the seven domains. However, factor analyses of responses to the seven items have typically identified either one or two factors reflecting the correlation among the responses to the seven items (Wong and Hickson, 2012).

International Classification of Functioning, Disability, and Health

The World Health Organization's International Classification of Functioning, Disability, and Health (ICF), endorsed in 2001, is considered the "international standard to describe and measure health and disability" (WHO, 2025). The framework is based on an integrated model that considers an individual's functioning and disability as well as their individual contextual factors, such as environmental factors (e.g., family attitudes, organizational policies) and personal factors (e.g., age, gender) (see Figure 3-2; Meyer et al., 2016).

Both comprehensive and brief core sets have been developed for a variety of health conditions based on the ICF framework. Danermark et al. found:

> A [comprehensive core set] includes as many categories as needed for describing the whole spectrum of problems for a certain condition. The [brief core set] is derived from the [comprehensive core set] and serves as a brief assessment of the functioning of a person with a certain condition. (Danermark et al., 2013, p. 324)

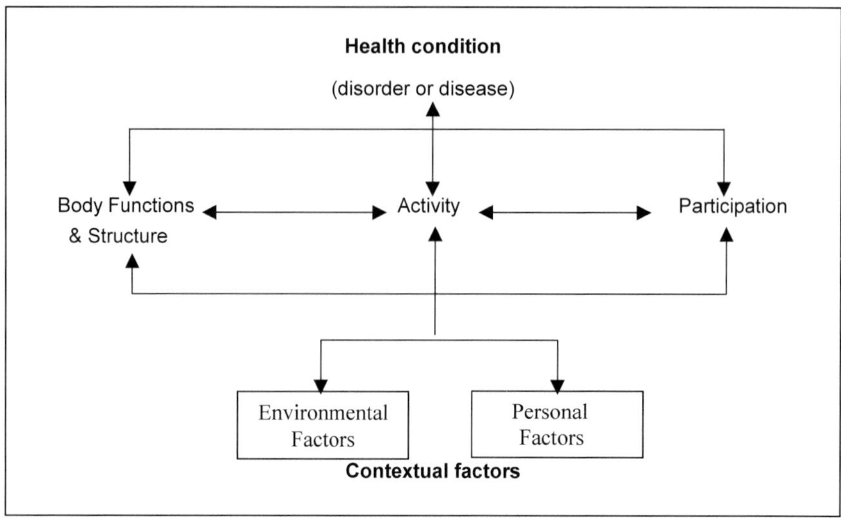

FIGURE 3-2 ICF model of functioning and disability.
NOTE: ICF = International Classification of Functioning, Disability, and Health.
SOURCE: Geneva, Switzerland: World Health Organization; 2002. CC BY-NC-SA 3.0 IGO.

Both ICF core sets for hearing loss include outcomes in the domains of body function (e.g., hearing functions), body structure (e.g., structure of external, middle, and inner ear), participation (e.g., handling stress and other psychological demands, conversation, community life), and environment (e.g., products and technology for communication, immediate family, health services and systems). However, it is important to note that unlike the focus of this report, these core sets are intended for a comprehensive description of the individual's hearing-related function, and not as a baseline for reporting outcomes.

Standardized Format for Reporting Hearing Outcomes in Clinical Trials

In 2012, with input from a range of hearing experts and organizations, the Hearing Committee of the American Academy of Otolaryngology-Head and Neck Surgery endorsed a standard for reporting hearing outcomes in clinical trials; it noted that "the lack of an adequate standardized method for reporting level of hearing function in clinical trials has hampered the ability of investigators to draw comparisons across studies" (Gurgel et al., 2012, p. 803). Over a 2-year period, the group developed a new hearing outcomes scale to reflect the function of patients across a wide range of audiometric loss. This scale consists of a scattergram that relates average pure-tone threshold to word recognition score. The group emphasized that "the new standards represent *minimal* reporting standards. Investigators are encouraged to consider and report additional hearing data if relevant and create innovative ways to assess and report hearing outcomes" (Gurgel et al., 2012, p. 806).

It is important to note that in response to this study, the American Academy of Audiology voiced concern about the applicability of these reporting standards to all clinical trials (Carlson, 2013). It argued that the use of the average pure-tone threshold would not be sensitive to noise-induced hearing loss or drug-induced ototoxicity and that word recognition tests would be problematic for "non-English speakers, pediatric populations, ill patients, and in situations when time constraints are necessarily imposed" (Carlson, 2013, p. 349).

In a subsequent response, Jackler and colleagues (2013) noted that "while we acknowledge that there is no such thing as an 'ideal' standard, we do believe that the formula adopted will substantially improve the value of our literature" (p. 350). They further noted that

> The standard merely defines a minimum dataset for comparison purposes and is not expected to be sufficient, unto itself, for many research purposes. Authors are encouraged to include additional data as needed to fully describe their study population.

Auditory Rehabilitation Outcomes Network

The Auditory Rehabilitation Outcomes Network (AURONET) is an international group established in 2014 to develop core sets of patient-centered hearing outcome measures for use in both clinical trials and individual practice settings based on the type of hearing loss (Tysome et al., 2015). The initiative focuses on four core areas: hearing (e.g., auditory perception, speech discrimination, sound localization), physical (e.g., pain, ear discharge), economic (e.g., cost to individual, society, and health care system), and psychosocial (e.g., relationships, quality of life, perception of self) (Tysome et al., 2015).

The group's first effort examined the treatment of conductive or mixed hearing loss (Hill-Feltham et al., 2021; Johansson et al., 2018; Tysome et al., 2015). As noted earlier in this chapter, a scoping review of the literature on the treatment of conductive and mixed hearing loss found 837 different outcomes were reported among the 278 papers reviewed (Hill-Feltham et al., 2021). Hill-Feltham and colleagues (2021) grouped these outcomes into nine domains of types of measures:

1. hearing threshold,
2. speech testing,
3. questionnaires,

4. immittance,[4]
5. binaural,
6. electrophysiology,
7. tinnitus, and
8. device output.

Hearing threshold measures (e.g., air–bone gap, pure-tone average, bone conduction thresholds, air conduction thresholds) accounted for about two-thirds (64.5 percent) of the reported outcomes. Speech testing accounted for about 20 percent of the reported outcomes, and the authors noted that the number of different measures used were too numerous to list them all in the study. Questionnaires (i.e., patient-reported outcome measures) accounted for only 8.8 percent of the measures reported. The researchers noted that "no single outcome measurement was reported in all studies" (Hill-Feltham et al., 2021, p. 244). They also noted that:

> In summary, the predominance of audiometry-based outcome measurements may have led to a comparative paucity of other outcome measurement being used. A [core outcome set] containing a broader range of outcome measurements with greater face validity to real-world situations would enhance the present evidence base, as well as moving away from a predominately clinician-[centered] approach, to a more patient-[centered] one. (p. 244)

Core Outcome Measures in the Tinnitus International Delphi Study

The TINnitus research NETwork (TINNET) is a European collaboration that focuses, in part, on developing "standards for tinnitus clinical trials and outcome measurements in clinical trials and everyday practice" (Hall et al., 2015, p. 4). Drawing on best practices described by COMET and COSMIN (earlier in this chapter), the Core Outcome Measures in Tinnitus International Delphi (COMiT'ID) initiative used a Delphi study process to propose core outcome sets for sound-based, psychology-based, and drug-based clinical trials of chronic subjective tinnitus in adults (see Table 3-1; Hall et al., 2018). The three core outcome sets share one common outcome: tinnitus intrusiveness. The initiative's next steps include determination of the best measure for each outcome.

Self-Report Core Outcome Domain Set

An Australian initiative noted that while there are a variety of outcome domains for hearing rehabilitation, "there is no consensus about which

---

[4] The domain of immittance contains objective outcome measurements of middle ear function (Hill-Feltham et al., 2021).

TABLE 3-1 COMiT'ID Core Outcome Sets by Intervention Type

Sound-Based Trials Core Set	Psychology-Based Trials Core Set	Drug-Based Trials Core Outcome Set
Tinnitus intrusiveness	Tinnitus intrusiveness	Tinnitus intrusiveness
Ability to ignore	Tinnitus acceptance	Tinnitus loudness
Concentration	Mood	
Quality of sleep	Negative thoughts and beliefs	
Sense of control	Sense of control	

NOTE: COMiT'ID = Core Outcome Measures in Tinnitus International Delphi.
SOURCE: Hall et al., 2018. CC BY 4.0.

outcome domains should be measured, when they should be measured, and how they should be measured" (Allen et al., 2022, p. 1). The consensus-based process engaged 79 hearing health professionals and 64 adults with hearing difficulties in a three-round Delphi process to identify the "most important" domains. This process resulted in seven potential domains, which were narrowed to four top domains by a group of 11 experts (including clinicians and patient advocates). These four domains (in rank order) were:

- communication ability,
- personal relationships,
- well-being, and
- participation restrictions.

The study reported that there was a dearth of measures for a wide variety of the domains deemed important.

FINDINGS

This section lists the committee's findings under their appropriate headings.

Core Outcome Sets

Finding 3-1: Core outcome sets represent the minimum set of data to be collected.

Finding 3-2: A lack of standard outcomes leads to multiple different outcomes being measured and reported for the same condition.

Finding 3-3: The use of core outcome sets can help enhance the consistency and quality of research, allow for meta-analysis of multiple smaller studies, and facilitate the comparison of effectiveness among different interventions.

Finding 3-4: While there is no single best method for developing a core outcome set, using a consensus process is important. Other key steps and best practices include:
- Define scope;
- Gather evidence to identify all potential outcomes;
- Group outcomes into domains;
- Determine which outcomes are most important to measure; and
- Provide transparency of the consensus process, including inclusion criteria and the steps for adding and dropping outcomes during the process.

Measuring Core Outcomes

Finding 3-5: Multiple measures often exist to evaluate a single, specific outcome.

Finding 3-6: The use of different measures for the same outcome contributes to the challenges in comparing interventions.

Finding 3-7: The COSMIN process for selecting measures mirrors the process for determining a core outcome set, including:
- Use of a consensus-based process;
- Definition of scope;
- Gathering of evidence to identify all potential measures;
- Grouping of outcomes into domains; and
- Selection of one measure for each core outcome.

Finding 3-8: Different measures may be needed by context, such as for specific subpopulations or settings.

Assessment of Outcome Measures

Finding 3-9: In practice, there is often a lack of evidence for the quality of measures.

Finding 3-10: Different methodologies exist to assess the quality of individual measures.

Finding 3-11: PQM uses five criteria to determine endorsement: importance, feasibility, scientific acceptability (including reliability and validity), use and usability, and equity.

Finding 3-12: Similar to the PQM approach, COSMIN's criteria for high-quality measurement properties consider reliability, validity, and responsiveness (i.e., the ability of the measure to detect change over time).

Core Outcome Sets for Hearing Health Interventions

Finding 3-13: No core outcome set has been broadly accepted by the hearing health community.

Finding 3-14: In addition to the lack of consensus for the most important outcomes, a variety of measures are being used to assess the same outcomes, which further contributes to the inability to compare studies or pool data.

Finding 3-15: Several efforts have sought to develop a core outcome set or define baseline outcome measures for hearing rehabilitation, either broadly or for more narrow aspects of hearing health.

REFERENCES

AHRQ (Agency for Healthcare Research and Quality). 2015. *Types of health care quality measures.* https://www.ahrq.gov/talkingquality/measures/types.html (accessed May 22, 2024).

Allen, D., L. Hickson, and M. Ferguson. 2022. Defining a patient-centred core outcome domain set for the assessment of hearing rehabilitation with clients and professionals. *Frontiers in Neuroscience* 16:787607.

Barker, F., E. MacKenzie, L. Elliott, and S. de Lusignan. 2015. Outcome measurement in adult auditory rehabilitation: A scoping review of measures used in randomized controlled trials. *Ear and Hearing* 36(5):567–573.

Carlson, D. 2013. American Academy of Audiology response to Gurgel et al. *Otolaryngology-Head and Neck Surgery* 149(2):349–350.

Chalmers, S., and P. Glasziou. 2009. Avoidable waste in the production and reporting of research evidence. *Lancet* 374(9683):86–89.

Chiarotto, A., R. W. Ostelo, D. C. Turk, R. Buchbinder, and M. Boers. 2017. Core outcome sets for research and clinical practice. *Brazilian Journal of Physical Therapy* 21(2):77–84.

Churruca, K., C. Pomare, L. A. Ellis, J. C. Long, S. B. Henderson, L. E. D. Murphy, C. J. Leahy, and J. Braithwaite. 2021. Patient-reported outcome measures (PROMs): A review of generic and condition-specific measures and a discussion of trends and issues. *Health Expectations* 24(4):1015–1024.

Clarke, M., and P. R. Williamson. 2016. Core outcome sets and systematic reviews. *Systematic Reviews* 5:11.

COSMIN (COnsensus-based Standards for the selection of health Measurement INstruments). n.d. *About COSMIN.* https://www.cosmin.nl/about (accessed June 25, 2024).

COSMIN. 2024b. Guideline for selecting instruments for a core outcome set. https://www.cosmin.nl/tools/guideline-selecting-proms-cos/ (accessed June 26, 2024).

Cox, R. 2000. Editorial. *Ear and Hearing* 21(4):1S.

Cox, R. M., and G. C. Alexander. 2002. The International Outcome Inventory for Hearing Aids (IOI-HA): Psychometric properties of the English version. *International Journal of Audiology* 41(1):30–35.

Cox, R., M. Hyde, S. Gatehouse, W. Noble, H. Dillon, R. Bentler, D. Stephens, S. Arlinger, L. Beck, D. Wilkerson, S. Kramer, P. Kricos, J. P. Gagné, F. Bess, and L. Hallberg. 2000. Optimal outcome measures, research priorities, and international cooperation. *Ear and Hearing* 21(4 Suppl):106s–115s.

CQMC (Core Quality Measures Collaborative). 2021. *CQMC core sets: Guiding principles and documents: Principles for core set measure selection.* https://www.qualityforum.org/CQMC_Core_Sets.aspx (accessed June 26, 2024).

Danermark, B., S. Granberg, S. E. Kramer, M. Selb, and C. Möller. 2013. The creation of a comprehensive and a brief core set for hearing loss using the International Classification of Functioning, Disability and Health. *American Journal of Audiology* 22(2):323–328.

Gargon, E., S. L. Gorst, K. Matvienko-Sikar, and P. R. Williamson. 2021. Choosing important health outcomes for comparative effectiveness research: 6th annual update to a systematic review of core outcome sets for research. *PLOS ONE* 16(1):E0244878.

Granberg, S., J. Dahlström, C. Möller, K. Kähäri, and B. Danermark. 2014. The ICF core sets for hearing loss—Researcher perspective. Part I: Systematic review of outcome measures identified in audiological research. *International Journal of Audiology* 53(2):65–76.

Gurgel, R. K., R. K. Jackler, R. A. Dobie, and G. R. Popelka. 2012. A new standardized format for reporting hearing outcome in clinical trials. *Otolaryngology—Head and Neck Surgery* 147(5):803–807.

Hall, D. A., H. Haider, D. Kikidis, M. Mielczarek, B. Mazurek, A. J. Szczepek, and C. R. Cederroth. 2015. Toward a global consensus on outcome measures for clinical trials in tinnitus: Report from the first international meeting of the COMIT initiative, November 14, 2014, Amsterdam, The Netherlands. *Trends in Hearing* 19:2331216515580272.

Hall, D. A., H. Smith, A. Hibbert, V. Colley, H. F. Haider, A. Horobin, A. Londero, B. Mazurek, B. Thacker, and K. Fackrell. 2018. The COMiT'ID study: Developing core outcome domains sets for clinical trials of sound-, psychology-, and pharmacology-based interventions for chronic subjective tinnitus in adults. *Trends in Hearing* 22:2331216518814384.

Hill-Feltham, P. R., M. L. Johansson, W. E. Hodgetts, A. V. Ostevik, B. J. McKinnon, P. Monksfield, R. Sockalingam, T. Wright, and J. R. Tysome. 2021. Hearing outcome measures for conductive and mixed hearing loss treatment in adults: A scoping review. *International Journal of Audiology* 60(4):239–245.

Hirsch, B. R., R. M. Califf, S. K. Cheng, A. Tasneem, J. Horton, K. Chiswell, K. A. Schulman, D. M. Dilts, and A. P. Abernethy. 2013. Characteristics of oncology clinical trials: Insights from a systematic analysis of ClinicalTrials.gov. *JAMA Internal Medicine* 173(11): 972–979.

Hopkins, J. C., N. Howes, K. Chalmers, J. Savovic, K. Whale, K. D. Coulman, R. Welbourn, R. N. Whistance, R. C. Andrews, J. P. Byrne, D. Mahon, and J. M. Blazeby. 2015. Outcome reporting in bariatric surgery: An in-depth analysis to inform the development of a core outcome set, the BARIACT study. *Obesity Reviews* 16(1):88–106.

ICHOM (International Consortium for Health Outcomes Measurement). n.d. *Why measure outcomes?* https://www.ichom.org/why-measure-outcomes (accessed November 12, 2024).

IOM (Institute of Medicine). 2001. *Crossing the quality chasm: A new health system for the 21st century.* Washington, DC: National Academy Press.

Jackler, R., R. Gurgel, R. Dobie, and G. Popelka. 2013. Reply to Dr. Carlson's letter: A new standardized format for reporting hearing outcome in clinical trials. *Otolaryngology-Head and Neck Surgery* 149(2):350.

Johansson, M. L., J. R. Tysome, P. Hill-Feltham, W. E. Hodgetts, A. Ostevik, B. J. McKinnon, P. Monksfield, R. Sockalingam, and T. Wright. 2018. Physical outcome measures for conductive and mixed hearing loss treatment: A systematic review. *Clinical Otolaryngology* 43(5):1226–1234.

Kirkham, J. J., and P. Williamson. 2022. Core outcome sets in medical research. *BMJ Medicine* 1(1):e000284.

Kirkham, J. J., K. Davis, D. G. Altman, J. M. Blazeby, M. Clarke, S. Tunis, and P. R. Williamson. 2017. Core Outcome Set-STAndards for Development: The COS-STAD recommendations. *PLoS Medicine* 14(11):e1002447.

Laird, E., C. Sucher, K. Nakano, and M. Ferguson. 2024. Systematic review of patient and service outcome measures of remote digital technologies for cochlear implant and hearing aid users. *Frontiers in Audiology and Otology* 2:1403814.

Meyer, C., C. Grenness, N. Scarinci, and L. Hickson. 2016. What is the International Classification of Functioning, Disability, and Health and why is it relevant to audiology? *Seminars in Hearing* 37(3):163–186.

Moberly, A. C., T. McRackan, and T. N. Tatami. 2023. *Expanding real-world outcomes in adults with hearing loss.* https://bulletin.entnet.org/clinical-patient-care/article/22873582/expanding-realworld-outcomes-in-adults-with-hearing-loss (accessed December 19, 2024).

Noble, W. 2002. Extending the IOI to significant others and to non-hearing-aid-based interventions. *International Journal of Audiology* 41(1):27–29.

NQF (National Quality Forum). 2013. *Patient reported outcomes (PROs) in performance measurement.* https://www.qualityforum.org/Publications/2012/12/Patient-Reported_Outcomes_in_Performance_Measurement.aspx (accessed June 26, 2024).

NQF. n.d. a. *NQF's history.* https://www.qualityforum.org/about_nqf/history/ (accessed June 26, 2024).

NQF. n.d. b. *Measure applications partnership.* https://www.qualityforum.org/setting_priorities/partnership/measure_applications_partnership.aspx (accessed June 26, 2024).

O'Connor, D. P., and M. R. Brinker. 2013. Challenges in outcome measurement: Clinical research perspective. *Clinical Orthopaedics and Related Research* 471(11):3496–3503.

PQM (Partnership for Quality Measurement). 2023. *Endorsement and maintenance (E&M) guidebook.* https://p4qm.org/sites/default/files/2023-10/Del-3-6-Endorsement-and-Maintenance-Guidebook-Final_0.pdf#page=40 (accessed June 26, 2024).

PQM. 2024a. *Endorsement & maintenance (E&M).* https://p4qm.org/EM (accessed June 26, 2024).

PQM. 2024b. *PQM measure evaluation rubric worksheet.* https://p4qm.org/media/3161 (accessed December 20, 2024).

Prinsen, C. A. C., S. Vohra, M. R. Rose, M. Boers, P. Tugwell, M. Clarke, P. R. Williamson, and C. B. Terwee. 2016a. *Guideline for selecting outcome measurement instruments for outcomes included in a core outcome set.* https://cosmin.nl/wp-content/uploads/COSMIN-guideline-selecting-outcome-measurement-COS.pdf (accessed June 25, 2024).

Prinsen, C. A. C., S. Vohra, M. R. Rose, M. Boers, P. Tugwell, M. Clarke, P. R. Williamson, and C. B. Terwee. 2016b. How to select outcome measurement instruments for outcomes included in a "core outcome set"—A practical guideline. *Trials* 17(1):449.

Sogi, G. M. 2023. Research waste. *Contemporary Clinical Dentistry* 14(3):179.

Tysome, J. R., P. Hill-Feltham, W. E. Hodgetts, B. J. McKinnon, P. Monksfield, R. Sockalingham, M. L. Johansson, and A. F. Snik. 2015. The Auditory Rehabilitation Outcomes Network: An international initiative to develop core sets of patient-centred outcome measures to assess interventions for hearing loss. *Clinical Otolaryngology* 40(6):512–515.

WHO (World Health Organization). 2002. *Towards a common language for functioning, disability and health (ICF).* Geneva, Switzerland: World Health Organization.

WHO. 2025. *International Classification of Functioning, Disability, and Health (ICF).* https://www.who.int/standards/classifications/international-classification-of-functioning-disability-and-health (accessed January 11, 2025).

Williamson, P. R., D. G. Altman, H. Bagley, K. L. Barnes, J. M. Blazeby, S. T. Brookes, M. Clarke, E. Gargon, S. Gorst, N. Harman, J. J. Kirkham, A. McNair, C. A. C. Prinsen, J. Schmitt, C. B. Terwee, and B. Young. 2017. The COMET handbook: Version 1.0. *Trials* 18:1–50.

Wong, L., and L. Hickson. 2012. *Evidence-based practice in audiology: Evaluating interventions for children and adults with hearing impairment.* San Diego, CA: Plural Publishing.

4

Meaningfulness and
Importance to Measure

As noted in Chapter 3, the initial steps of determining a core outcome set include identifying all potential core outcomes and then narrowing to a subset of outcomes that are significant in all contexts. The committee considered two main criteria for the first step in both identifying and narrowing these outcomes: meaningfulness of the outcome (with an emphasis on meaningfulness to adults with hearing difficulties and clinicians) and importance to measure (the ability of an intervention to affect the measured outcome). To achieve whole health, care systems must first understand what matters to people and then build around this to help achieve those goals (NASEM, 2023). This chapter gives an overview of the evidence on the meaningfulness of various outcomes and outcome domains in hearing health and introduces the concept of importance to measure. While all outcomes are meaningful for specific populations or purposes, the committee sought to understand which outcomes are most meaningful across contexts. Chapter 5 presents evidence on the connection between hearing health interventions and various outcomes, and Chapter 6 discusses the ability of individual measures to detect the changes in outcomes.

OVERVIEW OF MEANINGFULNESS

Traditionally, the hearing health field has relied on behavioral assessments of performance in unaided and aided conditions to evaluate success of the intervention (Moberly et al., 2023). Although measuring thresholds and word or sentence recognition is critical, these measures alone do not tell the whole story of an individual's real world communication abilities

77

(Moberly et al., 2023). There are serious concerns that these behavioral audiologic measurements do not accurately reflect everyday communication abilities because they are performed in highly constrained conditions in a lab or clinic and do not fully reflect the challenges of everyday listening environments (Moberly et al., 2023). Patient-reported outcome measures (PROMs) are standardized,[1] psychometrically valid questionnaires that collect data directly from patients about their health outcomes (Churruca et al., 2021). PROMs often ask patients about their "symptoms, health-related quality of life, and functional status" (Churruca et al., 2021, p. 1016). A breadth of research shows that objective audiologic measures poorly predict self-report measures (Cox et al., 2003; Dornhoffer et al., 2020; Fitzgerald, et al., 2024; Hoff et al., 2023; Wang et al., 2022).

At a public webinar of this committee, Russell Misheloff, an individual with hearing difficulties, shared:

> It would be useful to measure better speech perception in noise. I mean, typically, we know audiologists will do it in very quiet settings, and most of us do pretty well in very quiet settings, but that's not the real world and doesn't really have much sense of your quality of life living in the real world.

Similarly, as noted in Tysome and colleagues:

> Psychoacoustic measures of hearing such as pure-tone audiometry are most commonly used, as they are both objective and repeatable. They are of great importance in evaluating whether or not an intervention is successful from a technical point of view, and thus whether the goal of the intervention was met (e.g., closed air-bone gap or sufficient gain and output of hearing devices according to established targets). However, the ability to hear pure tones in quiet or speech in noise seldom reflects the overall effect of that hearing loss on the life of a patient, . . . nor does it act as a comprehensive measure of the therapeutic effect of any intervention to rehabilitate their hearing loss. (Tysome et al., 2015, p. 512)

As described in Chapter 3, an Australian initiative sought to identify outcomes for a self-report core outcome set for hearing rehabilitation (Allen et al., 2022). The primary outcome domains identified, in rank order from the consensus process, were:

1. communication ability: 10 of 11 ranked as first in importance;
2. personal relationships: 9 of 11 ranked as second or third in importance;

---

[1] The word *standardized* is used here in a broad sense to indicate that the same measures are being used for specific outcomes, and that there are prescribed materials and procedures for the use of these measures. The committee does not imply that the measures are part of national or international standards.

3. well-being: 5 ranked as second and 3 ranked as fourth in importance; and

4. participation restrictions: 5 ranked as fourth and 3 ranked as fifth in importance.

These results indicate that there are important consequences of hearing difficulties on speech communication, but that these consequences present only part of the picture regarding potential outcomes to assess. The remaining outcomes identified can all be described generally as assessing the social, emotional, and psychological consequences of hearing difficulties.

The committee identified three main questions to assess the meaningfulness of each outcome. First, is the outcome perceived as important by adults with hearing difficulties and clinicians to their hearing health? Next, is the prevalence of the difficulty in that outcome high? In other words, are many people experiencing this difficulty? And lastly, how severe is the difficulty? The following sections outline the evidence on the meaningfulness of various outcomes based on evidence from peer-reviewed literature, industry and consumer group surveys, testimony during committee webinars, and online platform submissions for this project.

PEER-REVIEWED LITERATURE ON MEANINGFULNESS

The Partnership for Quality Measurement identifies the meaningfulness of the outcome to the target population as the starting point in the development of outcome measures (PQM, 2024). Until recently, there have been few attempts to establish the meaningfulness of various outcomes to adults with hearing difficulties. However, researchers typically predetermine which outcomes they believe would be important to adults with hearing difficulties and then ask these individuals to respond to this limited list. In a recent review of the literature on how adults self-describe and communicate about the listening difficulties they experience, McNeice and colleagues concluded:

> Importantly, no study included in this review asked participants to describe their listening difficulties in their own words, nor did any study explore how participants choose to describe and communicate about their listening difficulties. (McNeice et al., 2024, p. 168)

Two older studies in the United Kingdom obtained responses to mailed questionnaires which instructed clinic patients to: "Please make a list of the difficulties you have as a result of your hearing loss. List them in order of importance, starting with the biggest difficulties. Write down as many as you can" (Tyler et al.,1983, p. 191; see also Barcham and Stephens, 1980). Questionnaires were completed at home and either mailed back or brought back to the clinic at the hearing-aid evaluation appointment. None of the respondents considered for analyses here had worn hearing aids previously and most were estimated to have at least moderate audiometric hearing loss (Tyler et al., 1983). Each team of investigators used slightly different categories to group the self-reported hearing difficulties listed by the participants. Despite this, there was generally good agreement between these two independent surveys. In both reports, difficulties in "general conversation" and in "group conservation" were among the four most prevalent and the four most important hearing difficulties reported.

Another way studies have examined meaningfulness for individuals with hearing difficulties is through the examination of patient satisfaction with specific hearing health interventions. For example, Manchaiah and colleagues surveyed hearing aid wearers about which functional aspects of hearing aids they prioritized when choosing a hearing aid (Manchaiah et al., 2021). In that survey, the top attributes deemed very or extremely important by at least 75 percent of respondents were "improved ability to hear friends and family in quiet and in noisy settings, physical comfort, and reliability" (Manchaiah et al., 2021, p. 540). (See later in this chapter for more evidence on patient satisfaction with specific hearing interventions as gathered from industry and consumer group surveys.)

Given the sparse evidence documenting directly reported meaningfulness of outcomes, the committee turned to indirect evidence on the meaningful outcomes. The committee identified studies with reasonably large samples of adults with hearing difficulties in which the prevalence and severity of various hearing difficulties had been reported. The committee used these studies to establish meaningfulness by addressing the following questions: (1) what are the hearing difficulties reported by adults; (2) how severe do they report these difficulties to be; (3) how prevalent are these difficulties; and (4) are there emotional, social, or psychological consequences of these difficulties? The committee identified two types of datasets identified in its review that addressed these questions: (1) clinical convenience samples and (2) population studies.

Conclusion 4-1: More direct evidence, including the use of open-ended questions asked of adults with hearing difficulties, is needed to build a more robust evidence base for the nature of hearing difficulties and which outcomes are most meaningful to adults with hearing difficulties.

Clinical Convenience Samples

Clinical convenience samples come from groups that are easy to access, such as patients who attend a clinic. These data are detailed, and the sample sizes can be large, but the population segment is biased because it is not a representative sample of the entire population. Examples of outcome measures evaluated using clinical convenience samples include the Communication Profile for the Hearing Impaired (CPHI), the Client-Oriented Scale of Improvement (COSI), the Glasglow Hearing-Aid Benefit Profile (GHABP), and the Profile of Hearing Aid Performance (PHAP). These questionnaires can provide insights into outcomes that are meaningful to adults with hearing difficulties.

Communication Profile for the Hearing Impaired

Perhaps the most comprehensive assessment of the communication difficulties experienced by adults with hearing difficulties is the CPHI (Demorest and Erdman, 1986, 1987; Erdman and Demorest, 1998a,b). The CPHI consists of 145 items that are reduced to 25 scale scores, 6 of which pertain directly to communication importance or performance. The psychometrics of the CPHI have undergone rigorous evaluation; both its validity and reliability have been well established.

Of the 25 scales of the CPHI, there are nine Personal Adjustment scales that address these consequences. The bulk of the CPHI assesses the personal adjustment to hearing difficulties, including scales assessing anger, discouragement, self-acceptance, stress, withdrawal, and denial, among others. Although the CPHI is comprehensive in its assessment of the problems experienced by those with hearing difficulties, it is not typically used as an outcome measure owing, in large part, to the length of the measure. Administration of the CPHI pre- and postintervention would be burdensome, although some researchers have done so (e.g., Chisolm et al., 2004). In addition, because of copyright protections and the requirements of special software for the scoring and generation of scale scores, its feasibility as a broadly used outcome measure is further reduced.

Client-Oriented Scale of Improvement

Rather than prescribe the communication scenarios and rate their importance, the COSI asks prospective hearing-aid wearers to identify the top five listening situations they would like to improve following hearing aid use (Dillon et al., 1997). Responses from 1,770 adults seen at various clinics across Australia were placed into one of 16 categories by Dillon and colleagues (1999). The five most frequently listed listening situations identified by these adults as in need of improvement were:

1. listening to television/radio at normal volume (74.8 percent),
2. conversation with one or two people in quiet (47.4 percent),
3. conversation with group in quiet (31.9 percent),
4. conversation with one or two people in noise (24.1 percent), and
5. conversation with a group of people in noise (23.5 percent).

Conversation with others in quiet and in noise represents four of the top five goals desired among these adults and can be considered meaningful to adults with hearing difficulties. The COSI also can be used for interventions beyond hearing aids (e.g., cochlear implants) (Warren et al., 2019).

Glasgow Hearing-Aid Benefit Profile

The GHABP questionnaire was developed from a large regional United Kingdom dataset (Gatehouse, 1999). Four listening situations were identified by the respondents in Gatehouse (1999) as both frequently occurring and difficult when unaided (without hearing aids):

1. listening to television when volume set by others;
2. conversing with one person in quiet;
3. conversing on a busy street or in a shop; and
4. group conversation.

These four prespecified listening situations were considered to be representative prototypes for outcome evaluation. Respondents can also identify up to four additional listening situations of importance representing patient-nominated goals.

Whitmer et al. (2014) reported results from 577 adults (with pure-tone average thresholds of 0 to 50 decibels hearing level for the frequencies of 0.5, 1, 2, and 4 kilohertz) who were not using hearing aids about their difficulty in each of the four GHABP prototypical listening situations. They were separately asked to indicate how much the difficulty in that situation worries, annoys, or upsets them. Respondents indicated either "no" or "slight" difficulty when conversing with one person in quiet, but this increased to "slight" or "moderate" difficulty for the other three listening situations. Difficulties increased as a function of hearing loss. In addition, frustration with those difficulties ranged from "little" to "moderate" for the three more difficult situations but from "none" to "little" for conversing with one person in quiet. Statistically significant main effects of hearing loss were observed in addition to statistically significant main effects of conversing with one person in quiet.

Profile of Hearing Aid Performance (and Benefit)

The PHAP is a 66-item survey assessing the frequency of difficulty in a variety of listening conditions (Cox and Gilmore, 1990; Cox, 1996). Of the 66 items, 48 focus on speech communication and the remainder focus on the loudness or aversiveness of environmental sounds. Cox and Gilmore (1990) reported results from 225 experienced hearing aid wearers with mild to moderate losses seen in the clinic. Among the 48 speech-communication items, the five with the highest frequency of difficulty (mean percentage) were as follows:

1. When I am in a room with the door closed and I want to overhear a conversation going on outside the door, I have to strain to listen (84.1 percent).
2. When I am listening to a speaker who is talking to a large group, and I am seated toward the rear of the room, I must make an effort to listen (78.1 percent).
3. When I am at a large, noisy party, conversation is very confusing (76.5 percent).
4. When I am in a crowd with a friend who does not want others to overhear our conversation, I have trouble hearing as well (72.9 percent).
5. When I am listening to the news on the car radio, and family members are talking, I have trouble hearing the news (71.8 percent).

Several of the situations in which respondents most frequently had difficulty involved listening to speech when others are talking in the background. Interestingly, the phrasing of the top two items of the PHAP listed above appears to tap listening effort rather than performance. Further, of these top five most-frequently difficult listening situations, only one, the last item shown above, is included in the 24-item abbreviated PHAP (APHAP) (Cox and Alexander, 1995; Cox, 1996). The PHAP and shortened APHAP focus on aided conditions (e.g., the perspective of the person wearing hearing aids). To assess the individual's perceived differences (i.e., with a hearing aid versus without a hearing aid) and compare differences over time, an expanded questionnaire was developed—the Profile of Hearing Aid Benefit (PHAB), which has the same items and subscales as the PHAP (Cox and Alexander, 1995; Cox, 1996). An abbreviated PHAB (APHAB) is commonly used as a self-report outcome today and is further discussed in Chapter 6.

Conclusion 4-2: Studies of clinical convenience samples of adults converged on similar conclusions. Specifically, adults with hearing difficulties have problems with communication, especially in groups, and these problems often lead to frustration. Frustration with hearing difficulties is considered a negative emotional reaction to those difficulties. Emotional and social difficulties are commonplace among those who have trouble hearing.

Population Studies

As compared to clinical convenience samples, population studies are conducted on a larger scale (capturing a community, region, or nation), making the data more representative. However, there is a limitation on how many questions can be asked and the level of detail of these surveys because of the burden on respondents. The following sections highlight population studies both within the United States, primarily the National Health and Nutrition Examination Survey (NHANES), as well as from other countries.

The National Health and Nutrition Examination Survey

NHANES is a national survey that collects data on a wide range of health concerns for different age distributions.[2] The 2017 to 2020 NHANES survey (NHANES, 2021) included three main items regarding perceived hearing difficulties for adults (age 20 and older): (1) the general condition of one's hearing with responses ranging from "excellent" to "deaf;" (2) the frequency of difficulties conversing in noise with responses ranging from "never" to "always;" and (3) the frequency of frustration when talking with friends and family, with responses again ranging from "never" to "always."

For the question on the general condition of one's hearing, 76.2 percent respondents rated their hearing as excellent or good, 21.2 percent rated it as having "a little trouble" or "moderate trouble," and 2.4 percent said they had "a lot of trouble" or were deaf (Humes, 2024). Humes (2024) analyzed data for the second two questions by large age groups (20–69 and over age 70) and by self-reported hearing difficulty. Figure 4-1 and Figure 4-2 show the population-weighted self-reported responses for the items related

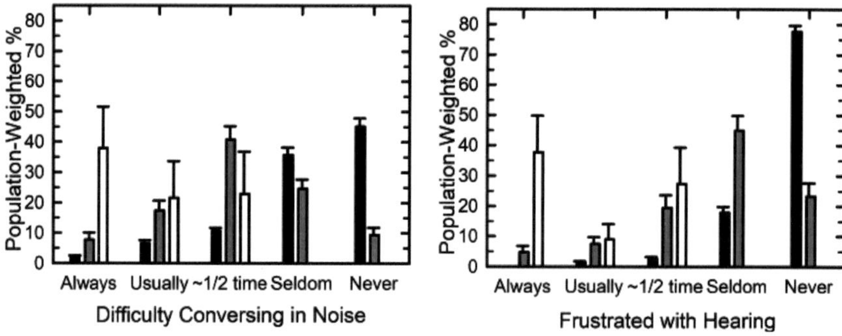

FIGURE 4-1 Population-weighted estimates of hearing difficulties ages 20–69 using 2017–2020 NHANES data.
NOTE: Black bars are for those with self-reported hearing difficulties rated as "excellent" or "good," gray bars are for those with self-reported hearing difficulties rated as "a little" or "moderate" trouble, and white bars are for those reporting "a lot" of hearing difficulties or deaf. NHANES = National Health and Nutrition Examination Survey.
SOURCE: Humes, 2024. CC BY-NC-ND.

---

[2] For more information, see https://www.cdc.gov/nchs/nhanes/index.html (accessed January 13, 2024).

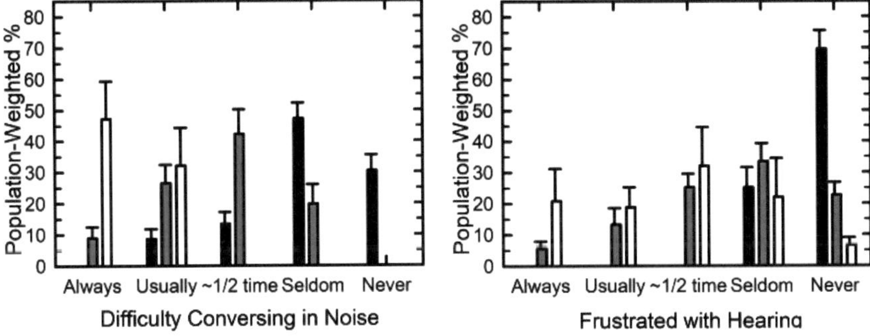

FIGURE 4-2 Population-weighted estimates of hearing difficulties ages 70 and older using 2017–2020 NHANES data.
NOTE: Black bars are for those with self-reported hearing difficulties rated as "excellent" or "good," gray bars are for those with self-reported hearing difficulties rated as "a little" or "moderate" trouble, and white bars are for those reporting "a lot" of hearing difficulties or deaf. NHANES = National Health and Nutrition Examination Survey.
SOURCE: Humes, 2024. CC BY-NC-ND.

to hearing difficulties in noise and frustration with hearing. Humes analysis revealed that overall, the prevalence of self-reported difficulty conversing in noise increased with the severity of the hearing condition; 19 to 22 percent of those with self-reported excellent or good hearing said they had difficulty conversing in noise at least half the time, while the percentage was 66 to 78 for those with a little or moderate trouble hearing, and 82 to 94 percent for those with more severe hearing difficulties (Humes, 2024).

Regarding the question of frustration when talking with friends and family, most (70 to 80 percent) adults with self-reported excellent or good hearing indicate they never feel frustrated. In comparison, 32 to 44 percent of those with a little or moderate trouble reported feeling frustrated at least half of the time (Humes, 2024). As noted by Humes,

> Frustration is an emotional reaction to the hearing difficulty and represents a more significant concern regarding negative impact of this difficulty on the individual's emotional wellness and overall well-being.

Overall, these analyses show difficulty conversing in noise and frustration with hearing as prevalent concerns among adults with hearing difficulties.

International Population Studies

Lutman and colleagues (1987) reported the results from 1,691 individuals who completed the second in-clinic stage of a two-stage random sampling process for the United Kingdom adult population (Davis, 1983; Lutman et al., 1987). A series of nine questions was asked of all in-clinic participants, who ranged in age from 17 to 89 years. Principal-components analysis by Lutman et al. (1987) of the response to these nine questions identified four components:

1. everyday speech;
2. speech in quiet;
3. sound localization; and
4. handicap.

"Everyday speech" represents speech communication in a background of competing sounds. The "handicap" outcome domain was based on the frequency with which hearing problems "restrict enjoyment of social and personal life," create "a feeling of being cut off from things," and "lead to embarrassment." Handicap captures social, emotional, and psychological consequences of hearing difficulties. Of these four principal components, approximately two-thirds of the variance was accounted for by "everyday speech communication" and "handicap" combined.

In the 1980s, the United Kingdom's (UK's) Medical Research Council National Study of Hearing was conducted to identify the prevalence and distribution of hearing loss in the UK (Akeroyd et al., 2019). The sample size and quality of the design made it particularly notable for the time, and since it was never repeated, it remains the "primary U.K. source for prevalence of auditory problems" (Akeroyd et al., 2019, p. 1). After an initial broad postal survey sent to 48,313 adults selected at random from the electoral registers, a representative sample of adults was selected for in-clinic follow-up using a custom set of survey questions. Some survey items inquired about the degree of difficulty experienced (e.g., a little, moderate, a lot) whereas others inquired about the frequency of occurrence of such difficulties (e.g., never, sometimes, always). The final in-person test sample included 2,578 adults. The study also collected data on "the prevalence and characteristics of both measured hearing impairment and self-reported hearing disability in adults (18–80 years) as a function of severity, age, gender, occupational group, and occupational noise exposure" (Akeroyd et al., 2019, p. 2).

Uchida and colleagues reported results from a population study in Japan of 2,150 adults 40 to 79 years of age; a total of 994 (45 percent) perceived that they had hearing loss (Uchida et al., 2003). Among these 994 adults, 83 percent responded "yes" or "occasionally" when asked whether their hearing difficulties resulted in speech-communication problems and 42 percent responded the same way when asked whether they had difficulty following conversations that included 4–5 people in a quiet room. Twenty-two percent responded similarly regarding experiencing restrictions to their daily life activities, and 20 percent indicated that their hearing difficulties led to a loss of self-confidence.

In an online survey of 2,352 Dutch volunteers, Boeschen-Hospers and colleagues (2016), using the Amsterdam Inventory for Auditory Disability and Handicap, asked how often the respondent could hear effectively in 29 different listening situations. Response options were: "almost always," "frequently," "occasionally," and "almost never." The top five listening situations with the highest response percentages of either "occasionally" or "almost never" hearing effectively were as follows:

1. follow the conversation among a few adults at dinner;
2. carry on a conversation with someone in a crowded meeting;
3. carry on a conversation with someone on a busy street;
4. carry on a conversation with someone in a bus or car; and
5. hear from what direction a question is asked during a meeting.

Of the next five listening situations, two had to do with difficulty understanding speech and the other three involved difficulties in localizing sound. Kramer and colleagues (1998) had previously used the same measure in a smaller convenience sample (239 people with hearing difficulties) and showed that "handicap resulting from the inability to understand speech in noise is most strongly felt" (p. 302).

A population study of 1,711 unaided adults 18 to 97 years of age by von Goblenz et al. made use of stratified random samples of residents in northwest Germany (von Gablenz et al., 2018). A brief 17-item version of the 49-item Speech, Spatial and Qualities of Hearing (SSQ) scale was used (Gatehouse and Noble, 2004). The SSQ provides a detailed description of a specific scenario and then asks a question such as "Can you follow the conversation?" or "Can you tell how far away a sound is?" An 11-point response scale ranging from 0 ("not at all") to 10 ("perfectly") is used. Results for the SSQ-17 were presented stratified by average pure-tone hearing loss but, regardless of hearing loss severity, the most commonly identified listening situations that were difficult were tasks that involved following conversations in noise including competing speech, discerning the distance and movement of sound sources, and listening effort required during conversations.

Conclusion 4-3: Population studies support the identification of several outcomes as being meaningful to adults with hearing difficulties: (1) communication performance, especially in groups, in background noise, and on the telephone; (2) sound localization; (3) identification or awareness of important environmental sounds (e.g., vehicles, warnings); and (4) psychosocial consequences of hearing difficulties. Listening effort emerged in one population study (von Gablenz et al., 2018) as well as in the Profile of Hearing Aid Performance (Cox and Gilmore, 1990) but this represents limited evidence regarding its importance at present.

OTHER SOURCES OF EVIDENCE ON MEANINGFULNESS

Apart from the peer-reviewed published literature, a variety of resources provide insights on outcomes that are meaningful to adults with hearing difficulties and clinicians. These sources include industry and consumer group surveys, testimony from this committee's public webinars, and comments received by this committee through its online platform.

Industry and Consumer Group Surveys

Some of the most direct evidence of the meaningfulness of specific outcomes and outcome domains is from surveys by industry and consumer groups that directly ask individuals with hearing difficulties about what matters the most to them regarding their hearing health. However, these types of surveys tend to ask about the effect of hearing loss itself or satisfaction with specific interventions rather than the meaningfulness of specific improvements to their hearing health.

MarkeTrak

MarkeTrak is a series of surveys conducted by the Hearing Industries Association to collect data on industry trends.[3] MarkeTrak 10 (completed in 2019) surveyed 3,132 individuals with hearing difficulties (Powers, 2020). The 969 hearing aid wearers within this group were directly asked about the factors that drove satisfaction with their hearing aids. The most highly ranked factors were hearing aid performance in quiet and noise, sound quality, and effectiveness of health care professionals (Appleton-Huber, 2022). When compared with other people with hearing difficulties in the survey, hearing aid wearers' satisfaction with their hearing in all listening situations was higher than those who did not wear hearing aids.

EuroTrak

In 2009, the European Hearing Instrument Manufacturers Association (EHIMA) created the EuroTrak (Hougaard and Ruf, 2011). This study was modeled after the MarkeTrak as a comprehensive study on hearing loss and hearing aids in Germany, France, and the UK. The EuroTrak has since been implemented in many countries across Europe and the Asia-Pacific region (EHIMA, n.d.). The survey is now the "largest comparative multicountry study on hearing loss and hearing aid usage" (EHIMA, n.d.). Both the MarkeTrak and the EuroTrak include common questions that make comparison across countries possible despite varying delivery systems for hearing aids (Powers and Bisgaard, 2022). A comparison between the 2022 MarkeTrak (MT2022),

---

[3] For more information see https://betterhearing.org/policy-research/marketrak/ (accessed May 13, 2024).

the 2022 EuroTrak in France (ET-F) and the 2022 EuroTrak in Germany (ET-G) found that all three countries have similar rates of self-reported hearing loss ranging from 10 to 13 percent (Powers and Bisgaard, 2022). Over 60 percent of the respondents in all three countries reported that they felt like they should have obtained hearing devices sooner because of the improvement of social interactions and the reduction of fatigue (Powers and Bisgaard, 2022). The EuroTrak not only collects valuable data about hearing impairment and the use of hearing aids in over a dozen countries but it also creates comparable data that show trends across countries.

In addition to the demographic data, the EuroTrak also collects information on patient satisfaction with hearing aids across a range of listening situations, as well as satisfaction with the dispenser, the sound quality and signal processing, and the product features (Hougaard and Ruf, 2011). Lastly, the EuroTrak asks, "Since you started using your hearing aid(s), please rate the changes you have experienced in each of the following areas, which you believe are due to your hearing aid(s)" (Hougaard and Ruf, 2011). When Germany, the United Kingdom, and France were compared, by percentage of people who noted improvement with hearing aids, the most common responses were effective communication (Germany 67 percent, United Kingdom 68 percent, France 79 percent), social life (Germany 53 percent, United Kingdom 57 percent, France 74 percent), relationships at home (Germany 47 percent, United Kingdom 53 percent, France 71 percent), and the ability to participate in group activities (Germany 58 percent, United Kingdom 60 percent, France 68 percent) (Hougaard and Ruf, 2011).

HLAA Voice of the Patient Report

In 2021, the Hearing Loss Association of America (HLAA) held an externally led patient-focused meeting on drug development for people living with sensorineural hearing loss and their families (HLAA, 2021). Subsequently, HLAA published a *Voice of the Patient* report with the findings from this meeting. As shown in Figure 4-3, when asked about hearing loss–related health concerns, meeting participants reported challenges hearing with background noise (92 percent), muffled sounds (66 percent), fatigue (62 percent), difficulty hearing consonants (51 percent), tinnitus (39 percent), trouble with balance or vertigo (30 percent), difficulty hearing higher-pitched voices (26 percent), headaches (10 percent), and other physical concerns (18 percent) (HLAA, 2021). The report also listed psychosocial health concerns with social isolation or avoidance (61 percent), depression or anxiety (35 percent), issues with verbal communication (35 percent), and loss of initiative in work and hobbies (24 percent) (HLAA, 2021).

Respondents identified difficulty hearing in background noise, social isolation or avoidance, and fatigue as the most troublesome hearing-related health concerns (HLAA, 2021). Eighty-eight percent of respondents reported

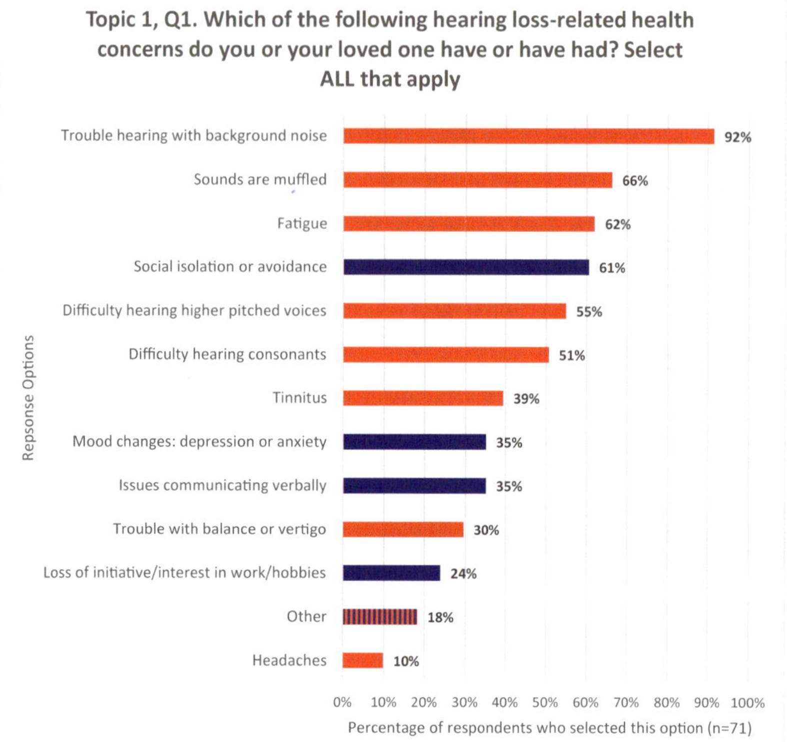

FIGURE 4-3 Hearing loss-related health concerns.
NOTE: orange bars = physical health concerns; purple bars = psychosocial health concerns.
SOURCE: HLAA, 2021. Reprinted with permission from HLAA, hearingloss.org.

that because of their hearing loss it is a struggle, or they are unable, to participate in social events (HLAA, 2021). Fifty-seven percent of respondents reported that their hearing loss made communication with family members difficult (HLAA, 2021). When it came to specific challenging listening environments the survey reflected that 43 percent of respondents felt there were barriers to attending concerts and events and 29 percent found school or work challenging (HLAA, 2021). Additional effects of hearing loss were difficulties accessing health care, safety, challenges running errands, and not being able to watch television. People with hearing loss reported worrying about future effects such as an increased risk of dementia (67 percent) and losing social connection with a spouse or child (60 percent) (HLAA, 2021).

Conclusion 4-4: Themes of meaningful outcomes among industry and consumer group surveys include speech communication (particularly speech in noise and other complex listening situations), social connection, psychological health, and listening fatigue.

Testimony from Public Webinars

The committee hosted two public webinars to hear directly from adults with hearing difficulties and clinicians about what outcomes are the most meaningful and therefore should be considered for a core set.[4] The quotes provided in this section were chosen to represent the range of individuals who testified to the committee and to highlight the most relevant issues raised during the webinars in response to the committee's questions and the statement of task.

The committee asked adults with hearing difficulties to share their goals for their hearing health (see Box 4-1). The most common goal noted by the panelists was that they wanted to improve their speech communication. In many cases, their personal challenges communicating with family

---

BOX 4-1
Hearing Health Goals

On a personal level I have a 3-year-old, almost 3-year-old, grandson and [I can maybe] understand half the time or a third of the time what he is saying because his voice is soft and the pitch . . . So that's what drives me to a more dramatic solution in my personal life.

—Kerry Sullivan

My goal is to be able to have the capacity to engage and actively participate one on one. And to attend performances and programs in public venues, including in environments that are less than ideal from a hearing perspective, and to do so without undue stress, inconvenience, fatigue, and embarrassment.

—Russell Misheloff

I think it would be useful to measure a better speech perception and in noise. I mean, typically, we know audiologists will do it in very quiet settings, and most of us do pretty well in very quiet settings, but that's not the real world and doesn't really have much sense of your quality of life living in the real world.

—Russell Misheloff

These quotes were collected from the committee's webinars.

---

[4] The webinar recordings can be accessed at https://www.nationalacademies.org/event/41996_02-2024_meaningful-outcome-measures-in-adult-hearing-health-care-webinar-1 and https://www.nationalacademies.org/event/42414_04-2024_meaningful-outcome-measures-in-adult-hearing-health-care-webinar-2.

members inspired them to seek out hearing health care. In particular, multiple panelists voiced that they were unable to understand young children and grandchildren because of the speed and high frequency of their speech, which was a major motivator toward getting hearing aids. Being able to hear with background noise was another significant challenge noted by participants. They noted that larger social gatherings usually take place in noisy environments making it very difficult for people with hearing loss to engage in conversation.

Several panelists shared how challenging their hearing loss made it for them to keep up in the workplace environment and the relief they experienced with hearing interventions. As shown in Box 4-2, multiple panelists

---

BOX 4-2
Effects of Hearing Loss in the Workplace

My ability to focus and concentrate in a business setting is so much greater now, and I just feel like I can process things so much more quickly and really follow what is going on. I had no idea that the hearing loss was holding me back from a professional standpoint.

—Chris Greame

I'm happy though to speak to some of those aspects of hearing loss that I think have not been addressed for me . . . which is the bigger picture of how it affects our work. In my case, I've had to change what I do because of my hearing loss. There are certain patients that it is very difficult for me to work with.

—Suzanne Johnston

I worked and still am working with executive leadership development. I made a conscious decision that I never talked about it. I can't be a trainer because I'm going to miss the jokes in the classroom to be able to interact and to work deeply with them and so that was a conscious choice because there is no solution for that. Instead, I went into curriculum development.

—Wynne Whyman

In my 60s working in nursing homes, in meetings I would remind people that I had hearing aids and I had difficulty hearing, but nobody paid attention. It didn't affect how anybody behaved in terms of making themselves accessible to me.

—Elizabeth Pentin

These quotes were collected from the committee's webinars.

BOX 4-3
Listening Effort and Listening Fatigue

Over the years what I found, and I didn't even realize this was going on, the amount of energy it takes in a social setting or in a business setting professionally to really communicate and process [. . . .] Because my energy levels were higher my productivity levels were higher, my ability to respond and think and process improved.

—Chris Greame

The thing I noticed when I put in these new hearing aids was that internally, I wasn't straining and putting my inner self out there to hear what people are saying. I didn't have to work so hard.

—Elizabeth Pentin

These quotes were collected from the committee's webinars.

---

said they had to shift their career paths because they could only perform specific roles with their hearing loss.

Multiple panelists expressed their struggles with listening fatigue as a consequence of their hearing loss. As shown in Box 4-3, the stress and exhaustion caused by hearing loss had a detrimental effect on their ability to fully participate and be productive in their daily lives.

During the second webinar, the committee also heard from hearing health professionals about their impressions of their patients' goals (see Box 4-4).

Online Platform Submissions

The committee invited members of the public to submit written comments answering a series of questions through an open platform. The following sections present samples from the 47 comments submitted to this committee by adults with hearing loss, their care partners, and hearing health professionals. Box 4-5 shows the range of concerns shared with the committee by adults with hearing difficulties.

Through the open platform, the committee asked clinicians about what they hear frequently from their patients as the most meaningful outcomes related to their hearing loss. Box 4-6 displays some of the responses. The overwhelming response was that their patients want to be able to understand speech in noisy environments.

BOX 4-4
Clinician Perspectives on Patient Goals

The common goals are understanding conversations, especially in background noise. Hearing grandkids, hearing soft speech, hearing at church.
—Lee Cottrell, Balance and Hearing Institute at Farragut ENT & Allergy

There's a difference between a new hearing aid user and an existing hearing aid user, and I think often that new users [don't] quite know what to expect. So, I think they have some shifting goals as their experience changes.
—Tim Steele, Associated Audiologists, Inc.

[Goals] change over time, but it is unbelievably critical to try to unearth those goals in the beginning because I may pick a different product or treatment option if it's a musician versus a car mechanic versus somebody else.
—Erika Person, Flex Audiology

These quotes were collected from the committee's webinars.

BOX 4-5
What Matters to Adults with Hearing Difficulties

My personal goal is to stay as fit, as active, and as engaged as I possibly can for the remainder of my life. This means physical health, mental health, and especially hearing health.
—Adult with hearing difficulties in Salem, OR

My goal: to fully participate in all aspects of life. That's more than just communication.
—Adult with hearing difficulties in Aurora, CO

Most important to me [. . .]: to again one day really hear without even thinking about it in all types of environments. This includes: one-on-one in restaurants; small groups of friends in restaurants; more than one other person in someone's home with typical noisy HVAC; meetings around a conference table with no hearing loop; lecture room with no hearing loop; theater with no hearing loop; movie theater with no technology or less than adequate technology and no open captioning.
—Adult with hearing difficulties in New York, NY

These quotes were collected from the committee's open platform. ·

BOX 4-6
What Clinicians Hear from Their Patients
About What Is Most Meaningful

Their stated primary desires are usually the benefit of speech in noise understanding, help with concentration, and better interactions with family/friends on a daily basis.

—Hearing Health Professional in Argyle, TX

The primary goal for most hearing aid wearers is improved speech perception, and while measures of audibility and subjective benefit are important, these measures fail to ascertain whether amplification has truly improved a patient's speech recognition ability.

—Hearing Health Professional in Tucson, AZ

Patients' primary concerns include speech intelligibility in noise.

—Hearing Health Professional in Cleveland, OH

Their main concerns have a lot to do with being able to hear in conversations, especially in background noise situations.

—Hearing Health Professional in Tucson, AZ

As a clinician in an ENT clinic, my patients often complained about their inability to understand speech in noise and quality-of-life issues due to hearing loss.

—Hearing Health Professional in Dorchester, MA

Quality of life; hearing/understanding speech better, especially in noisy environments; being able to effectively communicate while participating in social activities; cognitive decline.

—Hearing Health Professional in Orlando, FL

The most important outcome for people who need assistance is the ability to follow conversations in normal (noisy) environments. The resulting social connections are important for overall health. Audibility (and even words-in-noise recognition) are important, but follow a noisy conversation? How much listening effort does it take? How often does the patient have to ask for content to be repeated?

—Hearing Health Professional in Oakland, CA

These quotes were collected from the committee's open platform.

Conclusion 4-5: Themes of meaningful outcomes among the committee's public webinars and online platform submissions include speech communication (particularly speech in noise and other complex listening situations), social connection, participation, and listening fatigue.

IMPORTANCE TO MEASURE

The committee considered "importance to measure" as another factor in determining a core outcome set. First, importance to measure includes the extent to which the outcome is controllable, meaning that an intervention can change the outcome (Velentgas et al., 2013). This type of "importance" is distinct from the listening experiences considered by adults with hearing difficulties to be "important" to them. The concept is often associated with minimally clinically important differences (Velentgas et al., 2013). (See Chapter 6 for more on minimal clinically important differences.) Whereas an outcome may be very meaningful to adults with hearing difficulties and clinicians, a measure used for evaluating the core outcome set needs to be able to detect the smallest change deemed important to adults with hearing difficulties. Importance to measure also may be considered by whether the information gained by measurement helps inform treatment decisions (Velentgas et al., 2013).

The Partnership for Quality Measurement includes importance to measure as a criterion in their measurement endorsement process (PQM, 2023). It is outside of this committee's scope to conduct a full measure review, but the Partnership for Quality Measurement's comprehensive instructions on conducting measure evaluation greatly informed the committee's process. The rubric asks specific questions including whether use of the measure will lead to improved outcomes and whether there is credible evidence linking the intervention to improved outcomes. Importance to measure is further discussed in Chapters 5 and 6.

FINDINGS

Finding 4-1: Measurement of hearing ability in ideal listening conditions does not necessarily reflect real-world communication abilities or the outcomes that are most meaningful to adults with hearing difficulties.

Finding 4-2: The committee used three main questions to determine meaningfulness of outcomes:

1. Is the outcome perceived as essential by adults with hearing difficulties or clinicians?
2. Is the prevalence of the difficulty high?
3. How severe is the difficulty?

Finding 4-3: There is a significant lack of research that directly asks adults with hearing difficulties about what outcomes are most meaningful to them. Researchers tend to predetermine which outcomes they ask about rather than asking open-ended questions.

Finding 4-4: Surveys of adults with hearing loss tend to ask more about the effect of the hearing loss itself or their satisfaction with specific interventions rather than the meaningfulness of specific improvements (outcomes) of their hearing health.

Finding 4-5: Studies of clinical convenience samples show adults report problems with communication, especially in groups, and that these problems often lead to frustration. Hearing-related difficulties are common among those who have trouble hearing.

Finding 4-6: Population studies identify several outcome domains as being meaningful to adults with hearing difficulties: (1) communication performance, especially in groups, in background noise, and on the telephone; (2) sound localization; (3) identification or awareness of important environmental sounds (vehicles, warnings); and (4) the emotional and social consequence of hearing difficulties. Listening effort emerged as a meaningful outcome in one recent population study.

Finding 4-7: MarkeTrak 10 revealed that the most highly ranked factors for satisfaction among hearing aid wearers were hearing aid performance in quiet and noise, sound quality, and effectiveness of health care professionals. Hearing aid wearers had the least satisfaction with conversations in noise, talking on the phone, hearing over distance, and large group conversations.

Finding 4-8: A 2021 HLAA meeting of people living with sensorineural hearing loss found that their most troublesome concerns were hearing with background noise, social isolation or avoidance, and fatigue.

Finding 4-9: During public testimony to this committee, participants primarily noted challenges with speech communication (particularly understanding speech in a noisy environment and soft sounds). Other concerns were communicating with family, listening effort and fatigue, and having the ability to participate in their personal and professional lives.

Finding 4-10: Comments submitted on the committee's online platform by adults with hearing difficulties and clinicians primarily focused on the ability to understand speech in noise, as well as full participation in their desired activities.

Importance to Measure

Finding 4-11: Importance to measure is the extent to which the outcome is controllable, meaning that the intervention can change the outcome, or whether the information gained helps inform treatment decisions.

Finding 4-12: While an outcome may be very meaningful to adults with hearing difficulties and clinicians, if the intervention cannot significantly change the outcome, that outcome should not be included in a core set.

RECOMMENDATION

Limited *direct* research has been performed to determine which outcomes are most meaningful for adults with hearing difficulties and for clinicians. Existing evidence is mostly indirect, as it is usually derived from surveys of satisfaction with interventions or studies of the prevalence and severity of hearing difficulties that are typically based on (1) constrained surveys wherein the choices are developed by others (e.g., researchers and clinicians) and (2) varying degrees of direct input from those with hearing difficulties. More direct evidence, including answers to open-ended questions asked of adults with hearing difficulties, is needed to build a more robust evidence base concerning the nature of hearing difficulties and which outcomes are most meaningful to adults with hearing difficulties.

Recommendation 4-1: Sponsors of hearing health research should fund additional research to engage adults with hearing difficulties, their communication partners, and clinicians to determine the most meaningful outcomes based on direct evidence from adults with hearing difficulties.

Sponsors of hearing health research may include a wide variety of partners including federal agencies (e.g. the Centers for Disease Control and Prevention, the Department of Defense, the National Institutes of Health, the Veterans Administration), foundations, professional organizations, and industry.

REFERENCES

Akeroyd, M. A., G. G. Browning, A. C. Davis, and M. P. Haggard. 2019. Hearing in adults: A digital reprint of the main report from the MRC National Study of Hearing. *Trends in Hearing* 23:2331216519887614.

Allen, D., L. Hickson, and M. Ferguson. 2022. Defining a patient-centred core outcome domain set for the assessment of hearing rehabilitation with clients and professionals. *Frontiers in Neuroscience* 16:787607.

Appleton-Huber, J. 2022. *What is important to your hearing aid client...And are they satisfied?* https://hearingreview.com/hearing-loss/patient-care/counseling-education/what-important-to-your-hearing-aid-clients-are-they-satisfied (accessed May 22, 2024).

Barcham, L. J., and S. D. Stephens. 1980. The use of an open-ended problems questionnaire in auditory rehabilitation. *British Journal of Audiology* 14(2):49–54.

Boeschen-Hospers, J. M., N. Smits, C. Smits, M. Stam, C. B. Terwee, and S. E. Kramer. 2016. Reevaluation of the Amsterdam Inventory for Auditory Disability and Handicap using item response theory. *Journal of Speech, Language, and Hearing Research* 59(2):373–383.

Chisolm, T. H., H. B. Abrams, and R. McArdle. 2004. Short- and long-term outcomes of adult audiological rehabilitation. *Ear and Hearing* 25(5).

Churruca, K., C. Pomare, L. A. Ellis, J. C. Long, S. B. Henderson, L. E. D. Murphy, C. J. Leahy, and J. Braithwaite. 2021. Patient-reported outcome measures (PROMs): A review of generic and condition-specific measures and a discussion of trends and issues. *Health Expectations* 24(4):1015–1024.

Cox, R. M. 1996. *Phonak Focus 21: The Abbreviated Profile of Hearing Aid Benefit (APHAB)—Administration and application.* Stafa, Switzerland: Phonak AG.

Cox, R. M., and G. C. Alexander. 1995. The Abbreviated Profile of Hearing Aid Benefit. *Ear and Hearing* 16(2):176–186.

Cox, R. M., and C. Gilmore. 1990. Development of the Profile of Hearing Aid Performance (PHAP). *Journal of Speech, Language, and Hearing Research* 33(2):343–357.

Cox, R. M., G. C. Alexander, and C. M. Beyer. 2003. Norms for the International Outcome Inventory for Hearing Aids. *Journal of the American Academy of Audiology* 14(08):403–413.

Davis, A. C. 1983. 2 - Hearing disorders in the population: First phase findings of the MRC National Study of Hearing. In *Hearing science and hearing disorders*, edited by M. E. Lutman and M. P. Haggard. London, UK: Academic Press. Pp. 35–60.

Demorest, M. E., and S. A. Erdman. 1986. Scale composition and item analysis of the Communication Profile for the Hearing Impaired. *Journal of Speech, Language, and Hearing Research* 29(4):515–535.

Demorest, M. E., and S. A. Erdman. 1987. Development of the Communication Profile for the Hearing Impaired. *Journal of Speech and Hearing Disorders* 52(2):129–143.

Dillon, H., A. James, and J. Ginis. 1997. Client Oriented Scale of Improvement (COSI) and its relationship to several other measures of benefit and satisfaction provided by hearing aids. *Journal of the American Academy of Audiology* 8(1):27–43.

Dillon, H., G. Birtles, and R. Lovegrove. 1999. Measuring the outcomes of a national rehabilitation program: Normative data for the Client Oriented Scale of Improvement (COSI) and the Hearing Aid User's Questionnaire (HAUQ). *Journal of the American Academy of Audiology* 10(2):67–79.

Dornhoffer, J. R., T. A. Meyer, J. R. Dubno, and T. R. McRackan. 2020. Assessment of hearing aid benefit using patient-reported outcomes and audiologic measures. *Audiology and Neurotology* 25(4):215–223.

EHIMA (European Hearing Instrument Manufacturers Association). n.d. *Surveys.* https://www.ehima.com/surveys/ (accessed September 24, 2024).

Erdman, S. A., and M. E. Demorest. 1998a. Adjustment to hearing impairment I: Description of a heterogeneous clinical population. *Journal of Speech, Language, and Hearing Research* 41(1):107–122.

Erdman, S. A., and M. E. Demorest. 1998b. Adjustment to hearing impairment II: Audiological and demographic correlates. *Journal of Speech, Language, and Hearing Research* 41(1):123–136.

Fitzgerald, M. B., K. M. Ward, S. P. Gianakas, M. L. Smith, N. H. Blevins, and A. P. Swanson. 2024. Speech-in-noise assessment in the routine audiologic test battery: Relationship to perceived auditory disability. *Ear and Hearing* 45(4):816–826.

Gatehouse, S. 1999. Glasgow Hearing Aid Benefit Profile: Derivation and validation of a client-centered outcome measure for hearing aid services. *Journal of the American Academy of Audiology* 10(2):80–103.

Gatehouse, S., and W. Noble. 2004. The Speech, Spatial and Qualities of Hearing Scale (SSQ). *International Journal of Audiology* 43(2):85–99.

HLAA (Hearing Loss Association of America). 2021. *Voice of the patient report: HLAA's externally led patient-focused drug development (PFDD) meeting for people and families living with sensorineural hearing loss.* Rockville, MD: Hearing Loss Association of America.

Hoff, M., J. Skoog, T. H. Bodin, T. Tengstrand, U. Rosenhall, I. Skoog, and A. Sadeghi. 2023. Hearing loss and cognitive function in early old age: Comparing subjective and objective hearing measures. *Gerontology* 69(6):694–705.

Hougaard, S., and S. Ruf. 2011. *EuroTrak.* https://hearingreview.com/hearing-products/amplification/assistive-devices/eurotrak (accessed September 24, 2024).

Humes, L. E. 2024. Demographic and audiological characteristics of candidates for over-the-counter hearing aids in the United States. *Ear and Hearing* 45(5):1296–1312.

Kramer, S. E., T. S. Kapteyn, and J. M. Festen. 1998. The self-reported handicapping effect of hearing disabilities. *Audiology* 37:302–312.

Lutman, M. E., E. J. Brown, and R. R. A. Coles. 1987. Self-reported disability and handicap in the population in relation to pure-tone threshold, age, sex and type of hearing loss. *British Journal of Audiology* 21(1):45–58.

Manchaiah, V., E. M. Picou, A. Bailey, and H. Rodrigo. 2021. Consumer ratings of the most desirable hearing aid attributes. *Journal of the American Academy of Audiology* 32(08):537–546.

McNeice, Z., D. Tomlin, B. Timmer, C. E. Short, G. Nixon, and K. Galvin. 2024. A scoping review exploring how adults self-describe and communicate about the listening difficulties they experience. *International Journal of Audiology* 63(3):163–170.

Moberly, A. C., T. McRackan, and T. N. Tatami. 2023. *Expanding real-world outcomes in adults with hearing loss.* https://bulletin.entnet.org/clinical-patient-care/article/22873582/expanding-realworld-outcomes-in-adults-with-hearing-loss (accessed December 19, 2024).

NASEM (National Academies of Sciences, Engineering, and Medicine). 2023. *Achieving whole health: A new approach for veterans and the nation.* Washington, DC: The National Academies Press.

NHANES (National Health and Nutrition Examination Survey). 2021. *2017-March 2020 data documentation, codebook, and frequencies.* https://wwwn.cdc.gov/Nchs/Nhanes/2017-2018/P_AUQ.htm (accessed June 16, 2024).

Powers, T. A. 2020. MarkeTrak 10: Patients, providers, products, and possibilities. Guest editor Thomas A Powers, Ph.D. *Seminars in Hearing* 41(1).

Powers, T. A., and N. Bisgaard. 2022. MarkeTrak and EuroTrak: What we can learn by looking beyond the U.S. market. *Seminars in Hearing* 43(4):348–356.

PQM (Partnership for Quality Measurement). 2023. *Endorsement and maintenance (E&M) guidebook.* https://p4qm.org/sites/default/files/2023-10/Del-3-6-Endorsement-and-Maintenance-Guidebook-Final_0.pdf#page=40 (accessed June 26, 2024).

PQM. 2024. *Endorsement & maintenance (E&M).* https://p4qm.org/EM (accessed June 26, 2024).

Tyler, R. S., L. J. Baker, and G. Armstrong-Bednall. 1983. Difficulties experienced by hearing-aid candidates and hearing-aid users. *British Journal of Audiology* 17(3):191–201.

Tysome, J. R., P. Hill-Feltham, W. E. Hodgetts, B. J. McKinnon, P. Monksfield, R. Sockalingham, M. L. Johansson, and A. F. Snik. 2015. The Auditory Rehabilitation Outcomes Network: An international initiative to develop core sets of patient-centred outcome measures to assess interventions for hearing loss. *Clinical Otolaryngology* 40(6):512–515.

Uchida, Y., T. Nakashima, F. Ando, N. Niino, and H. Shimokata. 2003. Prevalence of self-perceived auditory problems and their relation to audiometric thresholds in a middle-aged to elderly population. *Acta Oto-Laryngologica* 123(5):618–626.

Velentgas, P., N. A. Dreyer, and A. W. Wu. 2013. Outcome definition and measurement. In *Developing a protocol for observational comparative effectiveness research: A user's guide.* Rockville, MD: Agency for Healthcare Research and Quality.

von Gablenz, P., F. Otto-Sobotka, and I. Holube. 2018. Adjusting expectations: Hearing abilities in a population-based sample using an SSQ short form. *Trends in Hearing* 22:2331216518784837.

Wang, X., Y. Zheng, G. Li, J. Lu, and Y. Yin. 2022. Objective and subjective outcomes in patients with hearing aids: A cross-sectional, comparative, associational study. *Audiology and Neurotology* 27(2):166–174.

Warren, C. D., E. Nel, and P. J. Boyd. 2019. Controlled comparative clinical trial of hearing benefit outcomes for users of the Cochlear Nucleus 7 Sound Processor with mobile connectivity. *Cochlear Implants International* 20(3):116–126.

Whitmer, W. M., P. Howell, and M. A. Akeroyd. 2014. Proposed norms for the Glasgow Hearing-Aid Benefit Profile (GHABP) questionnaire. *International Journal of Audiology* 53(5):345–351.

5

Outcomes for Hearing Health Interventions

While researchers and clinicians have examined a variety of outcomes for specific etiologies or interventions for hearing loss, no standardized set of outcomes has been defined or assessed consistently across the hearing health field. Over time there has been an evolution in which outcomes have been measured, based in part on what has been meaningful to individuals with hearing loss. (See Chapter 6 for a brief history of assessing hearing health outcomes.) This chapter describes the broad outcomes for the domain of hearing and communication as well as the relevant outcomes for domains beyond hearing and communication that were considered by the committee for inclusion in a core set. Several of the outcomes are overlapping and interdependent. For example, difficulties understanding speech in noise and decreased social activity can lead to mental health conditions such as depression; varying concepts of psychological health, social connection, and physical health contribute to quality of life. For each outcome the committee considered the evidence regarding the connection between hearing loss and the outcome as well as evidence for the ability of various interventions to affect the outcome at the individual level. The committee combined this evidence with evidence from Chapter 4 (for which outcomes are most meaningful to adults with hearing difficulties) to determine a final core outcome set. A high-level view of the ability to measure the outcome also was considered. Chapter 6 provides further detail on specific measures to assess the core outcome set.

PROXIMAL OUTCOMES OF HEARING HEALTH INTERVENTIONS

As a first step to determining a core outcome set, the committee needed to identify which outcomes to consider. The committee examined an extensive list of potential outcomes based on literature reviews of outcomes typically reported in studies of hearing interventions. The committee also hosted public webinars to hear directly from clinicians, professional groups, and adults with hearing difficulties. An online platform was established to invite members of the public to submit their comments as well. Based on this collective evidence, the committee conducted multiple iterative discussions to create a comprehensive set of outcomes to be considered for a core outcome set.

As shown in Figure 5-1, the committee considered both proximal and distal outcomes. Ultimately, the committee concluded that proximal outcomes are necessary precursors to outcomes of interest to individuals with hearing difficulties. Proximal outcomes are evaluated at the time of intervention. Distal outcomes are the outcomes that are typically most meaningful to adults with hearing difficulties. An overview of the key proximal outcome, audibility, is presented below.

Audibility

Audibility is defined as the ability to detect sound across a broad frequency range and across a range of input levels. Figure 5-2 illustrates the

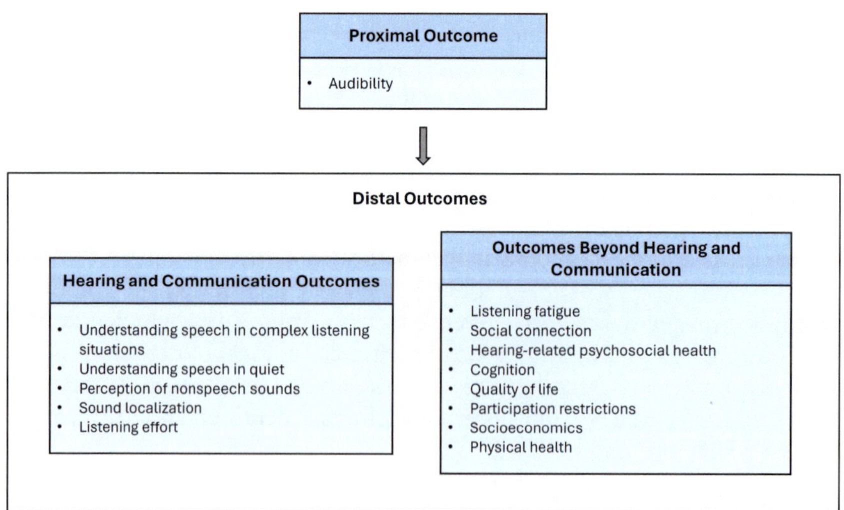

FIGURE 5-1 Proximal and distal outcomes of hearing health interventions.

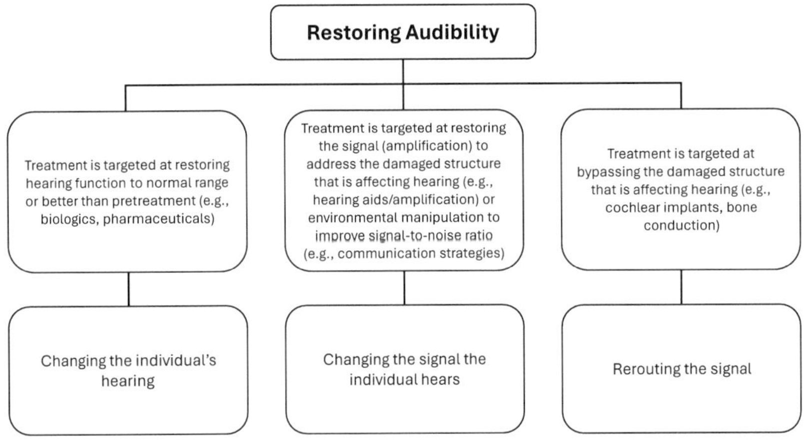

FIGURE 5-2 Restoring audibility.

approaches where maintenance or improvement of hearing, and therefore audibility, is the proximal outcome of the intervention. These approaches include interventions that use hearing aids (and other amplification devices), communication strategies that include environmental manipulation that improves signal-to-noise ratio, and biologic and pharmaceutical treatments. The proximal outcome is audibility, and an approach to improving audibility will be chosen depending on the individual's type, configuration, and degree of hearing loss and the target of the treatment. Improvement of audibility, which would be expected to be accomplished at the time of the intervention, is fundamental to the success of the intervention. However, given that the approach for improving audibility varies, the measurement of this proximal outcome cannot be achieved with a single approach for all contexts.

Restoring audibility through amplification has been the primary treatment for sensorineural hearing loss for decades (Ricketts, et. al., 2017). Although biologic, pharmaceutical, and genetic treatments of sensorineural hearing loss are being actively explored as investigational treatments, hearing aids remain the most widely available treatment (Isherwood et al., 2022; Le Prell, 2023). Audibility in the context of a hearing aid fitting requires frequency-specific manipulation of the incoming signal differentially as a function of input level (i.e., selective amplification). In this context, audibility is defined as the ability to detect sound across a defined frequency range (typically the range where speech sounds are expected to be prominent) and across a range of input levels (i.e., soft, moderate, and loud) while maintaining comfort related to the loudness of the amplified sounds. That is, the audibility of important sounds, such as speech over a wide range of levels, must be restored while also assuring that the sounds are not uncomfortably loud.

Otoprotective drugs have been assessed for threshold protection (i.e., prevention of the loss of audibility) (Brock et al., 2018; Kil et al., 2017; Kopke et al., 2015). In addition, in the case of biologics, improvement in threshold sensitivity has been a primary outcome of interest. In both cases, audibility continues to be the proximal outcome, but in these cases hearing sensitivity is being manipulated (i.e., the maintenance of current hearing or the restoration of hearing ability) rather than the incoming signal being manipulated, as is the case with hearing aid (amplification) interventions.

Approaches to the Measurement of Audibility

The difference among these interventions is not the proximal outcome (audibility) but the measurements used to verify that the intervention has been applied successfully (i.e., that audibility has been improved or maintained). The most common treatment for sensorineural hearing loss involves amplifying the incoming signal to improve hearing function. This is accomplished most often with an appropriate hearing aid fitting, but other devices such as assistive listening devices (including FM, infrared, and loop systems) also can amplify sounds of interest with or without the use of hearing aids. For hearing aids, the amplification is set in a manner that makes an incoming signal (e.g., speech) audible for quiet, moderate, and loud inputs across frequencies without being uncomfortable while realistically accounting for hearing thresholds (e.g., considering the level of gain needed or the expected distortion).

There are two evidence-based fitting formulas that provide targets to achieve this goal: the National Acoustic Laboratories Non-Linear 2 (NAL-NL2) and the Desired Sensation Level Version 5 (DSL v.5) (Keidser et al., 2012; Scollie et al., 2005). These targets are derived from the decibels hearing level (dB HL) pure-tone hearing thresholds of the individual. The output of the hearing aid as measured by a microphone in the ear canal is manipulated until the output matches the targets. Given that hearing threshold is displayed in dB HL, the transformation to decibels sound pressure level (dB SPL) required to derive targets will typically be obtained by measuring the individual's real-ear-to-coupler difference (Munro and Buttfield, 2005; Scollie et al., 2011; Vaisberg et al., 2018);[1] this supports transformation

---

[1] The real-ear-to-coupler difference is a real-ear measurement that is used as a part of hearing aid fittings. It measures the "difference in [decibels] across frequencies, between the SPL measured in the real-ear and in a 2cc coupler, produced by a transducer generating the same input signal" (Pumford and Sinclair, 2001).

from dB HL to dB SPL. The real-ear aided response measures output from the hearing aid in the individual's ear canal;[2] it is measured to verify that the incoming signal is matching targets and therefore audibility has been improved as much as possible given hearing loss constraints (Baker, 2017). This verification process (that the desired amplification has been achieved) is described in all available clinical practice guidelines from the audiology professional associations.

Rather than manipulating the incoming signal, the goal may be to maintain (e.g., with protective agents) or alter an individual's hearing (e.g., with pharmaceutical or gene therapy). In this case the signal is not being manipulated, rather the change is targeted at the individual's hearing function. This change will be measured either in terms of behavioral thresholds (e.g., measured with an audiogram) returning to the normal range of hearing (e.g., 0–20 dB HL across frequency) or as a decrease in the intensity level required for detection (across frequencies) (Carhart and Jerger, 1959). An audiogram is obtained in a soundproof booth with signals across frequencies being delivered to the individual through earphones in order to obtain ear-specific data. The individual responds whenever he or she hears a sound, with the clinician recording the lowest intensity level at each frequency where the signal is detected 50 percent of the time. The audiogram has been the clinical gold standard since the 1940s (Le Prell et al., 2022) and has served as the primary outcome measure in most investigations of possible otoprotective therapies (Le Prell, 2021).

In addition, when hearing sensitivity is the proximal outcome of interest, peripheral physiologic responses of auditory function that predict hearing thresholds may be applied. This may include the auditory brainstem response (ABR), among other peripheral physiologic measures. The ABR, along with similar peripheral electrophysiological measures, can be used to estimate thresholds and therefore verify the audibility of a signal. To perform these tests, clinicians place electrodes on the skin (e.g., forehead, earlobe, ear canal) that record brain wave activity in response to sound. This technique to verify audibility would most typically be applied to an individual who cannot voluntarily respond to a signal (e.g., young children, nonresponsive patients).

Of note, there are a variety of physiological measures that can be used in diagnosing hearing loss, assessing neural integrity, and evaluating more central auditory processing. In the case of this report, the committee is only

---

[2] The real-ear aided response is a real-ear measurement that is used as a part of hearing aid fittings. It measures the "frequency response of a hearing aid that is turned on, measured in the ear canal, for a particular input signal" (Pumford and Sinclair, 2001).

describing peripheral physiological measures as they relate to verification of audibility (threshold estimation). In emerging therapies, the restoration of hearing may be the initial (proximal) outcome that is targeted to prove that the treatment can work prior to addressing distal outcomes. However, the committee emphasizes the relevance of distal outcomes in the evaluation of pharmaceuticals and biologics, given that audibility (as a proximal outcome) is necessary but not sufficient to assure positive results with distal outcomes.

Although not the focus of this study, a third treatment strategy is to reroute the signal to achieve audibility. This is the case in treatments involving cochlear implants, auditory brainstem implants, midbrain implants, and bone-conducted signals. The treatment is verified by detecting a change in behavioral thresholds either with documented thresholds at lower levels or within the normal range of hearing.

Although it is a necessary precursor for desired outcomes of treatment, ensuring audibility alone does not guarantee desired distal outcomes. More distal outcomes would be measured as appropriate to the overarching goals of the treatment, regardless of the treatment modality. Whether a patient completes auditory training, receives hearing aids, or is treated with a pharmaceutical or biologic agent, distal outcomes are what patients identify as meaningful.

> *Conclusion 5-1: The improvement of audibility is a critical proximal outcome and requires verification. The methods for verification of audibility, however, vary depending on the intervention (e.g., changing hearing versus changing the incoming signal through amplification). As a result, the approach to measurement depends on the context, which does not align with the committee's approach to create a universally applicable core outcome set with consistent measures for all circumstances. Therefore, the verification of audibility is not included in the core set.*

> *Conclusion 5-2: Improvement in more distal outcomes may rely on improved audibility, but improved audibility does not guarantee desired distal outcomes. Therefore, improved audibility is a necessary precursor to attaining successful outcomes, but in most cases it is insufficient as a meaningful outcome for hearing health interventions.*

> *Conclusion 5-3: Use of improved audibility as the outcome of interest may be appropriate at early stages in the evaluation of novel interventions such as biologics, pharmaceuticals, and gene therapy. Even here, however, it is desirable that the evaluation of outcomes*

eventually progress to the inclusion of distal outcomes assessing every-day function.

HEARING AND COMMUNICATION OUTCOMES

As noted earlier, there is no consensus on core outcomes for hearing health interventions. As a result, a variety of outcome domains and individual outcomes have been defined in the literature to capture aspects of hearing and communication. Recent examples include:

- Speech in noise, speech in quiet, hearing thresholds, spatial hearing (localization), quality of hearing, hearing in reverberant conditions, binaural hearing and sound segregation, psychoacoustic performance, motion perception, hyperacusis, middle-ear function, softness of sound, and tinnitus perception, among others (Katiri et al., 2021).
- Communication ability (Allen et al., 2022).
- Clarity, sound distance, being aware of a sound, listening in complex situations, listening in reverberant conditions, group conversation in quiet, one-to-one conversation in general noise, group conversation in noisy social situations, sound localization, adverse listening environments, spatial orientation, one-to-one conversation in quiet, aversion to loud sounds (Katiri et al., 2022).
- Daily hours of hearing aid use, hearing handicap, hearing aid benefit, and communication and psychological outcome (Barker et al., 2015).

In its review of the literature and information gathered in public webinars and the committee's public platform, the committee considered the extensive list of potential outcomes and identified the following key outcomes for hearing and communication that are potentially meaningful to individuals with hearing difficulties:

- Understanding speech in complex listening situations;
- Understanding speech in quiet;
- Perception of nonspeech sounds;
- Sound localization; and
- Listening effort.

While the committee's overall conclusions regarding individual outcomes for hearing and communication are summarized in Table 5-1, the following sections elaborate on each of these outcomes and present evidence for inclusion of the outcome in the core set.

TABLE 5-1 Outcomes in Hearing and Communication Considered for Core Set

Outcome	Conclusion
Understanding speech in complex listening situations	Meaningful and a key complaint. Important to measure (intervention can impact outcome), and existing measures have a sufficient amount of psychometric data supporting the quality of the measures.
Perception of nonspeech sounds (e.g., music, nature)	Meaningful to specific subpopulations but not a key complaint. Psychometric data for existing measures are limited. Interventions meeting needs for speech in complex listening situations often meet needs for this outcome.
Understanding speech in quiet	Meaningful, but not a key complaint. Interventions meeting needs for speech in complex listening situations typically meet needs for this outcome.
Sound localization	Meaningful, but less frequently raised as a significant difficulty compared to other outcomes. Lack of feasible measures with a sufficient amount of psychometric data supporting the quality of the measures for sound localization specifically. Measurement development and refinement needed.
Listening effort	Meaningful, but outcome is not consistently defined. Measure development and refinement needed.

Understanding Speech in Complex Listening Situations[3]

Speech communication is defined as an exchange of information through the use of spoken words (Oxford Reference, n.d.). The ability to detect, discriminate, recognize, and identify speech is essential for effective spoken verbal communication (ASHA, n.d.). Impairments in speech communication, in turn, can cause a range of difficulties, from problems maintaining personal relationships and being able to participate in the workplace to navigating the health care system (Cunningham and Tucci, 2017). Individuals with hearing difficulties frequently need to ask people to repeat themselves or enunciate more clearly, and even then they may not be able to fully comprehend a conversation (Arlinger, 2003).

Everyday settings provide speech-communication challenges for many adults owing to the presence of competing sounds. Settings with background noise or reverberant acoustics degrade sound, making it very challenging for adults with hearing difficulties to understand speech (Contrera et al., 2016; Humes and Dubno, 2010; Mattys et al., 2012; Neal et al., 2022).

---

[3] While the term *speech in noise* is typically used, the committee prefers the use of *speech in complex listening situations*, which includes understanding speech in a variety of contexts including noisy environments, accented language, multiple speakers, with music playing, and other situations that complicate an individual's ability to understand speech.

Additional contextual obstacles to effective communication include distance from the sound source, intensity level of the speech, fast speech, shouting, unfamiliar accents, having the speaker's mouth covered, energy levels of the listener, and lack of awareness by a speaker of the listener's hearing loss (Hines, 2000; Mattys et al., 2012). Speech communication in these types of complex listening situations is particularly challenging because so many social interactions occur in adverse listening environments such as restaurants, parties, and noisy office settings (Bottalico et al., 2022; Bronkhorst, 2015; NASEM, 2016). People with hearing difficulties often avoid adverse or difficult listening environments because of the stress of not being able to communicate effectively and a fear of embarrassing oneself (Bennett et al., 2022). As a result, many people with hearing difficulties face activity limitations and participation restrictions and can become isolated and or lonely.

As noted in Chapter 4, multiple sources from the published literature, industry and consumer surveys, as well as evidence gathered by this committee indicate that many adults with hearing difficulties identify speech communication in noise as one of their most frequent and most severe hearing-related difficulties.

Conclusion 5-4: Evidence across the literature, in webinars, and from other sources shows that the ability to communicate in complex listening situations is the primary concern of most adults with hearing difficulties. Furthermore, the ability to understand speech in complex listening situations is an underlying factor for other outcomes, including psychological health, listening effort, and listening fatigue, since most social interactions occur in environments with competing background noise. Evidence also shows that the outcome is important to measure (i.e., intervention can significantly affect the outcome) and that existing measures have a sufficient amount of psychometric data supporting their quality.

Conclusion 5-5: Understanding speech in complex listening situations should be included in a core outcome set, meaning that it should be universally measured across settings and intervention types.

Understanding Speech in Quiet

Individuals with more severe hearing loss may have difficulties comprehending speech even in quiet settings (WHO, 2021). This outcome may be especially meaningful for these populations, as they may require the use of assistive devices to understand speech in quiet as well as noisy settings. Furthermore, understanding speech in quiet is essential for virtually all adults with hearing difficulties because if an individual cannot hear in a quiet environment, he or she will be even more challenged with background noise. However, examining the ability to detect and recognize speech in quiet alone is insufficient to evaluate the effect of hearing difficulties on everyday function. Data from a clinical convenience sample of 5,808 patients at Stanford Ear Institute revealed that many patients have significant challenges on the Quick Speech-in-Noise (QuickSIN) test despite normal word recognition in quiet (Fitzgerald et al., 2023). Effects of hearing loss on word recognition in quiet and in noise vary with hearing loss etiology, with sensorineural hearing loss and mixed hearing loss having greater effects on word recognition than conductive hearing loss, as shown in a second large convenience sample (5,593 patients at Stanford Ear Institute) (Smith, et al., 2024). More recent data from a smaller sample (1,633 patients at Stanford Ear Institute) revealed that word-in-quiet scores were not associated with disability measured using the 12-item Speech, Spatial and Qualities of Hearing Scale, but QuickSIN scores were associated with disability (Fitzgerald, et al., 2024). Data from a second clinical convenience sample of 3,400 patients seen in the audiology clinic at the Mountain Home, Tennessee, VA Medical Center similarly revealed many patients to have significant challenges on the Words-in-Noise (WIN) test despite normal word recognition in quiet (Wilson, 2011).

Conclusion 5-6: While understanding speech in quiet may be very meaningful to specific subpopulations (e.g., adults with more severe hearing loss), this outcome does not rise to the level of a core outcome because it is not identified by most adults with hearing difficulties as a frequently occurring or important difficulty. Furthermore, treatments meeting the needs for understanding speech in complex listening situations also typically meet the needs for this outcome.

Perception of Nonspeech Sounds

Individuals with hearing difficulties may not be able to detect, identify, locate, or appreciate nonspeech sounds, including alarms, sirens, traffic, music, and birds and other nature sounds (Arlinger, 2003; Bainbridge and Wallhagen, 2014). Many contextual factors make nonspeech sounds harder to identify and locate. In everyday listening, environmental sounds occur within the context of other sounds, and missing some auditory cues will make it more difficult to identify sounds of interest (Pichora-Fuller et al., 2016). The inability to identify and localize environmental sounds and safety signals is a safety concern and puts people with hearing loss at risk of physical injury (Dixon et al., 2020). For example, a dangerous situation may arise when a person is walking through a busy parking lot without the ability to hear a car approaching nearby.

The inability to perceive nonspeech sounds can have a range of consequences on one's everyday life and well-being. For example, many people with hearing difficulties cannot enjoy music like they did before their hearing loss (Dixon et al., 2020), as it may sound distorted and the chords and pitch may be indistinguishable (Leek et al., 2008). Music can even sound unpleasant, which can significantly impair quality of life for people who place a high value on listening to music. The committee recognizes that for subpopulations such as musicians, deficits related to perception of nonspeech sounds such as music can be career limiting, and supplemental measures for this outcome may need to be considered in such cases (Wartinger et al., 2019).

Conclusion 5-7: While the perception of nonspeech sounds (e.g., alerting signals, music, nature) may be very meaningful to specific subpopulations, this outcome does not rise to the level of a core outcome because it is not consistently identified by most adults with hearing difficulties as a frequently occurring or important difficulty, and few measures are available that have a sufficient amount of psychometric data supporting their quality. In addition, nonspeech sounds include a large range of signals making this difficult to apply across individuals with various listening needs. Furthermore, treatments meeting the needs for understanding speech in complex listening situations often meet the needs for this outcome in many contexts. Although not part of the core set, clinicians can target assessment of perception of specific nonspeech sounds depending on the needs and goals of an individual.

Sound Localization

The auditory system detects the location of sounds by analyzing spatial cues that are processed in the auditory portions of the central nervous system from the brainstem through the cortex (Middlebrooks, 2015). Sound localization involves the identification of the origin of sounds emanating from various locations in space and may include horizontal (left/right), vertical (up/down) and front/back locations as well as the perception of distance and motion of sound. Interaural timing differences and interaural level differences perceived by the auditory system are used to identify the location of sounds. Interaural timing difference (ITD) is the difference in the time it takes sound to reach one ear versus the other. Similarly, interaural level difference (ILD) is the difference in sound levels that reach the two ears. ITDs and ILDs are the primary cues for the localization of sounds in the horizontal plane.

As with most aspects of hearing, these cues become less salient for those with hearing loss and when background noise is present. High-frequency spectral energy provides key cues for the localization of sound in the horizontal (ILD) and vertical planes as well as for front/back distinctions. The latter two involve the shaping of sounds by the outer ear, primarily the pinna. Hearing loss, especially in higher frequencies (above about 1,500 Hz), and devices worn in the outer ear, such as hearing aids, can negatively affect the ability to localize sound.

People with untreated hearing loss have worse localization performance in both the horizontal and vertical planes than people with normal hearing (Noble and Byrne, 1990; Noble et al., 1994). Sound localization tests in hearing aid wearers have shown mixed results, with some studies showing poorer performance among hearing aid wearers than among individuals with hearing loss who are not hearing aid wearers, depending on the type of hearing aid and signal processing employed (Noble and Byrne, 1990; Zheng et al., 2022). Because sound localization relies on reliable and specific timing and intensity cues across the frequency domain (i.e., ITD, ILD, and spectral cues), these cues must be processed and reproduced accurately for hearing aid wearers to be able to correctly localize sounds.

The testing of sound localization by hearing health professionals may require equipment that is expensive and may not reflect real-world situations (Almeida et al., 2019). Given that sound localization ability is essential for the situational awareness and safety of military, law enforcement, and industrial workers, there have been some efforts to develop portable and affordable test systems (Thompson et al., 2024). In addition to the objective measurement of sound localization, several self-report measures seek to capture an individual's ability to localize sound (see Appendix B). Notably, the Speech, Spatial and Qualities of Hearing Scale includes items related to sound localization (i.e., directional and distance judgments) among many other items related to various outcomes (Gatehouse and Noble, 2004). However, current measures have not been validated specifically for sound localization, especially regarding sensitivity to change.

> *Conclusion 5-8: Sound localization, although an important ability, does not rise to the level of a core outcome. While difficulties with sound localization are a common complaint, they are raised less frequently than other outcomes.*

> *Conclusion 5-9: There is a lack of feasible measures validated for sound localization specifically. Current measures require the use of advanced equipment unavailable to many clinicians. Some self-report measures attempt to assess localization, but they have not been adequately validated for this outcome, especially regarding sensitivity to change following intervention.*

Listening Effort and Listening Fatigue[4]

People with hearing difficulties often report that they have to try harder to follow conversations, particularly when in complex listening situations; this can be taxing over time (McGarrigle et al., 2014). The phenomena of trying harder and being taxed by the effort are referred to as *listening effort* and *listening fatigue,* respectively. Listening effort has been defined as "a specific form of mental effort that occurs when a task involves listening," and listening fatigue has been defined as "simply fatigue resulting from the continued application of effort during difficult listening tasks" (Hornsby and Kipp, 2016; Pichora-Fuller et al., 2016). A significant amount of research has been conducted on listening effort and listening fatigue. However, inconsistencies in the definitions, populations, and methodologies have led to a lack of consensus on the best way to study and measure these constructs. The consensus-based, theoretical Framework for Understanding Effortful Listening (FUEL) was developed in 2015, and while it is complex and comprehensive, it has not been widely adopted in hearing health.

Listening Effort

Listening demand (also called *cognitive demand*) reflects the mental resources required to understand speech in acoustically challenging environments (Peelle, 2018). Factors such as background noise, reverberations, competing speakers, intensity, frequency, speed of speech, and accents or other speech differences all affect the quality of speech and can make it more challenging for people with hearing difficulties to comprehend that speech (Davis et al., 2021). Listening effort is a product of cognitive demand and the intensity level of motivation (see Figure 5-3). The motivational intensity theory acknowledges that listening effort is influenced by how important it is to the listener to comprehend the speech and how realistically the individual can understand it (Richter, 2016). If the listener does not deem the conversation important or possible to comprehend, then the individual may not be motivated to expend as much effort trying to understand it, thereby conserving cognitive energy but missing information. Adults with hearing difficulties, even when motivation is high, may encounter misperceptions that can lead to miscommunications and inaccuracies.

A 2017 systematic review demonstrated that while there was some evidence that listening effort increased more during speech tasks for listeners with hearing loss (as compared with listeners with normal hearing), there was insufficient evidence to conclude that amplification decreased listening

---

[4] While the committee discusses listening fatigue together with listening effort, the committee considers listening fatigue to be a downstream effect of hearing and communication difficulties, and therefore fatigue is designated as an outcome "beyond hearing and communication."

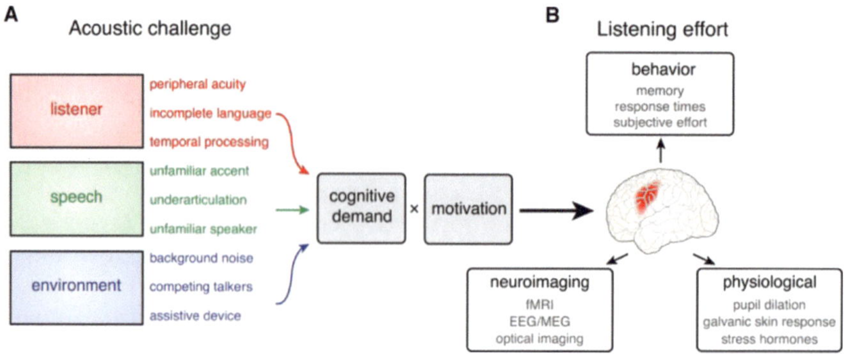

FIGURE 5-3 Acoustic challenge and listening effort.
NOTE: fMRI = functional magnetic resonance imaging; EEG/MEG = electroencephalography/magnetoencephalography.
SOURCE: Peelle, 2018. CC BY-NC-ND.

effort (Ohlenforst et al., 2017). Furthermore, the studies lacked consistency and standardization in measures and approach and lacked statistical power.

> *Conclusion 5-10: While listening effort is meaningful to adults with hearing difficulties, it does not rise to the level of a core outcome at this time because of inconsistencies with its definition.*

Listening Fatigue

Listening fatigue is thought to be a cumulative consequence of repeated encounters with effortful listening situations. Listening fatigue manifests as multiple types of symptoms, including headaches, increased need for sleep, and general low energy levels (Davis et al., 2021). Feeling mentally drained after a period of effortful listening is a common experience for many adults with hearing difficulties. Chronic listening fatigue has numerous consequences for an individual's quality of life, including lower productivity, mistakes in the workplace, social isolation, less physical activity, and depression (Davis et al., 2021). A theoretical framework developed by Davis and colleagues (2021) demonstrates the dynamic relationship between situational determinants of listening–related fatigue and experiences of fatigue, resulting in coping strategies to minimize the adverse effects of fatigue. Situational determinants include external factors (e.g., noisy conditions, listening in large groups or for a long period of time) and internal factors (e.g., relationship to the talker, importance of the listening situation). Experiences of fatigue include physical experiences (e.g., exhaustion, low energy), cognitive/mental experiences (e.g., difficulty thinking, inability to concentrate), social experiences (e.g., isolation), and emotional experiences (e.g., frustration, sadness, stress). Coping strategies can be behavioral (e.g., resting, use of hearing devices), social (e.g., avoidance of listening situations), or acceptance (e.g., "pushing through" fatigue).

More research is needed to determine if the use of hearing aids reduces listening fatigue, as current evidence shows there are large inconsistencies in both the types of populations that are studied and the self-reported measures used (Holman et al., 2021).

Conclusion 5-11: While listening fatigue is meaningful to adults with hearing difficulties, it does not rise to the level of a core outcome at this time because of inconsistencies with its definition.

Conclusion 5-12: Listening effort and listening fatigue are separate, yet potentially related, constructs. However, current definitions and theoretical approaches are not consistent. Future research is needed on the separate constructs of listening effort and listening fatigue themselves that incorporate a robust theoretical framework, a clear study population of adults with hearing loss (and a control group), and adequate statistical power.

Conclusion 5-13: More research is needed regarding if and how hearing health interventions reduce listening effort and/or listening fatigue in real-world conditions, in the short and long term.

The Current State of Measurement for Listening Effort and Listening Fatigue

Three main methods have been used for capturing listening effort: (1) physiological measures, (2) behavioral measures, and (3) self-report measures. Listening fatigue is most commonly captured via self-report measures (McGarrigle et al., 2014; Shields et al., 2023). Physiological measures capture autonomic responses from the body in situ (reactive) under various listening tasks and conditions; examples include pupillometry, skin conductance, heart rate, encephalography, and functional imaging. Behavioral measures or performance-based measures require patients to participate in a task; this commonly includes a dual-task paradigm with speech recognition as a primary task and a secondary task that results in a memory recall score or reaction time. Finally, self-report measures are often used and come in the form of a questionnaire with a set of items inquiring about effortful listening or fatigue or through the use of various visual analog scales administered in conjunction with a listening task (Alhanbali et al., 2017; Keur-Huizinga et al., 2024; McGarrigle et al., 2014; Shields et al., 2023).

A multitude of individual measures of listening effort exist. (See Appendix B for examples of each method.) Many measures are study specific, and currently there is no gold-standard measure. Most measures of listening effort, regardless of their method, have no or weak correlations, indicating that listening effort is a multidimensional construct (Keur-Huizinga et al., 2024; Shields et al., 2023).

> *Conclusion 5-14: Currently, there is not a single broadly accepted measure of listening effort or listening fatigue, yet some measures show promise. More research is needed to develop and refine measures in order to promote a standard way to measure listening effort and listening fatigue in clinical and research settings.*

OUTCOMES BEYOND HEARING AND COMMUNICATION

Examining outcomes beyond hearing and communication can help capture additional aspects of hearing health that are meaningful to adults with hearing difficulties. When considering a whole health approach, the person's needs are put at the center, shifting the focus from exclusively treating symptoms and disease-oriented medicine to recentering what matters to the individual (NASEM, 2023). Whole health takes into consideration "physical, behavioral, spiritual, and socioeconomic well-being as defined by individuals, families, and communities" (NASEM, 2023, p. 4). Improving hearing and communication is strongly correlated with improvement in outcomes beyond hearing and communication, such as social connection, education, quality of life, and occupational opportunities (Borre et al., 2023). Hearing-related social and emotional difficulties often are reduced following intervention with hearing aids (e.g., Chisolm et al., 2007). Therefore, measuring outcomes of hearing and communication alone may not fully capture an individual's hearing difficulties or the effect of hearing health intervention on those difficulties.

Similar to outcomes of hearing and communication, a variety of outcome domains and individual outcomes have been defined in the literature to capture outcomes of hearing health interventions beyond hearing and communication. Outcomes reported in the literature include:

- Personal relationships, well-being, and participation restrictions (Allen et al., 2022).
- Effects on individual activities, discomfort in listening situations, effect on learning, treatment satisfaction, device usage and malfunction, vulnerability, avoiding social situations, motivation, emotional distress, personal safety, self-stigma, dissatisfaction with life, balance problems, manual dexterity (Katiri et al., 2022).
- Global cognitive function, executive function, processing speed, and auditory and visual working memory (Glick and Sharma, 2020).
- Emotional/psychological impact, lifestyle impact, sleep, auditory perception, general health impact (Langguth and De Ridder, 2023).

In its review of the literature and information gathered in public webinars and the committee's public platform, the committee considered an extensive list of potential outcomes and identified the following key outcomes beyond hearing and communication:

- Listening fatigue,[5]
- Social connection,
- Hearing-related psychosocial health,
- Cognition,
- Quality of life,
- Socioeconomic effects;
- Participation restrictions; and
- Physical health.

The committee's overall conclusions regarding outcomes beyond hearing and communication are summarized in Table 5-2, while the following sections define each of these outcomes and present evidence for inclusion of the outcome in the core set.

Social Connection

Hearing loss among older adults affects speech communication and, as a result, alters social interactions (Shukla et al., 2020). As noted in the 2020 National Academies study *Social Isolation and Loneliness in Older Adults:*

> The broad, interdisciplinary scientific fields that together form the modern science of social relationships have used a variety of terms (e.g., *social isolation, social connection, social networks, social integration, social support, social exclusion, social deprivation, social relationships, loneliness*) to refer to empirical phenomena related to social relationships. Although there are important distinctions among these terms concerning what they describe or measure, they are often, incorrectly, used interchangeably. (NASEM, 2020, p. 28)

Some of the key terms include:

1. *Social support*—the actual or perceived availability of resources (e.g., informational, tangible, emotional) from others, typically one's social network
2. *Social isolation*—the objective lack of (or limited) social contact with others

---

[5] Listening fatigue is discussed in conjunction with listening effort in the previous section on hearing and communication outcomes.

TABLE 5-2 Outcomes Beyond Hearing and Communication Considered for Core Set

Outcome	Conclusion
Listening fatigue	Meaningful, but outcome is not consistently defined and measured. Measure development and refinement needed.
Social connection	Meaningful, but insufficient evidence that the intervention has a significant clinical effect on the outcome at the individual level.
Hearing-related psychosocial health	Meaningful, important to measure, existing measures have a sufficient amount of psychometric data supporting the quality of the measures.
Cognition	Meaningful, but there is inconsistency in the cognitive construct being measured. Insufficient evidence that the intervention has a significant clinical effect on the outcome at the individual level.
Quality of life	Meaningful, but there is inconsistency in the definition of the outcome and in the underlying constructs being measured. Many contributing factors to quality of life make measuring the direct effect of hearing intervention on the outcome difficult. Key constructs of psychological, social, and emotional health are covered by hearing-related psychosocial health.
Socioeconomic effects	Might be meaningful to specific subpopulations and types of research, but not a key complaint.
Participation restrictions	Outcome is inconsistently defined and measured.
Physical health	Not a key complaint. Insufficient evidence on the direct connection between hearing health interventions and physical health outcomes.

3. *Loneliness*—the perception of social isolation or the subjective feeling of being lonely
4. *Social connection*—an umbrella term that encompasses the structural, functional, and quality aspects of how individuals connect to each other (NASEM, 2020)

As illustrated in Figure 5-4, social connection consists of three components: structure, function, and quality.

Structure includes objective measures of connection, including the size and variety of one's social network and the frequency of interaction with others. An estimated 24 percent of older adults are socially isolated (Shukla et al., 2020). Rates of social isolation are consistently higher in adults with untreated hearing loss than in adults with normal hearing (Shukla et al., 2020). As noted earlier, a significant challenge with hearing loss is comprehending auditory information in real-world settings, which makes communication very difficult. Consequently, many individuals are less likely

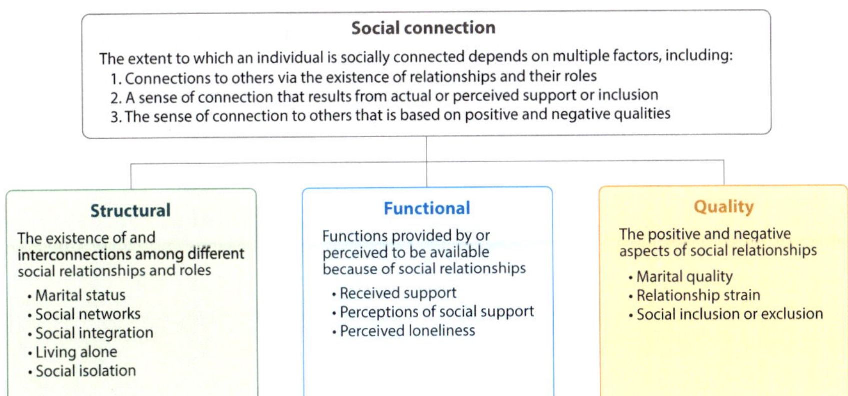

FIGURE 5-4 Social connection.
SOURCE: Holt-Lunstad, 2018. © Annual Reviews, used with permission.

to participate in social activities because of the fear of embarrassing themselves or not being able to fully engage with others (WHO, 2021).

Adults with hearing difficulties who participated in the committee's public webinars noted their inability to enjoy experiences like music, live performances, and movies.[6] Hearing loss contributes to challenges in communicating effectively with loved ones, which can cause frustration or resentment for both the individual with hearing difficulties and their family and friends. These factors shrink one's social network and can lead to social isolation, which in turn can contribute to a wide variety of negative health effects (NASEM, 2020).

The functional component of social connection reflects whether these relationships meet an individual's emotional support needs (Holt-Lunstad, 2018). This component encompasses loneliness and subjective satisfaction with one's social connections. Untreated hearing loss may make it more challenging to retain close relationships and build new ones; as such, it is plausible that people with hearing difficulties, especially and specifically late-onset hearing difficulties in adults without alternative language modes such as signed languages, may be less satisfied with their social networks than those with normal hearing ability.

One person may have a very small social network and be content and not feel lonely, while another person may have a large social network and still feel lonely. Social isolation can lead to loneliness either because

---

[6] The webinar recordings can be accessed at https://www.nationalacademies.org/event/41996_02-2024_meaningful-outcome-measures-in-adult-hearing-health-care-webinar-1 and https://www.nationalacademies.org/event/42414_04-2024_meaningful-outcome-measures-in-adult-hearing-health-care-webinar-2

someone's social network shrinks or because the hearing loss is infringing on the person's ability to engage (Jayakody et al., 2022). Loneliness is associated with depression, reduced physical activity, decreased satisfaction with life, and poor self-perceived well-being. Like social isolation, loneliness can contribute to a wide variety of negative health outcomes (NASEM, 2020).

The final component of social connection is quality, which involves satisfaction with existing relationships (Holt-Lunstad, 2018). Since effective communication is essential for all types of healthy relationships, untreated hearing loss can make it challenging to retain strong connections (Victory, 2021).

Recent systematic reviews suggest that hearing loss among older adults is consistently associated with loneliness and social isolation (Mick et al., 2014; Shukla et al., 2020). However, there is a paucity of longitudinal studies, and a major concern, especially with the social isolation measures, was a lack of consistency in the outcome measure used (Shukla et al., 2020). Indeed, some studies found positive associations but were limited to unvalidated questions and constructs of social isolation (Mick et al., 2014). When people with hearing difficulties do not seek treatment or develop coping mechanisms, they will likely avoid social situations and let relationships deteriorate, leading to more isolation and loneliness, which then causes poorer outcomes in other areas of health (Bennett et al., 2022). Social isolation and loneliness are both associated with a range of other health outcomes, including cognitive decline, depression, mortality, and coronary heart disease (NASEM, 2020; Shukla et al., 2020; Valtorta et al., 2016). Currently, the research is inconclusive about the degree to which interventions such as hearing aids can mitigate social isolation and loneliness (Ellis et al., 2021). Future research needs to be longitudinal, include a large sample size, and account for confounding variables to better understand this relationship.

> *Conclusion 5-15: While social connection is meaningful to virtually all adults with hearing difficulties, it does not rise to the level of a core outcome at this time because there is a lack of evidence that the intervention has a significant clinical effect on the outcome at the individual level. One reason for this is that many factors can influence social connection.*

> *Conclusion 5-16: There are issues with the inconsistent use of measures for different aspects of social connection and a lack of validation of the measures specific to hearing.*

Hearing-Related Psychological Health

The World Health Organization (WHO) defines mental/psychological health as "a state of mental well-being that enables people to cope with the stresses of life, realize their abilities, learn well and work well, and contribute to their community" (WHO, 2022b). Extensive research exists on the relationships between untreated hearing loss and psychological health, including depression, anxiety, and other aspects of mental, psychological, and emotional health (Laird et al., 2020). Adults report that the adverse effects of their untreated hearing loss on their psychological health include worsening depression, anxiety, paranoia, and suicidal ideation (Laird et al., 2020). Each of these domains of psychological health, with evidence on the impact of chronic hearing loss, is reviewed below.

Depression

A broad range of research shows an association between depression and hearing loss (Amieva et al., 2018; Armstrong et al., 2016; Brewster et al., 2018; Gosselin et al., 2023; Jayakody et al., 2018; Lawrence et al., 2020; Lee et al., 2010; Strawbridge et al., 2000).

Symptoms of depression include feeling sad, irritable, hopeless, having low self-worth and low energy, and thoughts about dying or suicide (WHO, 2022a). Hearing loss is associated with many depressive symptoms, including sadness, guilt, low self-worth, loss of interest in daily activities, change in appetite, and disturbed sleep (Lawrence et al., 2020). Some adults with hearing difficulties experience severe depression and suicidal ideation (Cosh et al., 2019). Untreated hearing loss is known to reduce social participation (in part because of the inability to participate in activities that were previously enjoyed) and increase loneliness, putting older adults with hearing difficulties at an increased risk of developing depression (Lawrence et al., 2020). This may be compounded by the individual's struggle to cope with the fact that hearing health interventions likely will not fully restore their hearing capacity (Laird et al., 2020). (See the previous section for more on social connection.)

However, whereas the majority of research finds an association between hearing loss and depression, several studies have not reached that same conclusion (Gopinath et al., 2009; Lawrence et al., 2020; Li et al., 2014; Mener et al., 2013). Comparison among studies is difficult because of the lack of standardized outcome measures for hearing loss or depression (Laird et al., 2020). For example, Armstrong and colleagues used both the Center for Epidemiologic Studies Depression Scale 5 (CESD-5) and the Patient Health Questionnaire (PHQ-9), which showed differences in the strength of the association depending on the measure (Armstrong et al., 2016). The types of depression examined also vary across studies. Cosh and colleagues, for example, found an association between hearing loss and depressive symptoms but not between hearing loss and major depressive disorder (Cosh et al., 2018).

Anxiety

Anxiety disorder is a highly prevalent chronic condition and is associated with untreated hearing loss (Cetin et al., 2010). However, as with the research on depression, because various definitions and outcome measures have been used in research on anxiety disorder it becomes difficult to form simple conclusions. One study demonstrated a statistically significant association between the prevalence of anxiety measured by the Hopkins Symptom Checklist and mild untreated hearing loss (Contrera et al., 2017). With more severe hearing loss, researchers found that hearing aids were not statistically significantly associated with lower odds of anxiety.

The relationship between anxiety and hearing loss may be bidirectional (NCOA, 2023). Untreated hearing loss can cause or worsen symptoms of anxiety. First, hearing loss strains communication and can cause anxiety around social interactions and the ability to carry out everyday life activities. Anxiety also can be triggered by "feelings of worry and unease around uncertain outcomes related to hearing loss that might creep into all areas of life: social, professional, physical, financial, and emotional" (NCOA, 2023).

Psychosis

There is a growing literature supporting a connection between hearing loss and psychosis disorders. A meta-analysis found increased risk of hearing impairment for a range of psychosis outcomes including hallucination, delusions, psychotic symptoms, and delirium (Linszen, 2016). Currently, there is insufficient evidence of a causal relationship between hearing loss and psychiatric disorders, but it is recommended that psychiatrists and mental health professionals look for signs of hearing loss and refer patients to hearing health care (or over-the-counter devices, if suitable) (Blazer, 2020).

Hearing-Related Psychosocial Health

The preceding paragraphs demonstrate associations between hearing difficulties and a variety of mental, psychological, and emotional health issues, although the inconsistent findings across studies for each health issue reflects the complex nature of these health conditions. The committee collectively refers to this group of health issues as psychological health issues. As noted in the earlier section on social connection, hearing difficulties also negatively affect social wellness. Psychological health and social wellness are often intertwined such that psychological difficulties, such as depression or anxiety, may negatively impact social wellness. The committee collectively refers to this combination as psychosocial health. Some available outcome measures, such as the longstanding Hearing

Handicap Inventory for the Elderly (HHIE) (see Chapter 6), measure the effect of hearing difficulties on psychosocial health. The HHIE includes items addressing the effect of hearing difficulties on feelings of embarrassment, irritability, frustration, nervousness, anger, and depression, among other outcomes. The HHIE also has several items addressing the social consequences of hearing difficulties. Although the committee noted that psychological and social wellness are separate dimensions of wellness, the prevailing audiological measure capturing these dimensions (the HHIE) has been found to be unidimensional in recent psychometric analyses (Cassarly et al., 2020; Heffernan et al., 2020). The HHIE shows sensitivity to change, implying that hearing-related psychosocial health has improved following the intervention. After considerable discussion, the committee opted to refer to this combination of psychological and social challenges experienced by those with hearing difficulties collectively as hearing-related psychosocial health.

Conclusion 5-17: Evidence across the literature, in webinars, and from other sources shows that hearing-related psychosocial health is meaningful to virtually all adults with hearing difficulties, and it is a key element of the concepts of overall quality of life and health-related quality of life. Evidence also shows that the outcome is important to measure (i.e., intervention can significantly affect the outcome) and that existing measures have a sufficient amount of psychometric data supporting their quality.

Conclusion 5-18: Hearing-related psychosocial should be included in a core outcome set, meaning that it should be universally measured across settings and intervention types.

Cognition

Researchers have proposed that hearing loss may be mechanistically associated with cognitive decline via several mediating pathways, including cognitive load, structural changes in the brain, and social isolation. One of the first studies of the association between peripheral measures of hearing loss (e.g., pure-tone audiometry) and cognitive dysfunction in older adults was a case–control study in 1989 that found a strong relationship between a hearing loss of 30 dB or greater and the risk of developing dementia (Uhlmann et al., 1989). Nearly two decades later, researchers began to revisit and more closely examine the association between hearing loss and cognitive outcomes (including dementia as well as cognitive function), which has culminated in a body of work that suggests a possible association between hearing loss in older adults and a decline in cognitive function.

The earliest studies of the recent wave of work verified an association between hearing loss and cognitive decline in cross-sectional datasets (Lin, 2011). Later, longitudinal studies found that hearing loss was associated with cognitive decline over multiple years and suggested a temporal effect that hearing loss preceded cognitive decline (Lin et al., 2013; Maharani et al., 2018). Two meta-analyses have concluded that the overall body of research to date suggests an association between hearing loss and performance on cognitive measures in older adults (Loughrey et al., 2018; Yeo et al., 2023). Various professional groups also have concluded that such a relationship exists (Lazar et al., 2021; Livingston et al., 2020). Research has culminated in the inclusion of hearing loss in the 2020 and 2024 Lancet Global Commission on Dementia reports (Livingston et al., 2020, 2024). Using meta-analyses and population attributable fraction models, the 2024 report suggests that 7 percent of all dementia cases are attributable to hearing loss. However, caution is needed when interpreting the figure as it assumes no unmeasured confounding. Moreover, the model highlights the importance of considering population- versus individual-level risk as hearing loss is extremely prevalent among older adults, so the effects may appear large at the population level but relatively smaller at the individual level. More work is needed to better understand individual-level risk for consideration in proposing a core set of outcome measures.

Another limitation of the research relevant to proposing a core set of outcome measures is that the studies use different measures of cognition and a large percentage of them are memory based, so it is difficult to definitively determine which cognitive functions are affected by hearing loss and whether others remain unaffected. A general concern in the cognition literature is that, beyond screening measures such as the Mini Mental State Examination and Montreal Cognitive Assessment, few tests are standardized or normed to the population and none are diagnostic, which limits external inferences beyond specific study populations.

Several studies suggest that the use of hearing aids may provide a certain amount of protection against cognitive losses in older adults whose hearing has gotten significantly worse. For instance, while the English Longitudinal Study of Ageing found poorer cognition among older adults with hearing loss relative to those with no hearing loss, the association was found only in those who did not use hearing aids; those with hearing loss who used hearing aids did not have significantly poorer cognition than those with no hearing loss (Ray et al., 2018). An analysis of data from the Health and Retirement Study, which has tracked a group aged 50 and older since 1992, found that the decline in episodic memory scores slowed significantly after people with hearing problems began using hearing aids (Maharani et al., 2018).

A large meta-analysis calculated that the use of hearing aids by individuals with hearing loss decreased the risks of long-term cognitive decline by 19 percent (Yeo et al., 2023). Furthermore, this same study noted that using hearing aids to restore hearing in those with hearing loss was associated in the short term with a 3 percent improvement in scores on tests assessing general cognition (Yeo et al., 2023). However, there are inherent limitations to using observational literature to explore the impact of hearing intervention on modifying the association between hearing loss and cognitive decline (Pichora-Fuller, 2023; Reuben et al., 2024). Hearing intervention is non-pharmacologic and requires counseling, consistent maintenance, and persistent use, which is difficult to capture in epidemiologic observational studies. More importantly, hearing aid ownership and use, even in countries that cover hearing care, is strongly associated with socioeconomic factors that are also protective from cognitive decline, including income, education level, and race/ethnicity (Bessen et al., 2024; Reed et al., 2021). Prospective intervention studies are required to balance confounding. A pilot study of adults randomized to either a best practices hearing intervention group, which received hearing aids and associated services, or an active-control aging intervention group found that there was not clear efficacy after 6 months and hypothesized that longer hearing treatment would be needed to see the full effects (Deal et al., 2017). The full-trial follow-on to that pilot, a large randomized controlled trial (n=977) of adults aged 70–84 with untreated hearing loss, found no difference in cognitive decline over a 3-year period between those given hearing aids and associative services compared with an active control group given health education (Lin et al., 2023). More trials are needed to understand if hearing intervention delays cognitive decline and in which populations it is most effective.

Despite the body of evidence suggesting a possible connection between hearing loss and cognitive decline, the potential mechanisms for mediating that connection have not been well studied (Lazar et al., 2021). One proposed model suggests a role for both social and physiological factors (Rutherford et al., 2018). At the social level, hearing loss could lead adults to avoid situations where they have difficulty hearing or communicating, and the resulting social isolation and loneliness could lead to cognitive decline (Rutherford et al., 2018). At the physiological level, the reduced neural activation in auditory pathways caused by hearing loss could lead to dysfunction in auditory–limbic connections and atrophy in certain frontal brain regions, which in turn could reduce cognitive reserve and increase executive dysfunction, resulting in cognitive decline (Rutherford et al., 2018). One group that carried out a meta-analysis of the connection between hearing loss and cognitive impairment pointed to impaired verbal communication and vascular dysfunction as potential contributing factors (Loughrey et al., 2018).

An analysis of data from the English Longitudinal Study of Ageing offered some support for the role of social effects (Maharani et al., 2019). Using episodic memory as a measure of cognitive function, the researchers found that hearing impairment had a significant effect on episodic memory and that this effect was partly mediated by loneliness and social isolation. However, further research will be required before it is clear how hearing loss in older adults may lead to cognitive decline, which older adults with hearing loss are most at risk, and whether hearing interventions can slow cognitive decline or reduce cognitive impairment. The connections among cognition, hearing loss, and hearing treatment are currently garnering a significant amount of attention by researchers, which may lead to more robust evidence for future consideration.

Conclusion 5-19: While recent literature suggests an association between hearing loss and cognition, cognition does not rise to the level of a core outcome at this time for several reasons. First, there is inconsistency in the cognitive construct being measured and the measures used in research. Second, potential concerns on the significance of risk and intervention effects at the individual versus population level exist. Third, cognitive decline is a distal outcome to hearing care, associated via proposed mediators that also could be measured (e.g., social connections, participation in activities), but there is a lack of key supporting data from mediation analyses and treatment effects on mediators. Fourth, questions remain on the effect of hearing intervention on cognitive decline, given the deep limitations of observational literature in this space and the null overall finding in the only powered randomized clinical trial.

Conclusion 5-20: Evidence on the connection between cognition and hearing intervention is evolving. While hearing care may cause minimal harm and could potentially benefit cognition, more research is needed to justify cognition as a core outcome. This includes studies with consistent definitions and measures, studies to determine the mechanism of impact, and studies that more consistently demonstrate the ability of interventions to reduce cognitive decline.

Quality of Life[7]

Quality of life (QoL) and health-related QoL are important to patients and individuals. QoL is a broad term that refers to an individual's subjective

---

[7] The committee emphasizes that this outcome is primarily focused on overall QoL and not the narrower health-related QoL, though both overlap with many other outcomes defined in this chapter.

well-being and ability to lead a fulfilling life. Teoli and Bhardwaj (2023) define it as "a concept which aims to capture the well-being, whether of a population or individual, regarding both positive and negative elements within the entirety of their existence at a specific point in time" and they note that common facets of QoL include such things as physical and mental health, relationships, work environment, social status, wealth, a sense of security and safety, freedom, social belonging, and physical surroundings. Their definition is just one among many that have been offered by various individuals and organizations (Barofsky, 2012; Boggatz, 2016; WHO, 2012). Health-related QoL refers to the aspects of QoL that relate only to health (Yin et al., 2016), and researchers have also developed various measures of QoL related to specific diseases or disorders, such as hearing-related QoL. This section focuses mainly on the overarching concept of QoL, with some additional consideration of health-related QoL and, specifically, hearing-related QoL.

For several decades researchers have studied the relationship between hearing loss and QoL and have generally found that hearing loss is associated with a decrease in QoL, while improved hearing through hearing aids and other hearing health interventions is associated with improved QoL (Borre et al., 2023; Brodie et al., 2018; Choi et al., 2024; Ciorba et al., 2012; Humes, 2021; Manrique-Huarte et al., 2016; Mulrow et al., 1990; Nordvik et al., 2018; Tseng et al., 2018). Intuitively that makes good sense, given the many important roles that hearing plays—in conversations with other people; in awareness of one's environment; in the enjoyment of music, movies, television shows, and other forms of entertainment; and so on. But on closer inspection, and for a number of reasons, the connection between hearing and QoL is not as clear as it would seem.

To begin with, there is no agreement on just what QoL means (Barofsky, 2012). It is an inherently subjective property, and two people in exactly the same circumstances may judge their QoL very differently, just as an individual's perception of his or her QoL may change over time as perceptions of what is important change. As Teoli and Bhardwaj (2023) commented, "While there is no shortage of textbook definitions, perhaps the most accurate meaning of QoL is the definition the patient provides when sitting across from their clinician."

A closely related issue—and one that is more relevant to this report—is that there is no agreement on the best way to measure QoL (Kaplan and Hays, 2022; Pequeno et al., 2020). Some of the earliest measures focused on generic QoL, asking individuals to rate their satisfaction with such things as marriage and family, work, housing, and leisure activities (Bunge, 1975; Gillingham and Reece, 1979; Liu, 1975). Over time, broader measures of QoL were developed that included such factors as economic, political, and social well-being (IOM, 1989). And by the 1980s medical and public health researchers were using more focused measures to study how overall health or issues related to specific diseases affected a patient's QoL (Guyatt et al., 1993).

General health-related QoL measures, which focus on the physical and mental health aspects of QoL, are frequently used in epidemiological studies, population studies, health services research, and randomized clinical trials as well as for economic analyses and calculation of quality-adjusted life years (Kaplan and Hays, 2022). Many measures of health-related QoL have been developed. However, unlike in Europe and Canada, researchers in the United States have not settled on a single measure of health-related QoL, so U.S. datasets often have different measures, making the data difficult to compare or combine (Kaplan and Hays, 2022).

QoL measures also have been developed specifically to focus on particular diseases or functional areas. In the case of hearing loss, three of the most common are the HHIE, the Hearing Handicap Inventory for Adults (HHIA), and International Outcomes Inventory—Hearing Aids (IOI-HA), which is used to measure improvement in QoL factors resulting from the use of hearing aids (Ciorba et al., 2012). Additionally, WHO's Disability Assessment Scale II (WHODAS II) assesses functioning across the following domains: communication, mobility, self-care, interpersonal, life activities, and participation (Chisolm et al., 2005). Convergent validity analysis found that WHODAS II was moderately correlated with the Abbreviated Profile of Hearing Aid Benefit, significantly correlated with the HHIE, and significantly correlated with the Short Form-36 for Veterans (SF-36 V). However, again, there is no agreed-upon standard. Two measures specific to hearing loss in adults include the Subjective Well-Being of Older Adults with Hearing Loss (SWB-HL) (Humes, 2021) and the Impact of Hearing Loss Inventory Tool (IHEAR-IT) (Stika and Hays, 2016). However, there has only been limited evaluation of these measures to date.

A major issue for hearing researchers is that different QoL measures vary in their ability to capture changes related to hearing interventions. A systematic review of research studying the effects of the treatment (i.e., hearing aids and cochlear implants) for hearing loss on health-related QoL showed that studies using certain measures—Health Utilities Index 2 and 3 (HUI2, HUI3), the Visual Analog Scale, and Time Trade-Off—generally found that treatment of hearing loss led to improvements in health-related QoL, while those using other measures, such as the European Quality of Life 5 Dimension (EQ-5D) and Short Form 6 Dimension (SF-6D), found little to no benefit (Borre et al., 2023). Borre and colleagues (2023) concluded,

> This suggests that the EQ-5D and SF-6D do not adequately detect benefits related to hearing and communication, especially considering several studies used multiple measures in the same patients and found disparate results between measures. (p. 477)

A key to this difference may be found in the domains covered by the different measures. For example, the HUI2 and HUI3 include elements of cognition and emotion (along with some other general measures). The self-administered Quality of Well-Being Scale (QWB-SA) includes social activity. Chisolm and colleagues (2007) found that "hearing aids improve health-related QoL by reducing psychological, social, and emotional effects of hearing loss" (p. 151). They conclude that more research is needed.

One thing that the research has made clear is that it is not possible to understand the effects of hearing loss on an individual's QoL without context; it is not enough to just know the details about the person's hearing. While measurement of QoL requires a clear definition and the development of measures that can achieve adequate psychometric properties for their intended purpose, understanding a person's level of QoL requires taking a number of factors into account whose importance will vary with the individual and with circumstances. One could list hundreds of these factors, but the following list assembled by WHO includes many, if not all, of the major ones, divided into six domains (WHO, 2012):

1. Physical: pain and discomfort, energy and fatigue, sexual activity, sleep and rest, sensory functions
2. Psychological: positive feelings; thinking, learning, memory, and concentration; self-esteem; bodily image and appearance; negative feelings
3. Level of independence: mobility, activities of daily living, dependence on medical substances and medical aids, dependence on nonmedicinal substances such as alcohol or tobacco or drugs, communication capacity, work capacity
4. Social relationships: personal relationships, social support, activities as provider or supporter
5. Environment: freedom, physical safety, and security; home environment; work satisfaction; financial resources; accessibility and quality of health and social care; opportunities for acquiring new abilities and skills; participation in and opportunities for recreation and leisure activities; the physical environment, including such things as climate, pollution, noise, and traffic; transport
6. Spirituality, religion, and personal beliefs

Conclusion 5-21: While QoL is meaningful for adults with hearing difficulties in both clinical and research settings, it is a complex outcome that is inconsistently defined and measured and therefore does not rise to the level of a core outcome at this time. Health-related QoL, a subset of QoL, is better defined and has been measured in many studies of hearing intervention, but the results of these studies are inconsistent. Therefore, health-related QoL does not rise to the level of a core outcome at this time. However, as noted earlier, the committee selected hearing-related psychosocial health, a key element of QoL and health-related QOL, as a core outcome.

Socioeconomic Effects

A small literature examines the socioeconomic effects of untreated hearing loss (beyond the cost of health care). The first area of research focuses on the effect on income. Socioeconomic factors in this context do not include the cost of treatment, but rather the socioeconomic status of the individual with hearing loss and those factors specifically related to the experience of hearing loss. The committee recognizes the many access issues related to the cost of hearing health interventions, but these concerns are beyond the scope of this report.

One nationally representative study including adults ages 20 to 69 found after controlling for education, age, sex, and race, individuals with hearing loss were 1.58 times more likely to have low income and 1.98 times more likely to be unemployed or underemployed than normal-hearing individuals (Emmett and Francis, 2015). The authors noted that these are cross-sectional data that cannot be used to establish causation and pointed to the need for longitudinal studies. This same study further found that individuals with hearing loss were 3.21 times as likely to have low educational attainment than those without hearing loss (Emmett and Francis, 2015). Adults with hearing loss retire earlier than adults without hearing loss, which can cause financial stress (Malcolm et al., 2022).

A second area of study focuses on direct and indirect health care costs. Wells and colleagues (2019) concluded that individuals with untreated severe hearing loss had higher annual medical costs ($14,349) than those without hearing loss ($12,118). These are medical costs separate from the cost associated with the treatment of hearing loss. Reed and colleagues found an association between untreated hearing loss and increased health care expenses at 2, 5, and 10 years after diagnosis (Reed et al., 2019). A longitudinal study that included individuals on private U.S. health insurance plans or Medicaid Advantage plans who had filed administrative claims found that at 10 years people with untreated hearing loss had 50 percent more hospital stays, 44 percent higher readmission rates (within 30 days), and attended on average 52 more outpatient visits over a 10-year period (Reed et al., 2019). Overall, individuals with hearing loss spent an average $22,434 more on health care than individuals without hearing loss over that 10-year period (Reed et al., 2019).

As noted in the 2016 National Academies study *Hearing Health Care for Adults:*

> Mohr and colleagues (2000) focused on severe to profound hearing loss and estimated the costs over a lifetime to an individual to be $297,000 (averaged across age at onset), with most of the losses (67 percent) due to reduced work productivity. . . . Ruben (2000) used several sources of labor and disability data to look at the economic effects of communications disorders, with some data focused on hearing loss, and found negative impacts of hearing loss on individual income and significant underemployment of individuals with hearing loss. Stucky and colleagues (2010) used a simulation model based on national estimates of the prevalence of hearing loss in individuals age 65 years and older across the range of hearing loss, as well as several sources of economic data, and estimated that the total costs of first-year treatment of hearing loss in 2002 were approximately $1,292 per person, or $8.2 billion nationally, and projected that by 2030 these costs would increase to approximately $51.4 billion nationally. They also estimated the 2002 lost productivity costs attributable to hearing loss in this age group to be approximately $1.4 billion nationally. Simpson and colleagues (2016) examined health care cost data from privately insured adults age 55 to 64 years and found higher health care costs for a number of chronic health conditions for individuals with a diagnostic code for hearing loss as compared with a matched group without that diagnostic code. (NASEM, 2016, p. 62–63)

Hearing loss has substantial economic consequences on a national and global level. A large systematic review concluded that in the United States "estimates of the economic cost of lost productivity varied widely, from $1.8 [billion] to $194 billion" (Huddle et al., 2017, p. 1040). Globally, in 2019, it was estimated that "total global economic costs of hearing loss exceeded $981 billion," which included health care costs, educational costs, productivity losses, and quality of life (McDaid et al., 2021). Other symptoms related to hearing loss may contribute to the estimation of the societal costs of untreated hearing loss. For example, depression is a common side effect of untreated hearing loss, which, as noted earlier, reduces the ability to participate in family events and affects familial relationships (Snow and Abrams, 2016). Costs of older adults' care also increase with more severe depressive symptoms and limit their ability to function independently (Snow and Abrams, 2016). Additionally, many older adults in good health assist with childcare in their families as unpaid caregivers (Snow and Abrams, 2016). Fifty percent of caregivers are age 50 and older, and 19 percent are 65 and older. Untreated hearing loss and its consequences can lessen their abilities to help their families in this way and is thus a productivity loss (Snow and Abrams, 2016).

Conclusion 5-22: While socioeconomic effects may be meaningful to specific subpopulations (e.g., adults in the workforce) or important for specific types of research, this outcome does not rise to the level of a core outcome at this time because it is not identified by most adults with hearing difficulties as a frequently occurring or important difficulty. The committee recognizes the many access issues related to the cost of hearing health interventions, but these concerns are beyond the scope of this report.

Participation Restrictions

As described in Chapter 3, Allen and colleagues (2022) conducted a study aimed at seeking consensus from a range of key stakeholders in Australia to define which client-centered outcome domains should be measured and when they should be measured. They queried 79 professional stakeholders involved in the delivery of hearing services in Australia and 64 hearing rehabilitation services' patients identified by not-for-profit consumer organizations. They concluded that, at a minimum, the core outcome domains to be measured for patients receiving hearing rehabilitation were communication ability, personal relationships, well-being, and participation restrictions.

"Participation restrictions have been defined as the difficulties an individual experiences with involvement in life situations" (WHO, 2001). Danermark and colleagues (2013) identified the following core set of participation domains relevant to hearing loss:

- Handling stress and other psychological demands
- Communicating with—receiving—spoken messages
- Conversation
- Using communication devices and techniques
- Family relationships
- School education
- Remunerative employment
- Community life

There are several challenges with this outcome, including the fact that there is no standardized definition of the concept. Additionally, the measures used are inconsistent, and there is insufficient evidence that existing measures are psychometrically accurate. Measures such as the HHI-based outcomes, however, include items on hearing-related social difficulties that can be considered participation restrictions. In fact, Cox and colleagues (2007) used the HHIE as a measure of participation restriction in a study of hearing-aid outcomes in 205 older adults.

Conclusion 5-23: While participation restrictions may be meaningful to adults with hearing difficulties, this outcome does not rise to the level of a core outcome at this time because of inconsistencies with its definition and measurement.

Physical Health

Hearing loss and physical functioning are independently associated in older adults (Chen et al., 2014). There is a dose–response relationship between hearing loss and physical function, meaning the more severe the hearing difficulties, the more severe the physical limitations. A number of factors may play a role in this association. First, as noted earlier, hearing loss often results in communication difficulties, increasing social isolation and loneliness (Shukla et al., 2020). Additionally, people with strong social networks are more likely to be informed about health care services and encouraged to maintain healthy behaviors (Shukla et al., 2020). They also receive emotional support, promoting robust mental health (Thoits, 2011; Unger et al., 1999).

One consequence of untreated hearing loss is low levels of physical activity (Gispen et al., 2014). Individuals with hearing loss have about a 60 percent increased odds of self-reporting low physical activity than individuals without hearing loss. Physical activity is essential for overall health and is proven to reduce all-cause mortality (Samitz et al., 2011). Hearing loss is significantly associated with self-reported falls even after adjustment for demographic factors, cardiovascular health, and vestibular function (Lin and Ferrucci, 2012). Damage to the cochlear and vestibular sense organs that cause hearing loss may worsen balance, leading to a higher risk of falls. Hearing loss also affects cognitive load, further impairing postural balance (Lin and Ferrucci, 2012). Lastly, an individual's reduced ability to pick up on environmental auditory cues and limited awareness of one's surroundings also increases the risk of falls (Lin and Ferrucci, 2012).

A study examining the association between hearing aids and falls within a population of older adults with hearing loss found 20 percent lower odds of falls for adults who used hearing aids than for adults who did not use hearing aids (Mahmoudi et al., 2019). Keeping the desire of reaching whole health in mind, physical health plays an essential role—along with behavioral, spiritual, and socioeconomic health—in achieving a complete sense of well-being (NASEM, 2023).

Another concern related to physical health is the individual's ability to communicate effectively with health care providers (Hines, 2000). In the primary care setting, a survey of 1,581 individuals with hearing loss found that the individuals reported moderate to significant challenges communicating with a variety of clinicians, including physicians, physician assistants, nurses, nurse practitioners, receptionists, and pharmacists (Stevens et al., 2019).

Individuals with hearing difficulties reported challenges with hearing their names called, privacy loss (from health care professionals having to raise their voices to communicate), scheduling, misunderstanding medical information, being unable to hear when a health care professional turns away, and difficulties with instructions on the phone (Stevens et al., 2019). The difficulties in navigating a primary care appointment as an adult with hearing loss threaten the quality of care, satisfaction with care, and, ultimately, health outcomes. Effective communication between health care professionals and patients is associated with improved adherence to treatment, which is essential for good overall health outcomes (DiMatteo et al., 2012; Haskard-Zolnierek and DiMatteo, 2009; Hays and Quigley, 2025).

Activities of Daily Living

Activities of daily living (ADLs) include walking, eating, dressing and grooming, toileting, bathing, and transferring (i.e., being able to move from one body position to another) (Kernisan, 2024). Instrumental activities of daily living (IADLs) include managing finances, transportation, shopping and cooking, house cleaning and home maintenance, communication, and taking medications. ADLs and IADLs are often used to assess individuals' physical functioning and ability to care for themselves independently as well as to diagnose and manage health issues. Perceived activity limitations have been significantly associated with hearing loss, and perceived participation restrictions have been significantly associated with general life satisfaction (Solheim et al., 2011). Humes, using national data from the National Health Interview Surveys, found that those who self-reported at least a little hearing trouble also reported significantly more hearing-related daily activity limitations (Humes, 2023).

One example related to hearing loss is driving (Hickson et al., 2010). Older adults are more likely to be involved in fatal car crashes than younger adults, and older adults with untreated hearing loss specifically have more challenges driving with distractions than people with good hearing ability (Hickson et al., 2010). Driving in complicated situations is a cognitive task requiring sign recognition and multitasking. The effortfulness hypothesis is that the combination of effortful listening and poor ability to recognize auditory signals harms other cognitive processes (Hickson et al., 2010).

> *Conclusion 5-24: Physical health does not rise to the level of a core outcome because it is not identified by most adults with hearing difficulties as a frequently occurring or important difficulty, although the degree to which adults with hearing difficulties are aware that physical health may be related to hearing difficulties is unclear. Furthermore, while there are several individual studies of evidence suggesting an association*

between hearing health interventions and specific individual physical health outcomes, there is insufficient evidence of the ability of hearing health interventions to affect physical health outcomes.

FINDINGS

Finding 5-1: No standardized set of outcome domains or individual outcomes has been defined or assessed consistently across the hearing health field.

Finding 5-2: Verification of the proximal outcome audibility is necessary but insufficient to assessing the distal outcomes associated with everyday function of hearing health interventions.

Finding 5-3: Individuals with hearing difficulties may not be able to detect or locate either speech or nonspeech sounds (e.g., alarms, sirens, traffic, birds, and music).

Finding 5-4: Many individuals with moderate hearing trouble may have difficulties comprehending speech even in quiet settings.

Finding 5-5: A significant amount of evidence shows that for most adults with hearing difficulties, it is both meaningful and important to measure how well an individual understands speech in complex listening situations.

Finding 5-6: Sound localization is meaningful to certain individuals, and several self-report measures have been designed to assess localization, but they have not been adequately validated.

Finding 5-7: While listening effort and listening fatigue are meaningful outcomes, inconsistencies in the definitions, populations, and methodologies have led to a lack of consensus on the best way to study these constructs.

Finding 5-8: Examining outcomes beyond hearing and communication can help capture additional aspects of hearing rehabilitation that are meaningful to individuals with hearing difficulties. However, many widely accepted constructs are overlapping (e.g., well-being, QoL, participation, psychosocial health).

Finding 5-9: Hearing loss has been associated with poorer social connection, but research is inconclusive about whether hearing interventions alone can mitigate these effects.

Finding 5-10: Research on the association between hearing loss and social connection has been limited by an inconsistent use of measures as well as by the fact that the measures have not been validated for use with hearing loss.

Finding 5-11: Hearing loss and hearing difficulties have been associated with psychosocial outcomes, including social isolation, loneliness, depression, and anxiety.

Finding 5-12: Hearing loss has been associated with cognitive decline, but a causal link in either direction has not been demonstrated.

Finding 5-13: There is no agreement on the definition of QoL, and there is inconsistency in the underlying constructs being measured.

Finding 5-14: Many factors contribute to QoL and health-related QoL, which makes measurement of the direct effect of hearing interventions difficult.

Finding 5-15: Studies of the impact of hearing interventions on health-related QoL are inconsistent.

Finding 5-16: A very small literature examines the socioeconomic effects of untreated hearing loss, mostly related to the effect on income and both direct and indirect health care costs.

Finding 5-17: Like QoL, the outcome of "participation restrictions" has been shown to be meaningful, but there is no standardized definition of the concept, the use of measures is inconsistent, and there is insufficient evidence that existing measures are of high quality.

Finding 5-18: Hearing loss and physical functioning are associated in older adults. However, research in this space is limited, particularly for the ability of hearing health interventions to affect physical outcomes.

RECOMMENDATIONS

In its review of the literature and information gathered in public webinars and the committee's public platform, the committee considered the extensive list of potential core outcomes and created a comprehensive and clearly defined set of outcomes to be considered for a core outcome set. Below, the committee provides recommendations on the core outcome set as well as areas of future research needed on individual outcomes.

Core Outcome Set

The use of a core outcome set will help standardize information gathered about the effect of interventions and allow for: (1) comparison of interventions across studies, clinics, populations, and time; (2) pooling of data from smaller studies for meta-analyses; and (3) focus on the outcomes that matter the most to individuals with hearing difficulties as well as to clinicians.

Significant literature supports several outcomes as being meaningful to adults with hearing difficulties and to clinicians, associated with hearing difficulties, and important to measure. These outcomes are well defined, and adequate measures exist that meet the committee's criteria to warrant their use in various contexts. The committee also considered factors that influence the burden of assessing the core outcome set overall (e.g., number of outcomes, availability of measures, mode of administration, time of administration). The committee determined that two outcomes have the strongest evidence for inclusion in a core outcome set: understanding speech in complex listening situations and hearing-related psychosocial health.

Recommendation 5-1: Individuals and organizations engaged in hearing health interventions should adopt the following outcomes as a core outcome set in both research and clinical settings:
a. Understanding speech in complex listening situations
b. Hearing-related psychosocial health

The committee notes that individuals and organizations engaged in hearing health interventions represent a wide variety of partners, including the academic and professional community of researchers and clinicians, federal agencies, industry, consumer groups, and individuals with hearing difficulties themselves and their care partners. The committee emphasizes that this core outcome set should be considered as a foundation for hearing-health outcome assessment following intervention—that is, this set represents the minimum that should be measured across settings and intervention types. This does not imply that other outcomes are not meaningful or should be unexamined. The committee further notes that the frequency and timing of the assessment of these outcomes may vary depending on the context.

Future Research on Outcomes

For many of the outcomes of interest, the committee found limited evidence and determined that more research is needed—both to better understand which outcomes are most meaningful for adults with hearing difficulties and for clinicians and also to better define and build the evidence base for these outcomes as potential candidates for an updated core outcome set.

Several meaningful outcomes need further research, for various reasons. For example, some outcomes are inconsistently defined, and measurement is inconsistent in terms of the underlying constructs examined. Furthermore, many of the outcomes considered by the committee lack robust evidence on the importance to measure—that is, whether the intervention itself can result in significant clinical change in the outcome, particularly at the level of the individual. The current literature is unable to support the inclusion of many of the outcomes considered for a core set; more research is needed to better define these outcomes and build evidence for their importance to measure.

Recommendation 5-2: Sponsors of hearing health research should fund research to build the evidence base on the clinical effect of hearing health interventions on key outcomes that are meaningful to adults with hearing difficulties and clinicians.

Examples of the types of research needed by outcome are provided in Table 5-3. This includes research on the outcome itself (e.g., improvements in definition) as well as on the impact of hearing interventions on the outcome.

TABLE 5-3 Areas of Needed Research by Outcome

Outcome	Research Needed on Outcome
Perception of nonspeech sounds (e.g., music)	Determine which subpopulations consider this most meaningful.
Listening effort and listening fatigue	Research on the separate constructs warranted. Currently, definitions and theoretical approaches are not consistent.
Social connection	Determine intervention's effect on clinical outcomes.
Hearing-related psychosocial health	Determine the differences of effects on social versus emotional health (currently not distinctly measured).
Cognition	Determine intervention's effect on clinical outcomes and also the mechanism for the effect.
Quality of life	Determine clear and consistent definition with common metrics across conditions.
Socioeconomic effects	Determine intervention's effect on the outcome.
Participation restrictions	Determine a consistent definition. Define the outcome independent of individual underlying constructs and overlapping outcomes.
Physical health	Determine intervention's effect on clinical outcomes.

Additional research will help determine which outcomes might be appropriate for an updated core outcome set. The committee recognizes that while this research is warranted, some outcomes may never rise to the level of a core set for use across hearing health interventions because the outcome may never be meaningful to all subpopulations. However, this type of research will be useful both for reconsideration of the outcome for an overarching core set and for understanding the outcomes' use as supplemental outcomes to be measured for specific populations.

The committee further emphasizes that research on these outcomes—and consideration for inclusion in an updated core outcome set—will require the development and use of clearly defined outcomes and high-quality measures. It is important to show that such measures are reliable and valid, including data defining a minimally important clinical difference. See Chapter 6 for evidence on the measurement of outcomes after hearing health intervention.

REFERENCES

Alhanbali, S., P. Dawes, S. Lloyd, and K. J. Munro. 2017. Self-reported listening-related effort and fatigue in hearing-impaired adults. *Ear and Hearing* 38(1):e39–e48.

Allen, D., L. Hickson, and M. Ferguson. 2022. Defining a patient-centred core outcome domain set for the assessment of hearing rehabilitation with clients and professionals. *Frontiers in Neuroscience* 16:787607.

Almeida, G. V. M., A. Ribas, and J. Calleros. 2019. Sound localization test in presence of noise (sound localization test) in adults without hearing alteration. *International Archives of Otorhinolaryngology* 23(3):e276–e280.

Amieva, H., C. Ouvrard, C. Meillon, L. Rullier, and J. F. Dartigues. 2018. Death, depression, disability, and dementia associated with self-reported hearing problems: A 25-year study. *Journal of Gerontology A Biological Sciences and Medical Sciences* 73(10):1383–1389.

Arlinger, S. 2003. Negative consequences of uncorrected hearing loss—a review. *International Journal of Audiology* 42(Suppl 2):2S17–2S20.

Armstrong, T. W., S. Surya, T. R. Elliott, D. F. Brossart, and J. N. Burdine. 2016. Depression and health-related quality of life among persons with sensory disabilities in a health professional shortage area. *Rehabilitation Psychology* 61(3):240–250.

ASHA (American Speech–Language–Hearing Association). n.d. *Aural rehabilitation.* https:// www.asha.org/practice-portal/professional-issues/aural-rehabilitation-for-adults/ #collapse_4 (accessed June 11, 2024).

Bainbridge, K. E., and M. I. Wallhagen. 2014. Hearing loss in an aging American population: Extent, impact, and management. *Annual Review of Public Health* 35:139–152.

Baker, S. 2017. Matching real-ear targets for adult hearing aid fittings: NAL-NL1 and DSL v5.0 prescriptive formulae. *Canadian Journal of Speech-Language Pathology & Audiology* 41(2):227–235.

Barker, F., E. MacKenzie, L. Elliott, and S. de Lusignan. 2015. Outcome measurement in adult auditory rehabilitation: A scoping review of measures used in randomized controlled trials. *Ear and Hearing* 36(5):567–573.

Barofsky, I. 2012. Can quality or quality-of-life be defined? *Quality of Life Research* 21(4): 625–631.

Bennett, R. J., L. Saulsman, R. H. Eikelboom, and M. Olaithe. 2022. Coping with the social challenges and emotional distress associated with hearing loss: A qualitative investigation using Leventhal's self-regulation theory. *International Journal of Audiology* 61(5):353–364.

Bessen, S., W. Zhang, E. E. G. Morales, E.-R. L. Akré, and N. S. Reed. 2024. Hearing aid use at the intersection of race, ethnicity, and socioeconomic status. Paper read at JAMA Health Forum.

Blazer, D. G. 2020. Hearing loss. *Geriatric Psychiatry, An Issue of Clinics in Geriatric Medicine* 36(2):201–209.

Boggatz T. 2016. Quality of life in old age—A concept analysis. *International Journal of Older People Nursing* 11(1):55–69.

Borre, E. D., K. Kaalund, N. Frisco, G. Zhang, A. Ayer, M. Kelly-Hedrick, S. D. Reed, S. D. Emmett, H. Francis, D. L. Tucci, B. S. Wilson, A. S. Kosinski, O. Ogbuoji, and G. D. Sanders Schmidler. 2023. The impact of hearing loss and its treatment on health-related quality of life utility: A systematic review with meta-analysis. *Journal of General Internal Medicine* 38(2):456–479.

Bottalico, P., R. N. Piper, and B. Legner. 2022. Lombard effect, intelligibility, ambient noise, and willingness to spend time and money in a restaurant amongst older adults. *Scientific Reports* 12(1):6549.

Brewster, K. K., A. Ciarleglio, P. J. Brown, C. Chen, H. O. Kim, S. P. Roose, J. S. Golub, and B. R. Rutherford. 2018. Age-related hearing loss and its association with depression in later life. *American Journal of Geriatric Psychiatry* 26(7):788–796.

Brock, P. R., R. Maibach, M. Childs, K. Rajput, D. Roebuck, M. J. Sullivan, V. Laithier, M. Ronghe, P. Dall'Igna, and E. Hiyama. 2018. Sodium thiosulfate for protection from cisplatin-induced hearing loss. *New England Journal of Medicine* 378(25):2376–2385.

Brodie, A., B. Smith, and J. Ray. 2018. The impact of rehabilitation on quality of life after hearing loss: A systematic review. *European Archives of Oto-Rhino-Laryngology* 275(10):2435–2440.

Bronkhorst, A. W. 2015. The cocktail-party problem revisited: Early processing and selection of multi-talker speech. *Attention, Perception, and Psychophysics* 77(5):1465–1487.

Bunge, M. 1975. What is a quality of life indicator? *Social Indicators Research* 2:65–79.

Carhart, R., and J. F. Jerger. 1959. Preferred method for clinical determination of pure-tone thresholds. *Journal of Speech and Hearing Disorders* 24(4):330–345.

Cassarly, C., L. J. Matthews, A. N. Simpson, and J. R. Dubno. 2020. The revised hearing handicap inventory and screening tool based on psychometric reevaluation of the hearing handicap inventories for the elderly and adults. *Ear and Hearing* 41(1):95–105.

Cetin, B., F. Uguz, M. Erdem, and A. Yildirim. 2010. Relationship between quality of life, anxiety and depression in unilateral hearing loss. *Journal of International Advanced Otology* 6:252–257.

Chen, D. S., D. J. Genther, J. Betz, and F. R. Lin. 2014. Association between hearing impairment and self-reported difficulty in physical functioning. *Journal of the American Geriatrics Society* 62(5):850–856.

Chisolm, T. H., H. B. Abrams, R. McArdle, R. H. Wilson, and P. J. Doyle. 2005. The WHO-DAS II: Psychometric properties in the measurement of functional health status in adults with acquired hearing loss. *Trends in Amplification* 9(3):111–126.

Chisolm, T. H., C. E. Johnson, J. L. Danhauer, L. J. Portz, H. B. Abrams, S. Lesner, P. A. McCarthy, and C. W. Newman. 2007. A systematic review of health-related quality of life and hearing aids: Final report of the American Academy of Audiology Task Force on the Health-Related Quality of Life Benefits of Amplification in Adults. *Journal of the American Academy of Audiology* 18(2):151–183.

Choi, Y., J. Go, and J. W. Chung. 2024. Association between hearing level and mental health and quality of life in adults aged > 40 years. *Journal of Audiology and Otology* 28(1):52–58.

Ciorba, A., C. Bianchini, S. Pelucchi, and A. Pastore. 2012. The impact of hearing loss on the quality of life of elderly adults. *Clinical Interventions in Aging* 7:159–163.

Contrera, K. J., M. I. Wallhagen, S. K. Mamo, E. S. Oh, and F. R. Lin. 2016. Hearing loss health care for older adults. *Journal of the American Board of Family Medicine* 29(3):394–403.

Contrera, K. J., J. Betz, J. Deal, J. S. Choi, H. N. Ayonayon, T. Harris, E. Helzner, K. R. Martin, K. Mehta, S. Pratt, S. M. Rubin, S. Satterfield, K. Yaffe, E. M. Simonsick, and F. R. Lin. 2017. Association of hearing impairment and anxiety in older adults. *Journal of Aging and Health* 29(1):172–184.

Cosh, S., I. Carriere, V. Daien, H. Amieva, C. Tzourio, C. Delcourt, and C. Helmer. 2018. The relationship between hearing loss in older adults and depression over 12 years: Findings from the three-city prospective cohort study. *International Journal of Geriatric Psychiatry* 33(12):1654–1661.

Cosh, S., C. Helmer, C. Delcourt, T. G. Robins, and P. J. Tully. 2019. Depression in elderly patients with hearing loss: Current perspectives. *Clinical Interventions in Aging* 14:1471–1480.

Cox, R. M., G. C. Alexander, and G. A. Gray. 2007. Personality, hearing problems, and amplification characteristics: Contributions to self-report hearing aid outcomes. *Ear and Hearing* 28(2).

Cunningham, L. L., and D. L. Tucci. 2017. Hearing loss in adults. *New England Journal of Medicine* 377(25):2465–2473.

Danermark, B., S. Granberg, S. E. Kramer, M. Selb, and C. Möller. 2013. The creation of a comprehensive and a brief core set for hearing loss using the International Classification of Functioning, Disability and Health. *American Journal of Audiology* 22(2):323–328.

Davis, H., D. Schlundt, K. Bonnet, S. Camarata, F. H. Bess, and B. Hornsby. 2021. Understanding listening-related fatigue: Perspectives of adults with hearing loss. *International Journal of Audiology* 60(6):458–468.

Deal, J. A., J. Betz, K. Yaffe, T. Harris, E. Purchase-Helzner, S. Satterfield, S. Pratt, N. Govil, E. M. Simonsick, and F. R. Lin. 2017. Hearing impairment and incident dementia and cognitive decline in older adults: The Health ABC study. *Journal of Gerontology Series A: Biological Sciences and Medical Sciences* 72(5):703–709.

DiMatteo, M. R., K. B. Haskard-Zolnierek, and L. R. Martin. 2012. Improving patient adherence: A three-factor model to guide practice. *Health Psychology Review* 6(1):74–91.

Dixon, P. R., D. Feeny, G. Tomlinson, S. Cushing, J. M. Chen, and M. D. Krahn. 2020. Health-related quality of life changes associated with hearing loss. *JAMA Otolaryngology—Head & Neck Surgery* 146(7):630–638.

Ellis, S., S. Sheik Ali, and W. Ahmed. 2021. A review of the impact of hearing interventions on social isolation and loneliness in older people with hearing loss. *European Archives of Oto-Rhino-Laryngology* 278(12):4653–4661.

Emmett, S. D., and H. W. Francis. 2015. The socioeconomic impact of hearing loss in U.S. adults. *Otology and Neurotology* 36(3):545–550.

Fitzgerald, M. B., S. P. Gianakas, Z. J. Qian, S. Losorelli, and A. C. Swanson. 2023. Preliminary guidelines for replacing word-recognition in quiet with speech in noise assessment in the routine audiologic test battery. *Ear and Hearing* 44(6):1548–1561.

Fitzgerald, M. B., K. M. Ward, S. P. Gianakas, M. L. Smith, N. H. Blevins, and A. P. Swanson. 2024. Speech-in-noise assessment in the routine audiologic test battery: Relationship to perceived auditory disability. *Ear and Hearing* 45(4):816–826.

Gatehouse, S., and W. Noble. 2004. The Speech, Spatial and Qualities of Hearing Scale (SSQ). *International Journal of Audiology* 43(2):85–99.

Gillingham, R., and W. S. Reece. 1979. A new approach to quality of life measurement. *Urban Studies* 16(3):329–332.

Gispen, F. E., D. S. Chen, D. J. Genther, and F. R. Lin. 2014. Association between hearing impairment and lower levels of physical activity in older adults. *Journal of the American Geriatrics Society* 62(8):1427–1433.

Glick, H. A., and A. Sharma. 2020. Cortical neuroplasticity and cognitive function in early-stage, mild-moderate hearing loss: Evidence of neurocognitive benefit from hearing aid use. *Frontiers in Neuroscience* 14:93.

Gopinath, B., J. J. Wang, J. Schneider, G. Burlutsky, J. Snowdon, C. M. McMahon, S. R. Leeder, and P. Mitchell. 2009. Depressive symptoms in older adults with hearing impairments: The Blue Mountains study. *Journal of the American Geriatrics Society* 57(7):1306–1308.

Gosselin, P., D. X. Guan, E. E. Smith, and Z. Ismail. 2023. Temporal associations between treated and untreated hearing loss and mild behavioral impairment in older adults without dementia. *Alzheimer's and Dementia* 9(4):e12424.

Guyatt, G. H., D. H. Feeny, and D. L. Patrick. 1993. Measuring health-related quality of life. *Annals of Internal Medicine* 118(8):622–629.

Haskard-Zolnierek, K. B., and M. R. DiMatteo. 2009. Physician communication and patient adherence to treatment: A meta-analysis. *Medical Care* 47(8):826–834.

Hays, R. D., and D. D. Quigley. 2025. A perspective on the use of patient-reported experience and patient-reported outcome measures in ambulatory healthcare. *Expert Review of Pharmacoeconomics & Outcomes Research.* January 17 [online ahead of print]. https//doi.org/10.1080/14737167.2025.2451749.

Heffernan, E., B. E. Weinstein, and M. A. Ferguson. 2020. Application of Rasch analysis to the evaluation of the measurement properties of the Hearing Handicap Inventory for the Elderly. *Ear and Hearing* 41(5):1125–1134.

Hickson, L., J. Wood, A. Chaparro, P. Lacherez, and R. Marszalek. 2010. Hearing impairment affects older people's ability to drive in the presence of distracters. *Journal of the American Geriatrics Society* 58(6):1097–1103.

Hines, J. 2000. Communication problems of hearing-impaired patients. *Nursing Standard* 14(19):33–37.

Holman, J. A., A. Drummond, and G. Naylor. 2021. The effect of hearing loss and hearing device fitting on fatigue in adults: A systematic review. *Ear and Hearing* 42(1):1–11.

Holt-Lunstad, J. 2018. Why social relationships are important for physical health: A systems approach to understanding and modifying risk and protection. *Annual Review of Psychology* 69:437–458.

Hornsby, B. W. Y., and A. M. Kipp. 2016. Subjective ratings of fatigue and vigor in adults with hearing loss are driven by perceived hearing difficulties not degree of hearing loss. *Ear and Hearing* 37(1):e1–e10.

Huddle, M. G., A. M. Goman, F. C. Kernizan, D. M. Foley, C. Price, K. D. Frick, and F. R. Lin. 2017. The economic impact of adult hearing loss: A systematic review. *JAMA Otolaryngology—Head and Neck Surgery* 143(10):1040–1048.

Humes, L. E. 2021. Development of the SWB-HL: A scale of the subjective well-being of older adults with hearing loss. *Frontiers in Psychology* 12:1–12.

Humes, L. E. 2023. U.S. population data on self-reported trouble hearing and hearing-aid use in adults: National Health Interview Survey, 2007–2018. *Trends in Hearing* 27: 23312165231160967.

Humes, L. E., and J. R. Dubno. 2010. Factors affecting speech understanding in older adults. In *The aging auditory system*, edited by S. Gordon-Salant, R. D. Frisina, A. N. Popper and R. R. Fay. New York: Springer New York. Pp. 211–257.

IOM (Institute of Medicine). 1989. *Quality of life and technology assessment.* Washington, DC: National Academy Press.

Isherwood, B., A. C. Gonçalves, R. Cousins, and R. Holme. 2022. The global hearing therapeutic pipeline: 2021. *Drug Discovery Today* 27(3):912–922.

Jayakody, D. M. P., O. P. Almeida, C. P. Speelman, R. J. Bennett, T. C. Moyle, J. M. Yiannos, and P. L. Friedland. 2018. Association between speech and high-frequency hearing loss and depression, anxiety and stress in older adults. *Maturitas* 110:86–91.

Jayakody, D. M. P., J. Wishart, I. Stegeman, R. Eikelboom, T. C. Moyle, J. M. Yiannos, J. J. Goodman-Simpson, and O. P. Almeida. 2022. Is there an association between untreated hearing loss and psychosocial outcomes? *Frontiers in Aging Neuroscience* 14:868673.

Kaplan, R. M., and R. D. Hays. 2022. Health-related quality of life measurement in public health. *Annual Review of Public Health* 43:355–373.

Katiri, R., D. A. Hall, D. J. Hoare, K. Fackrell, A. Horobin, N. Buggy, N. Hogan, and P. T. Kitterick. 2021. Redesigning a web-based stakeholder consensus meeting about core outcomes for clinical trials: Formative feedback study. *JMIR Formative Research* 5(8): e28878.

Katiri, R., D. A. Hall, D. J. Hoare, K. Fackrell, A. Horobin, N. Hogan, N. Buggy, P. H. Van de Heyning, J. B. Firszt, I. A. Bruce, and P. T. Kitterick. 2022. The Core Rehabilitation Outcome Set for Single-Sided Deafness (CROSSSD) study: International consensus on outcome measures for trials of interventions for adults with single-sided deafness. *Trials* 23(1):764.

Keidser, G., H. Dillon, L. Carter, and A. O'Brien. 2012. NAL-NL2 empirical adjustments. *Trends in Amplification* 16(4):211–223.

Kernisan, L. 2024. *What are activities of daily living (ADLs) & instrumental activities of daily living (IADLs)?* https://betterhealthwhileaging.net/what-are-adls-and-iadls (accessed May 22, 2024).

Keur-Huizinga, L., S. E. Kramer, E. J. C. de Geus, and A. A. Zekveld. 2024. A multimodal approach to measuring listening effort: A systematic review on the effects of auditory task demand on physiological measures and their relationship. *Ear and Hearing* 45(5): 1089–1106.

Kil, J., E. Lobarinas, C. Spankovich, S. K. Griffiths, P. J. Antonelli, E. D. Lynch, and C. G. Le Prell. 2017. Safety and efficacy of ebselen for the prevention of noise-induced hearing loss: A randomised, double-blind, placebo-controlled, phase 2 trial. *Lancet* 390(10098): 969–979.

Kopke, R., M. D. Slade, R. Jackson, T. Hammill, S. Fausti, B. Lonsbury-Martin, A. Sanderson, L. Dreisbach, P. Rabinowitz, and P. Torre III. 2015. Efficacy and safety of n-acetylcysteine in prevention of noise induced hearing loss: A randomized clinical trial. *Hearing Research* 323:40–50.

Laird, E. C., R. J. Bennett, C. M. Barr, and C. A. Bryant. 2020. Experiences of hearing loss and audiological rehabilitation for older adults with comorbid psychological symptoms: A qualitative study. *American Journal of Audiology* 29(4):809–824.

Langguth, B., and D. De Ridder. 2023. Minimal clinically important difference of tinnitus outcome measurement instruments—A scoping review. *Journal of Clinical Medicine* 12(22).

Lawrence, B. J., D. M. P. Jayakody, R. J. Bennett, R. H. Eikelboom, N. Gasson, and P. L. Friedland. 2020. Hearing loss and depression in older adults: A systematic review and meta-analysis. *Gerontologist* 60(3):e137–e154.

Lazar, R. M., V. J. Howard, W. N. Kernan, H. J. Aparicio, D. A. Levine, A. J. Viera, L. C. Jordan, D. L. Nyenhuis, K. L. Possin, and F. A. Sorond. 2021. A primary care agenda for brain health: A scientific statement from the American Heart Association. *Stroke* 52(6):e295–e308.

Le Prell, C. G. 2021. Investigational medicinal products for the inner ear: Review of clinical trial characteristics in ClinicalTrials.gov. *Journal of the American Academy of Audiology* 32(10):670–694.

Le Prell, C. G. 2023. Preclinical prospects of investigational agents for hearing loss treatment. *Expert Opinion on Investigational Drugs* 32(8):685–692.

Le Prell, C. G., C. C. Brewer, and K. C. Campbell. 2022. The audiogram: Detection of pure-tone stimuli in ototoxicity monitoring and assessments of investigational medicines for the inner ear. *Journal of the Acoustical Society of America* 152(1):470–490.

Lee, A. T. H., M. C. F. Tong, K. C. P. Yuen, P. S. O. Tang, and C. A. Vanhasselt. 2010. Hearing impairment and depressive symptoms in an older Chinese population. *Journal of Otolaryngology—Head & Neck Surgery* 39(5):498–503.

Leek, M. R., M. R. Molis, L. R. Kubli, and J. B. Tufts. 2008. Enjoyment of music by elderly hearing-impaired listeners. *Journal of the American Academy of Audiology* 19(06):519–526.

Li, C. M., X. Zhang, H. J. Hoffman, M. F. Cotch, C. L. Themann, and M. R. Wilson. 2014. Hearing impairment associated with depression in US adults, National Health and Nutrition Examination Survey 2005–2010. *JAMA Otolaryngology Head and Neck Surgery* 140(4):293–302.

Lin, F. R. 2011. Hearing loss and cognition among older adults in the United States. *Journal of Gerontology Series A: Biological Sciences and Medical Sciences* 66(10):1131–1136.

Lin, F. R., and L. Ferrucci. 2012. Hearing loss and falls among older adults in the United States. *Archives of Internal Medicine* 172(4):369–371.

Lin, F. R., K. Yaffe, J. Xia, Q. L. Xue, T. B. Harris, E. Purchase-Helzner, S. Satterfield, H. N. Ayonayon, L. Ferrucci, E. M. Simonsick, and Health ABC Study. 2013. Hearing loss and cognitive decline in older adults. *JAMA Internal Medicine* 173(4):293–299.

Lin, F. R., J. R. Pike, M. S. Albert, M. Arnold, S. Burgard, T. Chisolm, D. Couper, J. A. Deal, A. M. Goman, N. W. Glynn, T. Gmelin, L. Gravens-Mueller, K. M. Hayden, A. R. Huang, D. Knopman, C. M. Mitchell, T. Mosley, J. S. Pankow, N. S. Reed, V. Sanchez, J. A. Schrack, B. G. Windham, and J. Coresh. 2023. Hearing intervention versus health education control to reduce cognitive decline in older adults with hearing loss in the USA (ACHIEVE): A multicentre, randomised controlled trial. *Lancet* 402(10404):786–797.

Linszen, M. M., R. M. Brouwer, S. M. Heringa, and I. E. Sommer. 2016. Increased risk of psychosis in patients with hearing impairment: Review and meta-analyses. *Neuroscience & Biobehavioral Reviews* 62:1–20.

Liu, B.-C. 1975. Quality of life: Concept, measure and results. *American Journal of Economics and Sociology* 34(1):1–13.

Livingston, G., J. Huntley, A. Sommerlad, D. Ames, C. Ballard, S. Banerjee, C. Brayne, A. Burns, J. Cohen-Mansfield, and C. Cooper. 2020. Dementia prevention, intervention, and care: 2020 report of the Lancet Commission. *Lancet* 396(10248):413–446.

Livingston, G., J. Huntley, K. Y. Liu, S. G. Costafreda, G. Selbæk, S. Alladi, D. Ames, S. Banerjee, A. Burns, C. Brayne, N. C. Fox, C. P. Ferri, L. N. Gitlin, R. Howard, H. C. Kales, M. Kivimäki, E. B. Larson, N. Nakasujja, K. Rockwood, Q. Samus, K. Shirai, A. Singh-Manoux, L. S. Schneider, S. Walsh, Y. Yao, A. Sommerlad, and N. Mukadam. 2024. Dementia prevention, intervention, and care: 2024 report of the Lancet standing commission. *Lancet* 404(10452):572–628.

Loughrey, D. G., M. E. Kelly, G. A. Kelley, S. Brennan, and B. A. Lawlor. 2018. Association of age-related hearing loss with cognitive function, cognitive impairment, and dementia: A systematic review and meta-analysis. *JAMA Otolaryngology–Head & Neck Surgery* 144(2):115–126.

Maharani, A., P. Dawes, J. Nazroo, G. Tampubolon, and N. Pendleton. 2018. Longitudinal relationship between hearing aid use and cognitive function in older Americans. *Journal of the American Geriatrics Society* 66(6):1130–1136.

Maharani, A., N. Pendleton, and I. Leroi. 2019. Hearing impairment, loneliness, social isolation, and cognitive function: Longitudinal analysis using English Longitudinal Study on Ageing. *American Journal of Geriatric Psychiatry* 27(12):1348–1356.

Mahmoudi, E., T. Basu, K. Langa, M. M. McKee, P. Zazove, N. Alexander, and N. Kamdar. 2019. Can hearing aids delay time to diagnosis of dementia, depression, or falls in older adults? *Journal of the American Geriatrics Society* 67(11):2362–2369.

Malcolm, K. A., J. J. Suen, and C. L. Nieman. 2022. Socioeconomic position and hearing loss: Current understanding and recent advances. *Current Opinion in Otolaryngology & Head and Neck Surgery* 30(5):351–357.

Manrique-Huarte, R., D. Calavia, A. Huarte Irujo, L. Giron, and M. Manrique-Rodriguez. 2016. Treatment for hearing loss among the elderly: Auditory outcomes and impact on quality of life. *Audiology and Neurotology* 21(Suppl 1):29–35.

Mattys, S. L., M. H. Davis, A. R. Bradlow, and S. K. Scott. 2012. Speech recognition in adverse conditions: A review. *Language and Cognitive Processes* 27(7–8):953–978.

McDaid, D., A. L. Park, and S. Chadha. 2021. Estimating the global costs of hearing loss. *International Journal of Audiology* 60(3):162–170.

McGarrigle, R., K. J. Munro, P. Dawes, A. J. Stewart, D. R. Moore, J. G. Barry, and S. Amitay. 2014. Listening effort and fatigue: What exactly are we measuring? A British Society of Audiology Cognition in Hearing Special Interest Group 'white paper'. *International Journal of Audiology* 53(7):433–445.

Mener, D. J., J. Betz, D. J. Genther, D. Chen, and F. R. Lin. 2013. Hearing loss and depression in older adults. *Journal of the American Geriatrics Society* 61(9):1627–1629.

Mick, P., I. Kawachi, and F. R. Lin. 2014. The association between hearing loss and social isolation in older adults. *Otolaryngology—Head and Neck Surgery* 150(3):378–384.

Middlebrooks, J. C. 2015. Sound localization. *Handbook of Clinical Neurology* 129:99–116.

Mohr, P. E., J. J. Feldman, and J. L. Dunbar. 2000. The societal costs of severe to profound hearing loss in the United States. *Policy Analysis Brief H Series* 2(1):1–4.

Mulrow, C. D., C. Aguilar, J. E. Endicott, M. R. Tuley, R. Velez, W. S. Charlip, M. C. Rhodes, J. A. Hill, and L. A. DeNino. 1990. Quality-of-life changes and hearing impairment. A randomized trial. *Annals of Internal Medicine* 113(3):188–194.

Munro, K. J., and L. M. Buttfield. 2005. Comparison of real-ear to coupler difference values in the right and left ear of adults using three earmold configurations. *Ear and Hearing* 26(3):290–298.

NASEM (National Academies of Sciences, Engineering, and Medicine). 2016. *Hearing health care for adults: Priorities for improving access and affordability*. Washington, DC: The National Academies Press.

NASEM. 2020. *Social isolation and loneliness in older adults: Opportunities for the health care system*. Washington, DC: The National Academies Press.

NASEM. 2023. *Achieving whole health: A new approach for veterans and the nation*. Washington, DC: The National Academies Press.

NCOA (National Council on Aging). 2023. *Hearing loss and anxiety: Why it happens and how to cope*. https://www.ncoa.org/adviser/hearing-aids/hearing-loss-anxiety (accessed June 20, 2024).

Neal, K., C. M. McMahon, S. E. Hughes, and I. Boisvert. 2022. Listening-based communication ability in adults with hearing loss: A scoping review of existing measures. *Frontiers in Psychology* 13:786347.

Noble, W., and D. Byrne. 1990. A comparison of different binaural hearing aid systems for sound localization in the horizontal and vertical planes. *British Journal of Audiology* 24(5):335–346.

Noble, W., D. Byrne, and B. Lepage. 1994. Effects on sound localization of configuration and type of hearing impairment. *Journal of the Acoustical Society of America* 95(2):992–1005.

Nordvik, Ø., P. O. Laugen Heggdal, J. Brännström, F. Vassbotn, A. K. Aarstad, and H. J. Aarstad. 2018. Generic quality of life in persons with hearing loss: A systematic literature review. *BMC Ear, Nose and Throat Disorders* 18:1.

Ohlenforst, B., A. A. Zekveld, E. P. Jansma, Y. Wang, G. Naylor, A. Lorens, T. Lunner, and S. E. Kramer. 2017. Effects of hearing impairment and hearing aid amplification on listening effort: A systematic review. *Ear and Hearing* 38(3):267–281.

Oxford Reference. n.d. *Verbal communication*. https://www.oxfordreference.com/view/10.1093/oi/authority.20110803115457102 (accessed June 12, 2024).

Peelle, J. E. 2018. Listening effort: How the cognitive consequences of acoustic challenge are reflected in brain and behavior. *Ear and Hearing* 39(2):204–214.

Pequeno, N. P. F., N. L. A. Cabral, D. M. Marchioni, S. Lima, and C. O. Lyra. 2020. Quality of life assessment instruments for adults: A systematic review of population-based studies. *Health and Quality of Life Outcomes* 18(1):208.

Pichora-Fuller, K. 2023. *Is hearing loss in older adults predictive of later development of dementia and does hearing care modify dementia risk?* https://canadianaudiologist.ca/is-hearing-loss-in-older-adults-predictive-of-later-development-of-dementia-and-does-hearing-care-modify-dementia-risk (accessed March 11, 2025).

Pichora-Fuller, M. K., S. E. Kramer, M. A. Eckert, B. Edwards, B. W. Hornsby, L. E. Humes, U. Lemke, T. Lunner, M. Matthen, and C. L. Mackersie. 2016. Hearing impairment and cognitive energy: The Framework for Understanding Effortful Listening (FUEL). *Ear and Hearing* 37:5S–27S.

Pumford, J., and S. Sinclair. 2001. *Real-ear measurement: Basic terminology and procedures.* https://www.audiologyonline.com/articles/real-ear-measurement-basic-terminology-1229 (accessed March 31, 2025).

Ray, J., G. Popli, and G. Fell. 2018. Association of cognition and age-related hearing impairment in the English Longitudinal Study of Ageing. *JAMA Otolaryngology—Head & Neck Surgery* 144(10):876–882.

Reed, N. S., A. Altan, J. A. Deal, C. Yeh, A. D. Kravetz, M. Wallhagen, and F. R. Lin. 2019. Trends in health care costs and utilization associated with untreated hearing loss over 10 years. *JAMA Otolaryngology–Head & Neck Surgery* 145(1):27–34.

Reed, N. S., E. Garcia-Morales, and A. Willink. 2021. Trends in hearing aid ownership among older adults in the United States from 2011 to 2018. *JAMA Internal Medicine* 181(3):383–385.

Richter, M. 2016. The moderating effect of success importance on the relationship between listening demand and listening effort. *Ear and Hearing* 37:111S–117S.

Ricketts, T. A., R. Bentler, and H. G. Mueller. 2017. *Essentials of modern hearing aids: Selection, fitting, and verification.* San Diego, CA: Plural Publishing.

Reuben, D. B., S. Kremen, and D. T. Maust. 2024. Dementia prevention and treatment: A narrative review. *JAMA Internal Medicine* 184(5):563–572.

Ruben, R. J. 2000. Redefining the survival of the fittest: Communication disorders in the 21st century. *Laryngoscope* 110(2 Pt 1):241–245.

Rutherford, B. R., K. Brewster, J. S. Golub, A. H. Kim, and S. P. Roose. 2018. Sensation and psychiatry: Linking age-related hearing loss to late-life depression and cognitive decline. *American Journal of Psychiatry* 175(3):215–224.

Samitz, G., M. Egger, and M. Zwahlen. 2011. Domains of physical activity and all-cause mortality: Systematic review and dose–response meta-analysis of cohort studies. *International Journal of Epidemiology* 40(5):1382–1400.

Scollie, S., R. Seewald, L. Cornelisse, S. Moodie, M. Bagatto, D. Laurnagaray, S. Beaulac, and J. Pumford. 2005. The desired sensation level multistage input/output algorithm. *Trends in Amplification* 9(4):159–197.

Scollie, S., M. Bagatto, S. Moodie, and J. Crukley. 2011. Accuracy and reliability of a real-ear-to-coupler difference measurement procedure implemented within a behind-the-ear hearing aid. *Journal of the American Academy of Audiology* 22(9):612–622.

Shields, C., M. Sladen, I. A. Bruce, K. Kluk, and J. Nichani. 2023. Exploring the correlations between measures of listening effort in adults and children: A systematic review with narrative synthesis. *Trends in Hearing* 27:23312165221137116.

Shukla, A., M. Harper, E. Pedersen, A. Goman, J. J. Suen, C. Price, J. Applebaum, M. Hoyer, F. R. Lin, and N. S. Reed. 2020. Hearing loss, loneliness, and social isolation: A systematic review. *Otolaryngology–Head and Neck Surgery* 162(5):622–633.

Simpson, A. N., K. N. Simpson, and J. R. Dubno. 2016. Higher health care costs in middle-aged U.S. adults with hearing loss. *JAMA Otolaryngology—Head & Neck Surgery* 142(6):607–609.

Smith, M. L., M. B. Winn, and M. B. Fitzgerald. 2024. A large-scale study of the relationship between degree and type of hearing loss and recognition of speech in quiet and noise. *Ear and Hearing* 45(4):915–928.

Snow, C. E., and R. C. Abrams. 2016. The indirect costs of late-life depression in the United States: A literature review and perspective. *Geriatrics (Basel)* 1(4):30.

Solheim, J., K. J. Kvaerner, and E. S. Falkenberg. 2011. Daily life consequences of hearing loss in the elderly. *Disability and Rehabilitation* 33(23–24):2179–2185.

Stevens, M. N., J. R. Dubno, M. I. Wallhagen, and D. L. Tucci. 2019. Communication and healthcare: Self-reports of people with hearing loss in primary care settings. *Clinical Gerontologist* 42(5):485–494.

Stika, C. J., and R. D. Hays. 2016. Development and psychometric evaluation of a health-related quality of life instrument for individuals with adult-onset hearing loss. *International Journal of Audiology* 55(7):381–391.

Strawbridge, W. J., M. I. Wallhagen, S. J. Shema, and G. A. Kaplan. 2000. Negative consequences of hearing impairment in old age: A longitudinal analysis. *Gerontologist* 40(3):320–326.

Stucky, S. R., K. E. Wolf, and T. Kuo. 2010. The economic effect of age-related hearing loss: National, state, and local estimates, 2002 and 2030. *Journal of the American Geriatrics Society* 58(3):618–619.

Teoli, D., and A. Bhardwaj. 2023. Quality of life. In *Statpearls*. Treasure Island, FL: StatPearls Publishing. Pp. 435–441.

Thoits, P. A. 2011. Mechanisms linking social ties and support to physical and mental health. *Journal of Health and Social Behavior* 52(2):145–161.

Thompson, B. S., K. Lee, J. G. Casali, and K. M. Cave. 2024. Development and human factors evaluation of a portable auditory localization training system. *Human Factors* 66(10):2393–2408.

Tseng, Y. C., S. H. Liu, M. F. Lou, and G. S. Huang. 2018. Quality of life in older adults with sensory impairments: A systematic review. *Quality of Life Research* 27(8):1957–1971.

Uhlmann, R. F., E. B. Larson, T. S. Rees, T. D. Koepsell, and L. G. Duckert. 1989. Relationship of hearing impairment to dementia and cognitive dysfunction in older adults. *JAMA* 261(13):1916–1919.

Unger, J. B., G. McAvay, M. L. Bruce, L. Berkman, and T. Seeman. 1999. Variation in the impact of social network characteristics on physical functioning in elderly persons: MacArthur Studies of Successful Aging. *Journals of Gerontology. Series B, Psychological Sciences and Social Sciences* 54(5):S245–S251.

Vaisberg, J. M., P. Folkeard, J. Pumford, P. Narten, and S. Scollie. 2018. Evaluation of the repeatability and accuracy of the wideband real-ear-to-coupler difference. *Journal of the American Academy of Audiology* 29(06):520–532.

Valtorta, N. K., M. Kanaan, S. Gilbody, S. Ronzi, and B. Hanratty. 2016. Loneliness and social isolation as risk factors for coronary heart disease and stroke: Systematic review and meta-analysis of longitudinal observational studies. *Heart* 102(13):1009–1016.

Victory, J. 2021. *The impact of hearing loss on relationship*. https://www.healthyhearing.com/report/52619-The-impact-of-hearing-loss-on-relationships (accessed June 10, 2024).

Wartinger, F., H. Malyuk, and C. D. Portnuff. 2019. Human exposures and their associated hearing loss profiles: Music industry professionals. *Journal of the Acoustical Society of America* 146(5):3906–3910.

Wells, T. S., L. Wu, G. R. Bhattarai, L. D. Nickels, S. R. Rush, and C. S. Yeh. 2019. Self-reported hearing loss in older adults is associated with higher emergency department visits and medical costs. *Inquiry* 56:46958019896907.

WHO (World Health Organization). 2001. *International classification of functioning, disability, and health*. Geneva, Switzerland: WHO.

WHO. 2012. *Programme on Mental Health: WHOQOL user manual.* https://iris.who.int/handle/10665/77932 (accessed December 30, 2024).

WHO. 2021. *World report on hearing.* https://www.who.int/publications/i/item/9789240020481 (accessed December 27, 2024).

WHO. 2022a. *Mental disorders.* https://www.who.int/news-room/fact-sheets/detail/mental-disorders (accessed June 18, 2024).

WHO. 2022b. *Mental health.* https://www.who.int/news-room/fact-sheets/dtail/mental-health-strengthening-our-response (accessed June 11, 2024).

Wilson, R. H. 2011. Clinical experience with the Words-in-Noise test on 3430 veterans: Comparisons with pure-tone thresholds and word recognition in quiet. *Journal of the American Academy of Audiology* 22(07):405–423.

Yeo, B. S. Y., H. Song, E. M. S. Toh, L. S. Ng, C. S. H. Ho, R. Ho, R. A. Merchant, B. K. J. Tan, and W. S. Loh. 2023. Association of hearing aids and cochlear implants with cognitive decline and dementia: A systematic review and meta-analysis. *JAMA Neurology* 80(2):134–141.

Yin, S., R. Njai, L. Barker, P. Z. Siegel, and Y. Liao. 2016. Summarizing health-related quality of life (HRQoL): Development and testing of a one-factor model. *Population Health Metrics* 14:1–9.

Zheng, Y., J. Swanson, J. Koehnke, and J. Guan. 2022. Sound localization of listeners with normal hearing, impaired hearing, hearing aids, bone-anchored hearing instruments, and cochlear implants: A review. *American Journal of Audiology* 31(3):819–834.

6

Measurement of the Core Outcome Set

This report focuses on meaningful outcomes and the measures used to evaluate the efficacy and effectiveness of interventions, rather than focusing on the types of assessments used to diagnose hearing loss or determine candidacy for various devices. As part of its initial work in gathering evidence for potential core outcomes and importance to measure, the committee assembled a list of some of the most commonly used outcome measures across all the outcomes and outcome domains identified in Chapter 5 (see Appendix B). The committee used evidence of the existence and overall quality of measures to help determine the core outcome set (see Chapter 5). Then, the committee initiated a more in-depth analysis of individual measures for the core outcomes of understanding speech in complex listening situations and hearing-related psychosocial health. This chapter starts with a brief history of outcome measurement for hearing health interventions. Next the chapter details the committee's process and criteria for evaluating measures. Finally, the committee presents its individual analyses and recommendations regarding which measures should be used for each core outcome.

THE HISTORY OF ASSESSING HEARING HEALTH OUTCOMES

One of the earliest comprehensive protocols for the evaluation of hearing outcomes targeted veterans who returned from military service during World War II with hearing loss (Carhart, 1946). The hearing aid evaluation and fitting process included several steps and components, but two key elements were the measurement of speech understanding in noise under controlled conditions and the collection of self-report information from the hearing

151

aid wearer. For the next several decades, the focus of outcome measurement was confined to measuring the benefits of hearing aids using standardized measures of understanding speech in quiet and in noise. Typically, this involved obtaining percent-correct scores for standardized lists of words or sentences in quiet and in noise under controlled measurement conditions. Clinicians had to make several decisions regarding the speech materials, the speech presentation level, and the type and nature of the competing background noise. Recognizing that many standardized measures of speech understanding failed to capture the extent of communication difficulties (unaided) and the relative improvement with amplification, multiple self-report measures of hearing difficulties were developed in the 1980s (Erdman, 2014).

Walden (1997) described the rationale and procedures for a "model clinical trials protocol" to assess the benefits of hearing aid interventions. The protocol recommended that speech understanding be evaluated in the clinic at each of three speech levels, each with corresponding signal-to-noise ratios (SNRs) for that particular speech level. The speech levels and SNRs were designed to span the range likely to be encountered in everyday life (Pearsons et al., 1977). In addition to these measures of speech recognition, a self-report measure focused on speech communication in a variety of contexts, the 66-item Profile of Hearing Aid Benefit (PHAB), also was recommended (Cox and Gilmore, 1990). The model for a clinical trials protocol to evaluate the benefits of hearing aids proposed by Walden focused exclusively on speech communication, an important dimension of hearing-aid outcome, but certainly not the sole dimension of importance to those with hearing difficulties (Walden, 1997). The 66-item PHAB was quickly found to be too long for routine clinical application and an abbreviated PHAB, the 24-item Abbreviated PHAB (APHAB), was developed and evaluated (Cox and Alexander, 1995). (See later in this chapter for more on the APHAB.)

In the 1980s, additional self-report measures were developed recognizing the importance of the potential negative psychosocial consequences of hearing difficulties beyond those affecting communication directly. These include the Communication Profile for the Hearing Impaired (CPHI) (see Chapter 4), various versions of the Hearing Handicap Inventory (see later in this chapter), and the Glasgow Hearing Aid Benefit Profile (see Chapter 4). Recognizing that hearing difficulties entail more than problems with speech communication, the Speech, Spatial and Qualities of Hearing Scale (SSQ) was developed (Gatehouse and Noble, 2004). (See later in this chapter for more on the SSQ.)

Comparison of Measures

Throughout the proliferation of self-report hearing-aid outcome measures in the 1980s and 1990s, few studies compared the results across outcome measures to assess the independence of each. A series of studies sought to remedy this by obtaining multiple outcomes across several presumably independent outcome domains from a large number of adults fitted with hearing aids and then performed factor analyses on the results (Cox et al., 2007; Dillon et al., 1997; Humes, 1999, 2003; Humes and Krull, 2012; Humes et al., 2001, 2017). These analyses identified considerable redundancy among the outcome measures included, ranging from 10 to 26 in number across studies, with from 3 to 7 outcome dimensions identified in the ensuing factor analyses. The most common outcomes across all studies and analyses were clinically measured speech-understanding performance (aided only) or benefit (aided/unaided) most often measured in noise, self-reported benefit and satisfaction (always loaded together on a single factor), and daily usage (self-reported or data logging) (Humes and Krull, 2012). When measures of hearing-related social and emotional difficulties were included, this emerged as a separate outcome domain.

Among hearing aid wearers, behavioral measures are weakly correlated with self-report measures (Cox and Alexander, 1992; Cox et al., 2007; Dornhoffer et al., 2020; Humes et al., 2017; Stenbäck et al., 2023; Walden and Walden, 2004). Dornhoffer and colleagues (2020) suggested that the reason for these low correlations is that "hearing aid users' real-world listening environments [assessed with self-report measures] are more varied than can be predicted by simple audiologic measures [of speech understanding]" (p. 7). Overall, the evidence indicates that speech communication measured in the sound booth with standardized behavioral materials under controlled conditions and by self-report capture different aspects of speech communication.

On the surface, the self-report measures of speech communication would appear to be superior to those obtained behaviorally in the sound booth owing to their more direct connection to the everyday communication situations experienced by the individual with hearing difficulties, but these measures also are subject to bias. For example, individuals seeking treatment may want to feel good about the decision they have made or the time and money they have expended and therefore report more positive findings. A behavioral measure along with a self-report measure may provide a fuller picture of the outcome of interest, although the limited research available suggests both types of measures may be subject to placebo effects (Dawes et al., 2011, 2013). Generally, from the model clinical trial protocol of Walden (1997) to more recent comparative evaluations of hearing-aid technologies (e.g., Cox et al., 2014, 2016; Johnson et al., 2016, 2017), a combination of behavioral and self-report measures of outcomes has been implemented.

How and When to Measure Outcomes

Once core outcomes have been identified, decisions must be made about how and when to measure them (Clarke and Williamson, 2016;

Gatehouse, 2000). For many outcomes, one must choose among the many available measures for that outcome. In addition, some self-report measures require baseline and postintervention measurements separately whereas others can be administered postintervention only. For self-report measures, additional issues of how the survey is administered, paper-and-pencil versus electronically, as well as how they are scored, must be taken into consideration. For example, the mode of administration of the Hearing Handicap Inventory for the Elderly (HHIE) can affect the scores obtained as well as the test-retest reliability (Thorén et al., 2012; Weinstein et al., 1986).

The appropriate timing of outcome measurement will depend on the context, including the type of intervention. For example, various studies show that the intervals for measurement of outcomes after hearing aid intervention range from 1 week to 3 years postintervention; these assessments most commonly occur approximately 4 to 6 weeks after the hearing aid fitting (Bentler et al., 1993a,b; Cox and Alexander, 1992; Cox et al., 2007; Cox and Rivera, 1992; Dawes et al., 2014; Dawes and Munro, 2017; Humes et al., 1996, 2002, 2003; Saunders and Cienkowski, 1997; Surr et al., 1998; Wright and Gagné, 2021). As outcomes beyond hearing and communication are examined, longer periods of hearing-aid use may be required to achieve stable outcomes (Allen et al., 2022; Mulrow et al., 1992b). Additionally, other types of interventions such as pharmaceuticals and biologics may require different intervals to show effectiveness not only of the therapeutic substance at or immediately after the time of administration but also the sustained effects of the intervention after the prescribed period of treatment ends.

COMMITTEE PROCESS AND CRITERIA

As noted earlier, the committee created an inventory of measures for each of the candidate outcomes identified in Chapter 5 in order to inform its final conclusions for the core outcome set. Ultimately, the committee recommended that two outcomes should be included in the core outcome set: understanding speech in complex listening situations and hearing-related psychosocial health. For these outcomes, the committee prioritized in-depth evaluation for those measures with with a sufficient amount and quality of evidence regarding their development and testing. Several measures were ruled out of consideration for a range of reasons. For example, some measures were eliminated from consideration because they are primarily used for diagnostic assessment but are not appropriate as outcome measures. Others were eliminated because they are not broadly accessible. For example, some measures are subject to copyright restrictions (e.g., CPHI) or are currently not available for purchase for clinical use (e.g., the Hearing in Noise Test [HINT]). The committee focused on the in-depth evaluation of measures that were accessible to clinicians and researchers in both research and clinical settings.

The committee performed a comprehensive literature search for each remaining measure looking for studies related to the psychometric characteristics and scientific development of the measure. Overall, the committee considered descriptive elements of these studies for each measure (including population studied, number of participants, setting, and clinical unit of interpretation). Then, the committee assessed the strengths and weaknesses of each measure by examining evidence for two broad criteria: scientific acceptability (including reliability, validity, and sensitivity to change) and feasibility. While the committee recognizes that responsiveness (or sensitivity to change) may be viewed as a part of validity (rather than a distinct property) (Hays and Hadorn, 1992), the committee kept sensitivity to change as a separate criterion based, in part, on the criteria used in the COnsensus-based Standards for the selection of health Measurement INstruments (COSMIN) initiative described in Chapter 3. (See Appendix C for the committee's worksheet for evaluation of scientific acceptability.) The results of the individual analyses for the candidate outcome measures are presented later in this chapter. The committee notes that no single measure had robust evidence supporting all the criteria considered.

Scientific Acceptability

Scientific acceptability is the "extent to which the measure produces reliable and valid results about the intended area of measurement. These qualities determine whether use of the measure can draw reasonable conclusions about care in a given domain" (CMS, 2024). The definitions of the components of scientific acceptability that the committee adopted from COSMIN are displayed in Table 6-1 (COSMIN, 2024).

First the committee evaluated the measure's validity or the extent to which the results of a measurement reflect the construct or outcome of interest. In other words, does the test measure what it was intended to measure? Scientific acceptability was the first criterion because the measure needed to have evidence of at least face validity in order to continue with its consideration. The committee also looked for evidence of criterion validity, internal consistency, structural validity, areas of potential measurement error, and evidence that the measure is predictive of everyday performance.

Next, the committee evaluated the measure's reliability, which is the degree to which the result of a measurement, calculation, or specification is repeatable or consistent. The committee looked for evidence of test-retest reliability, meaning that the results were consistent when the measure was repeated, and interrater reliability, meaning that the results were consistent between different raters (people administering the measurement).

TABLE 6-1 Definitions of Scientific Acceptability

Measurement Property	Definition According to the COSMIN Taxonomy
Content validity (including face validity)	The degree to which the content of a measurement instrument is an adequate reflection of the construct to be measured
Reliability	The degree to which the measurement is free from measurement error
Responsiveness[a]	The ability of a measurement instrument to detect change over time in the construct to be measured
Internal consistency	The degree of interrelatedness among the items of the assessment
Structural validity	The degree to which the scores of a measurement instrument are an adequate reflection of the dimensionality of the construct to be measured
Measurement error	The systematic and random error of a patient's score that is not attributed to true changes in the construct to be measured
Criterion validity	The degree to which the scores of a measurement instrument are an adequate reflection of a "gold standard"

[a] Responsiveness is also known as sensitivity to change—the ability of the measure to accurately document a meaningful change in an outcome
NOTE: COSMIN = COnsensus-based Standards for the selection of health Measurement INstruments.
SOURCES: COSMIN, 2024; Prinsen et al., 2016. CC BY 4.0.

Finally, the committee considered the measure's responsiveness or sensitivity to change. In the context of health-related patient-reported outcome measures, sensitivity to change is the "ability of an instrument to detect significant change in health status over time" (Toussaint et al., 2020, p. 395). Where possible, the committee noted the percentage of participants whose scores were at ceiling and at floor. The committee deemed it to be critical that selected measures accurately reflect the change in an outcome resulting from the intervention. (See later in this chapter for a fuller discussion of interpreting changes in measure scores [i.e., statistical approaches for evaluating a measure's responsiveness].)

Feasibility

The feasibility of a measure is the extent to which the measure requires data, processes, or equipment that are readily available or easily performed without undue burden (CMS, 2024). The feasibility of a measure varies greatly by setting. The burden can fall on the patient as respondent fatigue from long questionnaires, on the clinician by requiring excessive time to administer (and score) the measure during a short appointment, or on researchers by requiring an unrealistic amount of time or money to implement. When performing its measure analyses, the committee considered three main criteria: (1) whether the data required for the measure are readily available (or easily captured) in both research and clinical settings; (2) whether there are clear instructions for administering, scoring, and interpreting the measure; and (3) the time needed for administration and scoring. The committee considered feasibility for each measure individually, but also collectively for the battery of core outcomes to be measured in a core set.

UNDERSTANDING SPEECH IN COMPLEX LISTENING SITUATIONS

Many measures exist for the evaluation of understanding speech in complex listening situations (primarily understanding speech in noise). The committee considered both behavioral measures as well as self-report measures. Behavioral measures capture outcomes in a controlled environment while self-report measures capture real-world experiences. However, before proceeding to a review of the specific measures, a general overview of these measures is provided.

Historically, a wide array of measures of speech understanding have been developed and evaluated. These measures are varied in the type of speech material used, with most using phonemes (distinct units of sound), nonsense syllables, words, or sentences. The measures also vary regarding the type of competition used, most frequently including various types of noise (e.g., white noise, speech-shaped noise) or competing speech (e.g., single-talker, multiple talker). These measures also employ a variety of response formats, including closed-set speech identification and open-set speech recognition as the most common alternatives. Finally, most of these measures fall into two general categories of procedure.

One option prescribes the speech and noise levels to be used and measures the percentage of test items correctly identified or recognized. In the other main approach, the speech or noise level is fixed, and the level of the other variable is varied adaptively to achieve a criterion level of performance. For example, the speech level may be fixed at 70 decibels (dB) sound pressure level and the competing noise or speech adjusted to bracket 50 percent correct, often referred to as the speech recognition threshold (SRT). Alternatively, the noise level may be fixed at 70 dB sound pressure level and the speech level adjusted to reach SRT. The measured SRT can be reported as the final value of the speech or noise level adjusted to achieve 50 percent-correct performance but, more often, it is reported as the relative difference in these two levels: the SNR in dB for 50 percent-correct performance.

Behavioral measures of understanding speech in complex listening situations were originally developed as efficient measures for use in diagnosis, including screening for hearing loss (e.g., Smits et al., 2006). To ensure consistency of results across time and clinics, the testing materials, conditions, and procedures have been highly standardized for each individual measure. Typically, testing is completed using earphones in a sound-treated test booth. Although desirable for consistency of results, this has often constrained the usefulness of such tests as measures of everyday hearing function. High and colleagues (1964) developed a self-report measure to capture hearing difficulties experienced in everyday life. Other self-report measures followed, many focused primarily on a detailed examination of speech communication in everyday situations (Cox and Alexander, 1995; Cox and Gilmore, 1990; Cox and Rivera, 1992; Demorest and Walden, 1984; Giolas et al., 1979; Johnson et al., 2010; Lamb et al., 1983).

In studies that have evaluated both behavioral and self-report measures of speech-understanding in adults, the correlations are typically weak to moderate, suggesting 16 to 36 percent overlap between these two types of measures for the same outcome; self-report measures appear to be as or more sensitive to the benefits provided by hearing intervention (e.g., Cox et al., 2003; Humes, 2003; Humes et al., 2017). In these studies, using both types of outcome measures, self-reported benefit was often significant in the absence of statistically significant differences in behavioral measures obtained in noise.

More recently, a study demonstrated that amplification provided clinically significant benefit on their behavioral measure of speech-in-noise performance for 53 percent of the participants in their randomized controlled trial. In contrast, the APHAB global benefit scores, their self-report measure, revealed statistically significant improvements in 77 percent of the participants (De Sousa et al., 2023).

Other studies contrast in that hearing aid benefit was shown in both self-report and behavioral outcome measures. For example, Perron and colleagues (2023) recently demonstrated statistically significant improvements in performance on the Quick Speech-in-Noise (QuickSIN) test with amplification relative to unaided performance, with a large effect size (0.53), and they also reported significant difference in self-reported listening effort ratings parallel to the QuickSIN differences. The clinical significance of the change must be considered for both behavioral and self-report measures. With respect to behavioral measures, McShefferty and colleagues (2016) demonstrated that, regardless of the specific SNR-based test used, the SNR change must be at least 3 dB to be detectable and at least 6 dB to be considered meaningful. Given that there are few data available that address the responsiveness of SNR-based speech-understanding measures like the QuickSIN and the Words-in-Noise (WIN) test to hearing-aid interventions, additional research is needed. Self-reported hearing difficulty and behavioral measures are correlated, although the significant individual variability in both may reduce sensitivity for measurement of intervention effects at the individual level (see, for example, Fitzgerald and colleagues [2024] who explored relationships between QuickSIN SNR and SSQ-speech scale scores).

Conclusion 6-1: Both a behavioral measure and a patient-reported outcome measure are needed to evaluate the core outcome of understanding speech in complex listening situations. While behavioral measures have face validity, are considered by some to be more objective, and are readily available, these measures lack data on their sensitivity to change and do not necessarily correlate with the individual's perception of their improvement.

Behavioral Measures

The following sections present evidence regarding behavioral (objective) measures of understanding speech in complex listening situations considered for in-depth analysis by the committee.

Audible Contrast Threshold Test

Given that most behavioral measures share a limitation with respect to the effects of native language, the committee was interested in options that are language agnostic. Few such tests are available, and data are limited for the emerging measures. The one commercially available test identified was the Audible Contrast Threshold (ACT) test. The ACT is a spectro-temporal modulation detection test; it uses modulated noise to determine the amount of contrast an individual needs to identify a difference between signals (Zaar et al., 2024). The committee reviewed two articles pertaining to the development and validation of the ACT (Zaar et al., 2023, 2024). The ACT strongly predicts other speech-in-noise measurements. This test is unique because it is language agnostic. The test requires less than 2 minutes on average to administer and currently is included on two commercially available audiometers. The test has moderate scientific acceptability and moderate test-retest data.

Conclusion 6-2: The ACT may be a promising measure, but it is new and lacks enough evidence to be recommended at this time.

AzBio Sentence Test

The AzBio Sentence Test has 33 lists of 20 recorded sentences in both male and female voices (Holder et al., 2018). The individual with hearing difficulties is presented these lists both in quiet and with a twenty-talker babble at SNR ratios of +10, +5, –, –5, and –10 dB. The individual is asked to repeat each sentence to the best of their ability. The sentences are more challenging than other tests, making them potentially more reflective of the patient's everyday experiences (Spahr et al., 2012). This test is appropriate for use in clinic and lab settings.

The committee reviewed six articles pertaining to the development and validation of the AzBio Sentence Test (Advanced Bionics LLC et al., 2011; Holder et al., 2018; Patro et al., 2024; Schafer et al., 2012; Spahr et al., 2012; Vermiglio et al., 2021). The scientific acceptability of this test is acceptable. In addition, the test-retest correlations were moderate. The Az-Bio requires 5 to 7 minutes to administer, somewhat limiting the feasibility. This test is most commonly used as a candidacy measure and for evaluating cochlear implants, which are outside the scope of this report. The committee concluded that the AzBio Sentence Test is not an appropriate outcome measure for evaluating the effectiveness of hearing interventions for the populations and treatments included in the scope of this report.

Conclusion 6-3: The AzBio Sentence Test has primarily been used as a candidacy measure and for evaluating cochlear implants. Additionally, the measure takes 5 to 7 minutes to administer making it less feasible than other behavioral measures. There is insufficient evidence to support the recommendation of the AzBio as an outcome measure for evaluating the effectiveness of hearing health interventions other than cochlear implants at this time.

Digits-in-Noise

The Digits-in-Noise (DIN) test was designed for clinical use and consists of digit triplets recorded by a male speaker measuring the speech reception threshold (the level of noise at which the person can no longer correctly repeat the digits). The committee reviewed 28 articles pertaining to the development and validation of DIN test (Armstrong et al., 2020; De Sousa et al., 2020a,b, 2023; Folmer et al., 2017, 2021; Hoth, 2016; Jansen et al., 2012, 2013; Koole et al., 2016; Kwak et al., 2022; Lyzenga and Smits, 2011; Melo et al., 2022; Motlagh Zadeh et al., 2021; Oremule et al., 2024; Potgieter et al., 2015, 2018a,b; Reynard et al., 2022; Roup et al., 2018; Schimmel et al., 2024; Śliwińska-Kowalska, 2020; Smits et al., 2013; Van den Borre et al., 2021; Wang and Wong, 2024; Watson et al., 2012; Wilson and Weakley, 2004; Wright and Gagné, 2021).

The DIN takes about 2 minutes to administer and is available in over a dozen languages making it highly feasible in the clinic and research settings. While there are some commonalities across tests in that the same digits are used across tests, it should be noted that not all studies use a standardized test. Digits are recorded with different speakers and used with different noise backgrounds across studies. The test has documented evidence of scientific acceptability, and DIN performance is strongly correlated with scores on word or sentence in noise tests. It is an effective screening tool for hearing loss. The greatest concern is that the test may not be sensitive to hearing interventions, including hearing aids, but this has not been studied frequently. Rather, most research on the DIN has been as an assessment of hearing sensitivity, substituting for measures like the audiogram. Without additional research, the committee concluded that the DIN is not an appropriate outcome measure for evaluating the effectiveness of hearing interventions.

Conclusion 6-4: The DIN has primarily been used as a diagnostic measure. There is insufficient evidence to support the recommendation of the DIN as an outcome measure for evaluating the effectiveness of hearing health interventions at this time.

Quick Speech-in-Noise Test

As the name implies, the QuickSIN estimates SNR hearing loss quickly (Killion et al., 2004). It consists of sets of six sentences, each sentence with five key words at a 70 dB hearing level presentation with a four-talker babble in the background; only repetition of the key words affects the score (Billings et al., 2023; Interacoustics, 2022; Killion et al., 2004). The level of the target speech remains constant while the level of the background babble increases by 5 dB after each sentence (Billings et al., 2023). The SNR's range from easy to difficult (i.e., 25, 20, 15, 10, 5 and 0) (Interacoustics, 2022). The QuickSIN is scored as an SNR deficit relative to normative population performance, with normative performance considered to be 2 dB SNR according to the QuickSin Instructions for Use (Interacoustics, 2022). The QuickSIN is only available in English at this time (Auditdata, n.d.).

The committee reviewed 15 articles pertaining to the development and validation of the QuickSIN (Bentler, 2000; Billings et al., 2023; De Sousa et al., 2023; Fitzgerald et al., 2023; Killion et al., 2004; Killion and Villchur, 1993; Kraus et al., 2011; McArdle and Wilson, 2006; McArdle et al., 2005; Mendel, 2007; Ou and Wetmore, 2020; Phatak et al., 2018; Sabin et al., 2020; Walden and Walden, 2004; Wilson et al., 2007b). The QuickSIN has strong criterion validity and correlates well with other measures of speech in noise. The test has strong homogeneity showing internal consistency. There is a lack of evidence on the reliability and consistency of the measurement over time. The minimal detectable difference is +/– 2.7 dB signal-to-babble ratio with a 95 percent confidence level when performance on two lists is averaged.

An analysis of the equivalency of the 18 QuickSIN lists revealed that "the psychometric functions for each list showed high-performance variability across lists for listeners with hearing loss but not for listeners with normal hearing" (McArdle and Wilson, 2006, p. 157). Furthermore, the analysis showed that 4 lists fell outside the critical difference for listeners with hearing loss, and 9 lists "provide homogenous results for listeners with and without hearing loss." The QuickSIN takes about a minute to administer each sentence set and two sentence sets are recommended, making it highly feasible (Mueller, 2016). Although the measure is familiar to clinicians, it is only available in English.

The committee noted weak evidence for the recommended 2-dB normative threshold value in its review of the evidence. Specifically, Killion and colleagues (2004) use the 2-dB normative threshold and attribute the 2-dB normative value to previous studies (Bentler, 2000; Killion and Niquette, 2000; Killion et al., 1996). However, the cited study by Killion and colleagues (1996) was not available to the committee as this was a conference proceedings, and a review of Bentler (2000) did not yield strong supporting evidence for the 2-dB SNR as a normative reference as Bentler's sample included only 40 adults (20 with normal hearing and 20 with sloping hearing loss, with equal numbers of males and females in the two groups).

Bentler (2000) does not explicitly report SNR threshold, but extrapolation of the data in Figure 4 of that report would yield a 50 percent threshold of approximately 2-dB for the subset of 20 participants with normal hearing. The committee additionally reviewed Killion and Niquette (2000) for supporting evidence for the 2-dB normative threshold. Killion and Niquette (2000) referenced Killion and Villchur (1993) as the source for the 2-dB reference value for normal hearing individuals. When reviewed, Killion and Villchur (1993) was found to include case data for 6 participants (3 younger adults and 3 older adults). A similarly sized cohort (18 women, 6 men) with normal hearing was evaluated by Wilson and colleagues (2007a,b) using the QuickSIN, WIN, the HINT, and the Bamford-Kowal-Bench Speech-in-Noise (BKB-SIN) test. The study found that the 50 percent point in the psychometric data for normal hearing listeners was 3.1 dB for list 1 and 4.1 dB for list 8, with an average threshold of 3.5 dB for those two lists. More recent data from Fitzgerald and colleagues (2023) demonstrate significant variability in Quick-SIN dB SNR loss scores across patients with normal audiometric thresholds. Although the QuickSIN test appears well suited for use in clinical and research settings, additional research with larger samples would be helpful in evaluating whether 2-dB is representative of a larger normal-hearing cohort.

Conclusion 6-5: The QuickSIN is a good candidate to consider for inclusion in a core outcome set.

Words-in-Noise Test

The WIN provides a dB signal-to-babble ratio threshold based on percent correct performance during administration of prerecorded monosyllabic words presented against a multitalker babble background (Wilson et al., 2005, 2007a). The test was originally developed with 70-word lists (Wilson and Strous, 2002; Wilson et al., 2003). Later, to improve efficiency, the test was modified to consist of trials with lists each containing 35 words (Wilson, 2003; Wilson and Burks, 2005). First, the words are presented at 84 dB hearing level with a background six-person babble at 60 dB hearing level. Every five words, the signal level drops 4 dB while the background stays constant, thus the SNR becomes poorer (more difficult) as the test progresses. Each word is scored as correct or incorrect. A stopping rule is implemented when all words are missed at a given SNR, decreasing the total test time for patients with significant functional deficits (Wilson and Burks, 2005). The WIN takes from 4 to 6 minutes to administer and has been recommended for clinical use (Mueller, 2016; Toolbox Assessments, Inc., 2024; Wilson and McArdle, 2007).

The committee reviewed 17 articles pertaining to the development and validation of the WIN (Billings et al., 2023; McArdle et al., 2005; McLean et al., 2021; Mehrkian et al., 2019; Wilson, 2003, 2011; Wilson et al., 2003, 2005, 2006, 2007a,b, 2012; Wilson and Burks, 2005; Wilson and Cates, 2008; Wilson and McArdle, 2007; Wilson and Strouse, 2002; Wilson and Watts, 2012). The WIN has strong criterion validity and correlates well with other measures of speech in noise. It has been benchmarked relative to the BKB-SIN, the HINT, and QuickSIN (Wilson et al., 2007b), digit triplets in noise (Wilson et al., 2006), and the Speech Recognition in Noise Test (Wilson and Cates, 2008).

The psychometric development of the WIN was very strong, and test-retest reliability for each of the word lists is well documented, in addition to documentation of the equivalency of the difficulty of the word lists. Participants with hearing loss typically have WIN thresholds that are 7 to 10 dB poorer than participants with hearing thresholds that are 20 to 25 dB hearing level or better (Wilson et al., 2007b). Based on test-retest data and 95 percent confidence intervals for true change, the minimal detectable difference is 3.5 dB signal-to-babble ratio (Wilson and McArdle, 2007).

A shortcoming of the WIN is that the majority of the development of the WIN was based on data from a largely male veteran population. A strength of the WIN is that it is included in the NIH (National Institutes of Health) ToolBox (Toolbox Assessments, Inc., 2024). The WIN is also available on the VA CD and comes preloaded onto some audiometers (Wilson, 2006). An additional strength of the WIN is the availability of a Spanish test form (Fox et al., 2021), although additional validation of the Spanish WIN is warranted. The NIH Toolbox for Assessment of Neurological and Behavioral Function was explicitly developed in both English and Spanish. An initial assessment of the psychometric properties of the Spanish-language version of the WIN showed that test-retest reliability was poor relative to prior literature using the English-language version, with no statistically significant correlations across test and retest data (Fox et al., 2021). However, the sample size was small, with only 9 to 10 participants contributing test-retest data.

Conclusion 6-6: The WIN is a good candidate to consider for inclusion in a core outcome set.

QuickSIN vs. WIN

The committee compared the two best candidates for a behavioral measure for the core outcome of understanding speech in complex listening situations—the QuickSIN and the WIN—using its predetermined criteria (see Appendix D for a side-by-side comparison of the psychometric evidence for the WIN and QuickSIN). Discussions of these two candidate measures considered several factors, including content validity. Word-based (WIN) and sentence-based (QuickSIN) testing in a background of competing talkers both have ecological validity for the assessment of function in a standardized representation of many everyday listening situations, but a sentence-based test is probably more representative of communication in such situations (e.g., Neal et al., 2022). In addition, some sentence-based tests draw on more top-down resources and may tap broader aspects of speech perception and listening than word-based tests (Neal et al., 2022). In addition, the committee notes that the QuickSIN, which evaluates an individual's ability to understand sentences, may be more familiar to audiologists and somewhat shorter to administer. However, psychometric evaluation of the QuickSIN shows a lack of evidence on the reliability and consistency of the measurement over time with moderate test-retest reliability. On the other hand, the WIN, which evaluates an individual's ability to understand single words, has had a much more rigorous psychometric development and evaluation (including strong test-retest reliability), is currently used as part of the NIH Toolbox, and is available in Spanish (although the committee notes that additional validation of the Spanish WIN is needed).

Conclusion 6-7: The WIN is the strongest candidate for use as a behavioral outcome measure for understanding speech in complex listening situations at this time.

Self-Report Measures

The following sections present evidence regarding self-report (subjective) measures of understanding speech in complex listening situations considered for in-depth analysis by the committee.

Abbreviated Profile of Hearing Aid Benefit

As discussed in Chapter 4, the 66-item PHAB was developed as a self-report measure of the speech-communication benefits of hearing aids in real-world situations. The measure was quickly found to be too long for routine clinical application and an abbreviated 24-item PHAB (APHAB) was developed and evaluated (Cox and Alexander, 1995). Both the PHAB and the APHAB use a 7-item response scale that asks the frequency with which the respondent experiences various hearing difficulties with responses ranging from "never (1 percent)" to "always (99 percent)," with higher scores reflecting more frequently experienced difficulties. Despite the name (due to the origin of the measure), both the PHAB and APHAB are applicable for all types of hearing interventions.

Factor analyses of PHAB scores led to the development of seven PHAB subscales, five pertaining to communication difficulties in a variety of listening conditions (i.e., ease of communication, familiar talkers, background noise, reverberation, and reduced cues) and two pertaining to the distortion and aversiveness of environmental sounds (Cox and Alexander, 1995). The APHAB retained four of the original seven PHAB subscales, but each scale was limited to 6 items; three scales pertain to communication difficulties (familiar talkers, background noise, reverberation) and one focuses on the aversiveness of environmental sounds. Several subsequent studies found the communication subscales of the APHAB to be strongly correlated and these subscales are often averaged to form a single APHAB-global score (Chisolm et al., 2005; Dornhoffer et al., 2020; Kochkin, 1997; Sabin et al., 2020). The APHAB-global scores are reliable and sensitive to change (from the use of hearing aids) (Chisolm et al., 2005; Cox and Alexander, 1995).

Although, as noted, the shorter APHAB is widely used clinically, the longer PHAB has been used frequently in clinical research, including several clinical trials comparing technologies (Haskell et al., 2002; Walden, 1997) and recent randomized controlled trials evaluating fitting methods (Humes et al., 2017; Sabin et al., 2020). The test-retest correlation was estimated to be approximately 0.85 for the PHAB- and APHAB-global baseline scores (Cox and Gilmore, 1990; Cox and Rivera, 1992; Cox and Alexander, 1995).

Overall, the committee examined nine articles pertaining to the development and validation of the PHAB and APHAB (Chisolm et al., 2005; Cox and Alexander, 1995; Cox and Gilmore, 1990; Cox and Rivera, 1992; Dornhoffer et al., 2020; Kam et al., 2011; Kochkin, 1997; Löhler et al., 2017; Sabin et al., 2020). The measure has strong psychometric evidence of reliability and validity, and there is some evidence for its sensitivity to change. The APHAB is also available in at least 20 languages (Srinivasan and O'Neill, 2023). The APHAB requires around 10 minutes or less to complete.

This is feasible for the research context but is a time commitment in the clinic; however, since it is a self-report measure, it can be completed by the patient prior to an appointment to save time. As noted, the measure has good test-retest reliability for ease of communication, reverberation, and background noise (the scales comprising the global score), and is sensitive to change, making the APHAB-global score a good candidate given its focus on the core outcome, strong psychometrics, and relative feasibility.

> *Conclusion 6-8: The APHAB-global score is a good candidate to consider for inclusion in a core outcome set.*

Speech, Spatial and Qualities of Hearing Scale

The SSQ49 is a 49-item questionnaire "designed to measure a range of hearing disabilities" including speech, spatial ability, and qualities of hearing (Gatehouse and Noble, 2004, p. 1). The SSQ49 is meant to reflect real-world hearing performance by assessing the ability to segregate sounds and understand simultaneous speech (Gatehouse and Noble, 2004). Unlike other measures that focus solely on the measurement of hearing and communication ability, the SSQ49 additionally assesses spatial hearing via ratings of ability to detect the direction, distance, and movement of speech. Of the 49 items in the original SSQ, 14 pertained to speech understanding in a variety of situations, 17 assessed spatial hearing and sound localization, and the remaining 18 items assessed various hearing abilities including sound segregation, music and voice identification, and sound source identification.

Although the developers did not perform factor analysis of the item scores, they did note that many of the SSQ items were intercorrelated both within subscales and across subscales (Gatehouse and Noble, 2004). Akeroyd and colleagues (2014) subsequently administered the 49-item SSQ to 1,220 adults and performed factor analysis (Akeroyd, 2014). Three factors were identified in that analysis, each factor largely supporting the three scales of the SSQ. Importantly, oblique rotation of factors was used, which allows for correlations among the factors in the solution; the authors reported interfactor correlations ranging from about 0.5 to 0.7. The results of this factor analysis, including the interfactor correlations, were replicated using a French version of the measure (Moulin et al., 2015). The presence of moderate to high interfactor correlations suggests considerable shared variance among the three scales of the SSQ. Consistent with this, Humes and colleagues (2013) reported that a single factor emerged in their factor analysis of the full SSQ.

To improve the efficiency of the SSQ, a variety of shortened versions have been developed and evaluated, including a 5-item screener (SSQ5) and 12-item version (SSQ12) (Demeester et al., 2012; Noble et al., 2013).

The SSQ12 was developed as a more feasible alternative to capture spatial hearing and real-world hearing more quickly, making it well suited for clinical practice; the measure is only 12 questions long and is well correlated with the SSQ49 (Noble et al., 2013). A limitation of the SSQ12 is that the subscales of the measure are not preserved; the SSQ12 yields a single overall score. Additionally, validation is limited because the 12 items were extracted from the full survey.

A newer version (French SSQ15, or 15iSSQ) contains 5 questions on each of the three subscales (Moulin et al., 2019). This version has been psychometrically evaluated on its own and verified that the scale scores, as well as the total score, were reliable and valid in adults with hearing difficulties (Moulin et al., 2019). The French SSQ15 is distinct from a German SSQ15 (Kiessling et al., 2011); the German SSQ15 does not have three distinct factors,[1] whereas the French SSQ15 does (Moulin et al., 2019).

The committee reviewed 10 articles pertaining to the development and validation of the SSQ49, SSQ12, and SSQ15 (Akeroyd et al., 2014; Banh et al., 2012; Demeester et al., 2012; Fitzgerald et al., 2024; Gatehouse and Noble, 2004; Moulin et al., 2019; Noble et al., 2012, 2013; Singh and Pichora-Fuller, 2010; Wyss et al., 2020). Six additional articles related to the validation of the SSQ49 were reviewed (Motlagh Zadeh et al., 2021; Sanchez-Lopez et al., 2022; Saxena et al., 2022; Srinivasan and O'Neill, 2023; Stenbäck et al., 2023; Utoomprurkporn et al., 2021). Major strengths of the SSQ are that the psychometric structure of both the original 49-item survey and the French 15-item survey have been carefully studied with cluster and factor analysis. The tests have good test-retest reliability, and while the tests are the most reliable when administered in interview format, reliability is still excellent when administered using paper and pencil, computer, or online formats. Use of an interview format takes more time. The test is sensitive to change and has been used to measure the effects of hearing aid and cochlear implant interventions on speech in noise and other hearing subscales.

The SSQ49 and SSQ12 are available in multiple languages including Colombian Spanish (Sanchez-Lopez et al., 2022), Turkish (Kılıç et al., 2021), Dutch (Batthyany et al., 2023), Brazilian Portuguese (Aguiar et al., 2019), Iranian (Lotfi et al., 2016), Norwegian (Myhrum et al., 2024), French (Moulin and Richard, 2016; Moulin et al., 2015), Romanian (Radulescu et al., 2024), Spanish (Cañete et al., 2022), Arabic (Alkhodair et al., 2021), and Chinese (Meng et al., 2024). The rigor of the translation and validation process was not considered as part of the review process; compliance with best practices for translating and adapting hearing-related questionnaires

---

[1] The German SSQ15 was unable to be reviewed by this committee as the full study was not translated into English (Kiessling et al., 2011).

will need to be considered if foreign language versions are used (Hall et al., 2018).

> *Conclusion 6-9: The SSQ is a good candidate to consider for inclusion in a core outcome set.*

APHAB vs. SSQ

The committee compared the two best candidates for a self-report measure for the core outcome of understanding speech in complex listening situations—the APHAB and the SSQ—using its predetermined criteria. Both measures have good evidence for reliability and validity, with some evidence for sensitivity to change, and both are available in multiple languages. One of the brief versions of the SSQ would be more feasible to administer than the full 49-item SSQ and because the French SSQ15 maintains a 5-item SSQ-Speech score, it would appear to be the best candidate for use as an outcome measure among the available SSQ measures. Compared to the APHAB-global, however, much less information is available for the French SSQ15 at this time. Both the APHAB and SSQ can take a relatively long time to administer, but as self-report measures, they could be filled out in advance by the patient. They also would not necessarily have to be administered at every visit. Overall, the 18-item APHAB-global score focuses on the scales related to scenarios of complex listening alone, which is the core outcome. The SSQ, on the other hand, includes a mix of speech, spatial location, and sound quality that are incorporated into the final score and the shorter 5-item SSQ-Speech score requires further psychometric evaluation as an outcome measure.

> *Conclusion 6-10: The APHAB-global score is the strongest candidate for use as a self-report outcome measure for understanding speech in complex listening situations at this time.*

> *Conclusion 6-11: The SSQ is a good candidate to consider for supplemental measurement (beyond the core set) when sound quality and localization are also of interest.*

HEARING-RELATED PSYCHOSOCIAL HEALTH

The following sections present evidence regarding self-report measures of hearing-related psychosocial health considered by the committee. The committee considered many measures but ultimately zeroed in on variations of the Hearing Handicap Inventory (HHI).

Hearing Handicap Inventories

The HHIE was the original 25-item self-report measure of HHI (Ventry and Weinstein, 1982, 1983). The HHIE measures emotional consequences and social/situational effects of hearing difficulties in adults 65 years of age and older. Soon after the original HHIE was published, a brief 10-item screening version, the HHIE-S was developed (Weinstein and Ventry, 1983). Subsequently, the original measure was modified to develop the HHI for adults (HHIA), which targeted adults under the age of 65 years (Newman et al., 1990). Emotional and social subscales were recommended for both the HHIE and the HHIA based primarily on the content validity of the test items. After elimination of 9 of the original 25 items of the HHIE to optimize measurement properties, Heffernan et al. (2020) found the remaining 16 items of the shortened HHIE to be unidimensional.

In 2020, two detailed psychometric item analyses of the HHIE and HHIA were published, each recommending an overall reduction in the number of questions (Cassarly et al., 2020; Heffernan et al., 2020). Cassarly and colleagues (2020), using a large community-based convenience sample, referred to their new 18-item scale as the Revised Hearing Handicap Inventory (RHHI) and developed a shorter 10-item screener as well (RHHI-S). Social and emotional subscales were not supported for the abbreviated HHI measures in either analysis. More evaluations of the RHHI measures have been completed since 2020 (Dillard et al., 2024a,b; Humes, 2021).

The committee reviewed 25 articles pertaining to the development and validation of the HHIE and HHIA (Chisolm et al., 2005; Dillon et al., 1997; Heffernan et al., 2020; Humes, 2021; Humes et al., 1996, 2001, 2002, 2003, 2017; Jerger et al., 1996; Malinoff and Weinstein, 1989; McArdle et al., 2005; Mulrow et al., 1990a,b, 1992a,b; Newman et al., 1990; Newman and Weinstein, 1988, 1989; Öberg et al., 2007; Stark and Hickson, 2004; Taylor, 1993; Ventry and Weinstein, 1982; Weinstein et al., 1986; Weinstein and Ventry, 1983), 8 articles pertaining to the development and validation of the HHIE-S (Humes, 2021; Lichtenstein et al., 1988; Lin et al., 2023; Mulrow et al., 1990b; Newman et al., 1991; Sanchez et al., 2024; Tomioka et al., 2013; Ventry and Weinstein, 1983), and 3 articles pertaining to the development and validation of the RHHI or RHHI-S (Cassarly et al., 2020; Dillard et al., 2024a,b).

In terms of administration efficiency, the HHIE requires about 10 minutes to complete, compared to the HHIE-S which takes 2–3 minutes, the RHHI which takes 5–7 minutes, and the RHHI-S which takes about 2–3 minutes.

Generally, the HHIE had the most evidence supporting sensitivity to change, including three randomized controlled trials, and both the HHIE and the HHIE-S had considerable evidence supporting adequate test-retest reliability. On the other hand, the RHHI and RHHI-S are probably the most psychometrically sound based on the item analyses by Cassarly and colleagues (2020). Given that the RHHI-based measures are a verbatim subset of original HHIE items, it is assumed here that the sensitivity to change and the test-retest reliability observed for the HHIE-based measures apply to the corresponding RHHI-based measures.

Overall, despite the absence of direct information on the reliability and sensitivity of the RHHI-based measures, the RHHI is the strongest candidate for use as an outcome measure for hearing-related psychosocial health at this time. Generally, a self-report measure comprised of 18 items would be expected to be a little more reliable than a 10-item RHHI-S score. Further, given that the minimum detectable difference is closely tied to test-retest reliability, the RHHI would be expected to be more sensitive to postintervention change than the shorter 10-item RHHI-S. Finally, to the extent that assessment of the measure relies primarily on data regarding the reliability and sensitivity to change reported for the 25-item HHIE, it is perhaps more appropriate to assume these results apply to the 18-item RHHI, which includes 72 percent of the items common to the HHIE.

Conclusion 6-12: The RHHI is the strongest candidate for use as a self-report outcome measure for hearing-related psychosocial health at this time.

STATISTICAL APPROACHES FOR FUTURE RESEARCH

Strengthening hearing health care outcome measurement will require research in several areas and various new approaches, including better research on evaluating a measure's responsiveness, linking currently available measures, and using item response theory.

Evaluating a Measure's Responsiveness

One of the key challenges the committee faced when assessing measures was determining the responsiveness of these measures. Responsiveness (also known as sensitivity to change) can be thought of as the degree to which a measure accurately documents a meaningful change in an outcome, or, in the words of the COSMIN initiative, responsiveness is "the ability of an [health-related patient-reported outcomes] instrument to detect change over time in the construct to be measured" (Mokkink et al., 2010, p. 742). The general consensus is that the best way to assess responsiveness is with a longitudinal study in which at least some of the patients are known to change on the construct of interest (Crosby et al., 2003).

The measurement literature commonly discusses two complementary types of methods for evaluating the responsiveness of a measure, one of which is based only on the data accumulated on the measure of interest, while the other evaluates those data relative to an outside standard. The first type, distribution-based methods, expresses change scores "in terms of an underlying sampling distribution, whether in between-person standard deviation units, within-person standard deviation units, or some variation of the standard error of measurement" (Haley and Fragala-Pinkham, 2006, p. 737), which is an absolute reliability coefficient that quantifies the consistency of measured values in the same units of the original measurement. Distribution-based methods "are based on statistical significance, sample variability, and measurement precision. In contrast, anchor-based approaches require an external, independent standard to 'anchor' the meaning of clinical importance, one that is itself interpretable and at least moderately correlated with the test or measure of interest" (Haley and Fragala-Pinkham, 2006, p. 737).

Distribution-Based Methods

As noted above, distribution-based methods rely on statistical evaluations of the data of interest, without bringing in outside values. To evaluate the size of the effect from a particular treatment, for instance, the typical approach would be to compare the average before-treatment and after-treatment scores of a group of patients, with the effect size being the difference of the two means ("after" minus "before"), with this number divided by a standardizing value intended to account for the choice of scaling. (For instance, changes in effect scored on a scale of 0 to 10 would appear to be twice the size of changes in effect scored on a scale of 0 to 5 even if the absolute change in effect was exactly the same.) In other words, the effect size would be expressed as a fraction whose numerator is the difference between the two means and the denominator is a standardizing factor, typically a standard deviation of one of the distributions under consideration (de Vet et al., 2011). Cohen (1988) defined the "standardized effect size" as being an effect size whose denominator is the standard deviation of the collection of scores on the outcome measure at baseline. Cohen also suggested how to interpret effect sizes: 0.20 should be considered a small effect size, 0.50 a moderate effect size, and 0.80 and greater should be considered a large effect size. A decade later Samsa and colleagues (1999) carried out a comprehensive literature review and, based on its results, suggested that an effect size of 0.20 should be considered the hallmark of a minimal clinically important difference.

Samsa and colleagues (1999) argued that effect sizes calculated with distribution-based methods can be used effectively in determining when treatments result in clinically important differences (CIDs). "First, the effect size approach is efficient—implementation merely requires: (1) selecting the effect size benchmark; and (2) estimating the standard deviation . . . relevant to the population under study. This standard deviation can usually be obtained from the literature or extant data bases—if not, a small observational study (using a group which is representative of the trial's target population) should suffice" (Samsa et al., 1999, p. 144). Second, researchers in a variety of areas have used effect size benchmarks in their work, with reasonable results. Samsa and colleagues (1999) also noted that Cohen's suggestion for the cutoffs for small, moderate, and large effect sizes was based on the analysis of data distributions for a large variety of characteristics. However, the researchers ultimately concluded that the ideal approach would be to use effect sizes for an initial estimate of the CID but then to check that result using at least one anchor-based method (Samsa et al., 1999).

If one is to use effect size to evaluate the effectiveness of a treatment, it is important to keep in mind some of the method's limitations. One of the most important of these limitations is, as Crosby and colleagues (2003) noted, the way that the "characteristics of the distribution, particularly at baseline, may strongly influence the effect size" (p. 400). For example, the more heterogeneous a sample is at baseline, the larger the standard deviation of that sample—and the smaller the effect size—will be. "Thus, the same amount of individual change produces different effect sizes depending upon the heterogeneity of the sample at baseline" (Crosby et al., 2003, p. 400).

Another way to measure response to treatment which is closely related to the effect size is the standardized response mean (SRM), which is also known as the efficacy index or the responsiveness–treatment coefficient. Like the effect size, the SRM is a ratio whose numerator is the change in a measure, but its denominator, instead of being the standard deviation of the baseline measurement, is the standard deviation of the changes in the measure in the population that was studied. Thus, the SRM takes into account the variation in the measured changes; it is smaller when the variation in changes is larger and larger when the variation is smaller. Researchers have suggested assessing SRM values in the same way that effect size values are typically assessed, with 0.20 representing a small change, 0.50 a medium one, and 0.80 a large change. While the SRM, by taking into account the variation in the measured changes, can be a useful way to characterize responses in a population, it is less valuable for individuals, as their SRM score will vary depending on how heterogeneous the population response is (Crosby et al., 2003).

The standard error of measurement (SEM) offers an alternative approach to determining clinically meaningful differences—and one that is relatively independent of the population sample being measured. The SEM, which provides a measure of how precise a given test or measure is for a given sample, is a function of both the standard deviation of that sample and the sample's reliability coefficient (Crosby et al., 2003). Both values vary according to the sample, but because the relationship between the two remains relatively stable from sample to sample, the SEM also remains relatively constant across samples. Thus, as Crosby and colleagues note, "the SEM is considered to be an attribute of the measure and not a characteristic of the sample per se" (Crosby et al., 2003, p. 402). Different authors have suggested different SEM threshold values as indicating clinically meaningful differences, including 1 SEM (Wolinsky et al., 1998), 1.96 SEM (McHorney and Tarlov, 1995), and 2.77 SEM (McHorney and Tarlov, 1995; Wyrwich et al., 1999). Among the limitations of using the SEM approach is that it is based on the assumption that measurement error does not vary from score to score and thus the SEM remains fixed across scores—an assumption that is not borne out in practice (Crosby et al., 2003).

The SEM is used in the calculation of the minimal detectable change (MDC), which is, as the name suggests, the smallest change that can be detected by a measure, given the measurement error of the instrument being used to make the measurements. It is referred to by a variety of other names as well, including the smallest detectable change, the smallest real difference, and the reliable change index (Beckerman et al., 2001; Streiner et al., 2015). The MDC can be calculated in a variety of ways and will depend not only on the SEM but also the desired confidence level. For a 95 percent confidence level, for instance, $MDC = 1.96 \times \sqrt{2} \times SEM$ (de Vet et al., 2006). This has often been referred to as "95 percent critical differences" in audiology (Demorest and Walden, 1984; Demorest and Erdman, 1988).

Generally speaking, distribution-based methods of assessing responsiveness have a number of limitations. As noted above, for instance, the effect size varies according to the heterogeneity of the baseline sample; thus, a change of a certain magnitude may be considered important if it is observed in a homogeneous study population but not important if it were observed in a heterogeneous study sample. Similarly, the SRM varies with heterogeneity in the population response. Furthermore, while distribution-based methods can reliably detect change over time in a measure, "these methods do not in themselves provide a good sense of the clinical relevance of the change" (Crosby et al., 2003). Thus, they may require additional comparisons to interpret their clinical meaning.

Crosby and colleagues (2003) concluded that "[t]he distribution-based measures that seem most promising for establishing clinically meaningful change are those based on the measurement precision of the instrument," such as the SEM (p. 402).

Anchor-Based Approaches

A major advantage of anchor-based methods over distribution-based methods is that the use of an anchor in the method makes it possible to look for changes that are clinically relevant or important to the patient rather than simply being statistically significant; in particular, the anchor is chosen to reflect the changes that patients and clinicians find to be most valuable or important to study. One important use of anchor-based methods is to determine the "minimal clinically important difference" (MCID), which was defined by Jaeschke and Guyatt (1989) as the "smallest difference in score in the domain of interest which patients perceive as beneficial and which would mandate, in the absence of troublesome side effects and excessive cost, a change in the patient's management" (p. 408; see also Zhang et al., 2023). The MCID differs from the MDC in that there is no consideration in the MDC that a change is clinically important—only that it can be detected—whereas the MCID is specifically focused on changes that are both detectable and clinically relevant.

Researchers have used various types of anchor-based approaches in establishing an MCID, and there is no consensus on which is the best to use. One anchor-based approach that is commonly used in longitudinal studies to establish which changes are clinically meaningful is the global rating of change scale, which has patients rate their degree of overall health improvement or deterioration over time (Kamper et al., 2009). The mean change method determines the MCID by calculating the mean change in score on the relevant measure among a group of patients who have rated themselves as "a little better" on a global rating of change (Dekker et al., 2024).

Crosby and colleagues (2003) offered the following conclusion about the use of anchor-based approaches in determining the responsiveness of a measure. Their conclusion dealt specifically with measures of health-related quality of life but also applies to hearing measures:

> The clear advantage of anchor-based approaches is that change in [health-related quality of life] is linked to a meaningful external anchor. Lydick and Epstein (1993) have likened this approach to establishing the construct validity of a measure. The most notable advantage of global ratings, particularly patient ratings, is that they provide the single best measure of the significance of change from the individual perspective. They also have the potential to take into account more information (e.g., other life circumstance) that may affect [health-related quality of life] than other methods for assessing clinically meaningful change. (p. 399)

From the perspective of what the clinician, rather than the individual patient, finds most meaningful, Crosby and colleagues (2003) recommended the use of clinician global ratings and longitudinal disease-related measures of outcome.

Anchor-based methods that depend on global ratings have a number of limitations. One of these is that they depend upon patient reporting, which can be biased in various ways, including by inaccurate memory (recall bias). Since memory tends to become less accurate with time, recall bias is a particular issue when there is an extended period of time between the measures. Thus, researchers who use global ratings of change need to be careful to assess how reliable the ratings are (Crosby et al., 2003).

In light of the different types of limitations that affect distribution-based and anchor-based measures, Crosby and colleagues (2003) recommended an integrated approach that uses information from both approaches to arrive at a reliable evaluation of clinically meaningful change. When the two approaches provide answers that agree relatively well with one another, researchers can have reasonable confidence in that answer, and when the two approaches disagree, researchers need to look more closely to determine which answer should be judged more reliable.

MCIDs for Outcome Measures in Hearing Health

The committee particularly notes that MCIDs do not currently exist for the RHHI, APHAB-global, QuickSIN, SSQ, and WIN. Distribution-based MDCs, in the form of 95 percent critical differences, however, have been published for the parent HHI measure of the RHHI, the HHIE (Weinstein, 1986). They also have been published separately for the scales that make up the APHAB global score, but not for the APHAB global outcome measure itself (Cox and Alexander, 1995). In addition, all MDCs published for these outcome measures have been presented as a single value to be applied across all baseline scores, a practice that is not supported by research (Crosby et al., 2003).

For hearing-aid patient-reported outcome measures, MDCs or critical differences most often have been reported as single values, and this holds for the PHAB-based measures reviewed here. For the APHAB measures, Cox and Alexander (1995) reported 95 percent critical differences of 26 percent for both unaided and aided APHAB scores and 33 percent for the APHAB benefit score, for all individual subscales. These values were subsequently confirmed by Haskell and colleagues (2002). For the APHAB global score, Chisolm and colleagues (2005) reported 95 percent critical-difference values of 17.8 percent and 15.9 percent for test–retest intervals of 2 or 10 weeks, respectively. Much additional research is needed to establish MDCs and MCIDs for the recommended outcome measures.

Conclusion 6-12: Statistical approaches such as distribution-based methods and anchor-based approaches could help develop more robust evidence on the sensitivity to change of various outcome measures relative to hearing interventions.

Linking

Linking is a statistical process that makes it possible to directly compare two measures that are similar but not identical; their differences can be of various types—e.g., the measures may have different content or different construct severity levels (Brady et al., 2022). To carry out a linking analysis, one first determines a "target measure" and an "anchor measure" to which the target measure will be linked. The two measures should be quantifying essentially the same construct. Next, using a statistical analysis one establishes a relationship between the target measure and the anchor measure that maps scores on the target measure onto equivalent scores on the anchor measure. The resulting links between scores on the two measures are referred to as *crosswalks*, and they make it possible to compare results from different measures of similar constructs. For example, linking might allow one clinician to use the QuickSIN and another to use the WIN and still be able to compare their scores. Similarly, linking could provide the ability to use any of the HHI variations.

Conclusion 6-13: Linking could be useful to determine comparable scores among various outcome measures for hearing interventions.

Item Response Theory

Item response theory (IRT) is an approach used both in the design of tests and in the analysis and scoring of the responses on tests. IRT differs from classical test theory in its focus on how an individual answers individual items on a test rather than on the overall score from the test. An individual's response on a particular item is assumed to be a function both of that individual's overall latent ability or performance on the construct the test was designed to measure and of the characteristics of the particular item. In particular, the theory does not assume that each item in a measure is equally difficult for an individual to answer or equally informative about the construct being tested. Instead, the theory focuses on how individual items on a test contribute to measuring a construct rather than just looking at an overall test score.

IRT allows for more precise measurement by considering the difficulty of each item and the individual's ability level, making it possible to make comparisons between different versions of the same measure even if they have different sets of questions. An example of the application of IRT in the development of tests can be found in the design of computer adaptive testing (Benton, 2021). Computer adaptive testing is an administration method that uses test software to adjust the difficulty of questions presented to an individual based on that person's response to previous questions. The test software selects questions for each individual based on how they answered previous questions. Correct answers lead to more difficult questions, while incorrect answers lead to less difficult questions. By tailoring the difficulty of questions presented to an individual based on their performance, computer adaptive testing software can make the assessment more efficient to administer. It should be noted that a version of IRT was applied to the development of the RHHI, one of the core outcome measures (Cassarly et al., 2020).

> *Conclusion 6-14: Item response theory may be useful in making outcome measurement more precise, making the administration of measures more efficient, and allowing for the comparison of different versions of the same measure.*

FINDINGS

Finding 6-1: The committee used two overarching criteria to assess measures: (1) scientific acceptability—including reliability, validity, and sensitivity to change and (2) feasibility—including burden on individuals, clinicians, and researchers.

Finding 6-2: Many measures have been used primarily for diagnostic assessment, but not for outcome measurement.

Finding 6-3: Some measures are not broadly accessible.

Finding 6-4: No measure had robust evidence for all criteria examined by the committee.

Finding 6-5: The ACT is a newer, language-agnostic measure that strongly predicts other speech-in-noise measurements. However, there is limited evidence on the measure.

Finding 6-6: The AzBio Sentence Test has limited evidence for its development and validation. The test is most commonly used as a candidacy measure and for evaluating cochlear implants.

Finding 6-7: The DIN test focuses on repeating digits (rather than words or sentences), takes about 2 minutes to administer, and is available in multiple languages. The test is primarily used as a screener for hearing loss, and most research has been using the test as a substitution for measures like the audiogram.

Finding 6-8: The QuickSIN takes about a minute to administer and is familiar to clinicians. However, there is a lack of evidence on the reliability of the measure and consistency of the measurement over time, and the test is only available in English.

Finding 6-9: The WIN takes 4–6 minutes to administer. There is a significant amount of psychometric data supporting the quality of the measure, and test-retest reliability for each of the word lists is well documented, in addition to documentation of the equivalency of the difficulty of the word lists. A Spanish version is available, but it has not been sufficiently validated.

Finding 6-10: The APHAB is a self-report measure that includes three subscales pertaining to communication difficulties in various situations (familiar talkers, background noise, reverberation) and one subscale on the aversiveness of environmental sounds.

Finding 6-11: The APHAB has a sufficient amount of psychometric data supporting the reliability and validity of the measure, and there is some evidence for its sensitivity to change. The measure is available in at least 20 languages and takes around 10 minutes to complete.

Finding 6-12: The communication subscales of the APHAB are often averaged to form a single APHAB-global score, which has been shown to be reliable and sensitive to change.

Finding 6-13: The SSQ examines speech, spatial abilities, and qualities of hearing. The measure has a sufficient amount of psychometric data supporting the reliability and validity of the measure, with some evidence for sensitivity to change, and is available in multiple languages.

Finding 6-14: Behavioral measures capture outcomes in a controlled environment while self-report measures capture real-world experiences.

Finding 6-15: The HHIE requires about 10 minutes to complete, compared to the HHIE-S which takes 2–3 minutes, the RHHI which takes 5–7 minutes for completion, and the RHHI-S which takes about 2–3 minutes.

Finding 6-16: The HHIE has the most evidence supporting sensitivity to change, and there is a sufficient amount of psychometric data supporting the test-retest reliability of the measure.

Finding 6-17: The RHHI includes items that are a verbatim subset of the HHIE.

Finding 6-18: Several statistical methods can help improve the evidence base for measures' sensitivity to change including distribution-based methods and anchor-based approaches. More research is needed to develop appropriate MCIDs for all outcome measures used to assess hearing interventions.

Finding 6-19: Linking is a statistical process that makes it possible to create an equivalency mapping between the scores from two different measures of the same construct. With this technique, researchers can directly compare the scores from various tests that measure the same, or approximately the same, characteristic. These links are known as crosswalks.

Finding 6-20: IRT is a statistical approach used to understand how individual items on a test contribute to measuring a construct rather than just looking at the overall score. Broader application of IRT to measuring outcomes of hearing interventions is desirable.

RECOMMENDATIONS

Many outcome measures have been developed to assess the outcomes of understanding speech in complex listening situations and hearing-related psychosocial health. The committee focused on the measures with the most available information concerning their psychometric development and use. First, the committee documented descriptive characteristics of the studies used in each measure's development, including the population studied, the number of participants, the setting, and how the measure is scored. Next the committee evaluated each measure according to a series of criteria—scientific acceptability (including reliability, validity, and sensitivity to change) and feasibility (by setting). Overall, current outcome measures are imperfect, but there is adequate evidence to support the standard use of specific measures at this time.

Standardized[2] Outcome Measures

For the assessment of the outcome of understanding speech in complex listening situations, the committee considered both behavioral measures and self-report measures and concluded that both types of measures are necessary. While behavioral measures have face validity, are considered by some to be more objective, and are readily available, these measures often lack data on their sensitivity to change and do not necessarily correlate with an individual's perception of their improvement.

---

[2] The word *standardized* is used here in a broad sense to indicate that the same measures are being used for specific outcomes, and that there are prescribed materials and procedures for the use of these measures. The committee does not imply that the measures are part of national or international standards.

For the self-report measure, the committee narrowed the candidates down to the APHAB and the SSQ. While both measures have good evidence for psychometric strength and both are available in multiple languages, the APHAB (and the APHAB-global score in particular) has a greater focus on scenarios of complex listening situations, whereas the SSQ includes a mix of speech, spatial location, and sound quality. Therefore, the committee concluded that the APHAB-global score currently is the best candidate for assessing an individual's experience with understanding speech in complex listening environments.

For the behavioral measure, the committee narrowed the candidates down to the QuickSIN and the WIN. The QuickSIN, which evaluates an individual's ability to understand sentences, may be more familiar to audiologists and somewhat shorter to administer. However, psychometric evaluation of the QuickSIN shows a lack of evidence on the reliability and consistency of the measurement over time with moderate test-retest reliability. The WIN, which evaluates an individual's ability to understand single words, has had a much more rigorous psychometric development and evaluation (including significant evidence for test–retest reliability), is currently used as part of the NIH Toolbox, and is available in Spanish (although the committee notes that additional validation of the Spanish WIN is needed). The committee emphasizes that measures for understanding speech in complex listening situations need to be implemented as recommended by the developers in order to avoid variability and allow for comparison across studies.

For hearing-related psychosocial health, the committee ultimately zeroed in on variations of the HHI. The committee concluded that the 18-item RHHI is the best current candidate. The well-studied HHIE was eliminated primarily because of its length and because psychometric analyses favor the RHHI. The shorter screening version (RHHI-S) had less robust research on psychometrics. The RHHI, a relatively new measure, has undergone rigorous item analysis but lacks explicit data regarding reliability and sensitivity to change following intervention. Given that 18 of the 25 items included in the HHIE are common to the RHHI, the committee relied on evidence regarding reliability and sensitivity to change for the HHIE when considering the RHHI.

Recommendation 6-1: When assessing outcomes in hearing health, clinicians, researchers, and individuals should use the following outcome measures for each of the outcomes in the core outcome set:
a. **Understanding speech in complex listening situations**
    i.   **Abbreviated Profile of Hearing Aid Benefit global score (APHAB-Global)**
    ii. **Words-in-Noise (WIN) test**
b. **Hearing-related psychosocial health**
    i.   **Revised Hearing Handicap Inventory (RHHI)**

The committee recognizes the potential burden of assessing outcomes with three different measures and emphasizes that it will be important to determine the timing and frequency of the outcome measurements that will deliver optimal information. Additionally, it will not necessarily be required to evaluate each measure at each encounter, and self-report measures could be completed by the adult with hearing difficulties in advance of a clinical or research encounter. Finally, the committee reemphasizes that supplemental measures will likely be needed, depending on the specific context of the outcome measurement, including verification of audibility as appropriate.

Measure Development and Refinement

The committee recognizes that the measurement of hearing health outcomes requires an improvement in psychometric rigor overall. Research on measure development and refinement is needed to improve the quality of existing measures, including the previously recommended measures. For example, statistical approaches such as IRT and linking may help with refinement of existing measures. In particular, creating links between the two behavioral measures of speech understanding in complex listening situations, the WIN and QuickSIN, and among alternate forms of the HHI measures would be of value. Additionally, research on sensitivity to change, associations among core outcomes, and variations of existing measures may also help with measure choice and refinement.

Recommendation 6-2: Sponsors of hearing health research should fund further psychometric evaluation of the measures recommended for the core outcome set. Specific areas of research include the following:
a. Development of links and crosswalks
   i.   Words-in-Noise (WIN) test versus Quick Speech-in-Noise (QuickSIN) test
   ii. Among different variations of the Hearing Handicap Inventory (HHI)
b. Establishment of the sensitivity to change relative to intervention (including minimal detectable change and minimal clinically important difference) for the WIN, the global score from the Abbreviated Profile of Hearing Aid Benefit (APHAB-global), the Revised HHI (RHHI), and the screening (RHHI-S)
c. Development of WIN (and QuickSIN) in other languages
d. Assessment of associations among the set of core outcomes to further establish the independence and uniqueness of each measure
e. Application of item response theory to further develop and refine the recommended outcome measures

Research beyond the currently recommended measures is needed to build evidence for the use of measures not recommended by this committee that might be reconsidered for an updated core outcome set.

Recommendation 6-3: Sponsors of hearing health research should fund research to develop and refine hearing health outcome measures beyond the currently recommended measures, including:
a. **Broader psychometric development of the Quick Speech-in-Noise (QuickSIN) test;**
b. **Exploration of the use of the digits-in-noise test as an outcome measure; and**
c. **Exploration of the usefulness of high-quality language agnostic tests for sound processing in complex listening situations.**

REFERENCES

Advanced Bionics LLC, Cochlear Americas, and M.-E. Corporation. 2011. *Minimum speech test battery (MSTB) for adult cochlear implant users 2011.* https://www.auditorypotential.com/MSTBfiles/MSTBManual2011-06-20%20.pdf (accessed November 7, 2024).

Aguiar, R. G. R., K. de Almeida, and E. C. de Miranda-Gonsalez. 2019. Test-retest reliability of the Speech, Spatial and Qualities of Hearing scale (SSQ) in Brazilian Portuguese. *International Archives of Otorhinolaryngology* 23(04):e380-e383.

Akeroyd, M. A. 2014. An overview of the major phenomena of the localization of sound sources by normal-hearing, hearing-impaired, and aided listeners. *Trends in Hearing* 18:2331216514560442.

Akeroyd, M. A., F. H. Guy, D. L. Harrison, and S. L. Suller. 2014. A factor analysis of the SSQ (Speech, Spatial, and Qualities of Hearing Scale). *International Journal of Audiology* 53(2):101–114.

Alkhodair, M. B., T. A. Mesallam, A. Hagr, and M. F. Yousef. 2021. Arabic version of short form of the Speech, Spatial, and Qualities of Hearing scale (SSQ12). *Saudi Medical Journal* 42(11):1180.

Allen, D., L. Hickson, and M. Ferguson. 2022. Defining a patient-centred core outcome domain set for the assessment of hearing rehabilitation with clients and professionals. *Frontiers in Neuroscience* 16:787607.

Armstrong, N. M., B. C. Oosterloo, P. H. Croll, M. A. Ikram, and A. Goedegebure. 2020. Discrimination of degrees of auditory performance from the Digits-in-Noise test based on hearing status. *International Journal of Audiology* 59(12):897–904.

Auditdata. n.d. What is Quick-SIN? https://www.auditdata.com/audiology-solutions/measure/hearing-assessment/quicksin/#:~:text=The%20sentences%20are%20presented%20at,available%20in%20the%20English%20Language (accessed March 4, 2025).

Banh, J., G. Singh, and M. K. Pichora-Fuller. 2012. Age affects responses on the Speech, Spatial, and Qualities of Hearing Scale (SSQ) by adults with minimal audiometric loss. *Journal of the American Academy of Audiology* 23(2):81–91.

Batthyany, C., A.-R. Schut, M. van der Schroeff, and J. Vroegop. 2023. Translation and validation of the Speech, Spatial, and Qualities of Hearing scale (SSQ) and the Hearing Environments and Reflection on Quality of Life (HEAR-QL) questionnaire for children and adolescents in Dutch. *International Journal of Audiology* 62(2):129–137.

Beckerman, H., M. E. Roebroeck, G. J. Lankhorst, J. G. Becher, P.D. Bezemer, and A. L. M. Verbeek. 2001. Smallest real difference, a link between reproducibility and responsiveness. *Quality of Life Research* 10:571–578.

Bentler, R. A. 2000. List equivalency and test-retest reliability of the Speech in Noise test. *American Journal of Audiology* 9(2):84–100.

Bentler, R. A., D. P. Niebuhr, J. P. Getta, and C. V. Anderson. 1993a. Longitudinal study of hearing aid effectiveness. I: Objective measures. *Journal of Speech and Hearing Research* 36(4):808–819.

Bentler, R. A., D. P. Niebuhr, J. P. Getta, and C. V. Anderson. 1993b. Longitudinal study of hearing aid effectiveness. II: Subjective measures. *Journal of Speech and Hearing Research* 36(4):820–831.

Benton, T. 2021. Item response theory, computer adaptive testing, and the risk of self-deception. *Research Matters* 32:82–100. Available at https://files.eric.ed.gov/fulltext/EJ1317443.pdf (accessed March 27, 2025).

Billings, C. J., T. M. Olsen, L. Charney, B. M. Madsen, and C. E. Holmes. 2023. Speech-in-noise testing: An introduction for audiologists. *Seminars in Hearing* 45(1):55–82.

Brady, K. J. S., P. Ni, L. Carlasare, T. D. Shanafelt, C. A. Sinsky, M. Linzer, M. Stillman, and M. T. Trockel. 2022. Establishing crosswalks between common measures of burnout in U.S. physicians. *Journal of General Internal Medicine* 37(4):777–784.

Cañete, O. M., D. Marfull, M. C. Torrente, and S. C. Purdy. 2022. The Spanish 12-item version of the Speech, Spatial and Qualities of Hearing scale (SP-SSQ12): Adaptation, reliability, and discriminant validity for people with and without hearing loss. *Disability and Rehabilitation* 44(8):1419–1426.

Carhart, R. 1946. Selection of hearing aids. *Archives of Otolaryngology (1925)* 44:1–18.

Cassarly, C., L. J. Matthews, A. N. Simpson, and J. R. Dubno. 2020. The Revised Hearing Handicap Inventory and screening tool based on psychometric reevaluation of the Hearing Handicap Inventories for the elderly and adults. *Ear and Hearing* 41(1):95–105.

Chisolm, T. H., H. B. Abrams, R. McArdle, R. H. Wilson, and P. J. Doyle. 2005. The WHO-DAS II: Psychometric properties in the measurement of functional health status in adults with acquired hearing loss. *Trends in Amplification* 9(3):111–126.

Clarke, M., and P. R. Williamson. 2016. Core outcome sets and systematic reviews. *Systematic Reviews* 5:11.

CMS (Centers for Medicare & Medicaid Services). 2024. *Measure testing.* https://mmshub.cms.gov/measure-lifecycle/measure-testing/evaluation-criteria/overview (accessed March 6, 2024).

Cohen, J. 1988. *Statistical power analysis for the behavioral sciences, 2nd edition.* New York: Academic Press.

COSMIN (COnsensus-based Standards for the selection of health Measurement INstruments). n.d. *Guideline for selecting instruments for a core outcome set.* https://www.cosmin.nl/tools/guideline-selecting-proms-cos (accessed June 26, 2024).

Cox, R. M., and C. Gilmore. 1990. Development of the Profile of Hearing Aid Performance (PHAP). *Journal of Speech and Hearing Research* 33(2):343–357.

Cox, R. M., and I. Rivera. 1992. Predictability and reliability of hearing aid benefit measured using the PHAB. *Journal of the American Academy of Audiology* 3(4):242–254.

Cox, R. M., and G. C. Alexander. 1992. Maturation of hearing aid benefit: Objective and subjective measurements. *Ear and Hearing* 13(3):131–141.

Cox, R. M., and G. C. Alexander. 1995. The Abbreviated Profile of Hearing Aid Benefit. *Ear and Hearing* 16(2):176–186.

Cox, R. M., G. C. Alexander, and C. M. Beyer. 2003. Norms for the international outcome inventory for hearing aids. *Journal of the American Academy of Audiology* 14(08):403–413.

Cox, R. M., G. C. Alexander, and G. A. Gray. 2007. Personality, hearing problems, and amplification characteristics: Contributions to self-report hearing aid outcomes. *Ear and Hearing* 28(2):141–162.

Cox, R. M., J. A. Johnson, and J. Xu. 2014. Impact of advanced hearing aid technology on speech understanding for older listeners with mild to moderate, adult-onset, sensorineural hearing loss. *Gerontology* 60(6):557–568.

Cox, R. M., J. A. Johnson, and J. Xu. 2016. Impact of hearing aid technology on outcomes in daily life I: The patients' perspective. *Ear Hear* 37(4):e224–e237.

Crosby, R. D., R. L. Kolotkin, and G. R. Williams. 2003. Defining clinically meaningful change in health-related quality of life. *Journal of Clinical Epidemiology* 56(5):395–407.

Dawes, C., D. Cesarini, J. H. Fowler, M. Johannesson, P. K. Magnusson, and S. Oskarsson. 2014. The relationship between genes, psychological traits, and political participation. *American Journal of Political Science* 58(4):888–903.

Dawes, P., and K. J. Munro. 2017. Auditory distraction and acclimatization to hearing aids. *Ear and Hearing* 38(2):174–183.

Dawes, P., S. Powell, and K. J. Munro. 2011. The placebo effect and the influence of participant expectation on hearing aid trials. *Ear and Hearing* 32(6):767–774.

Dawes, P., R. Hopkins, and K. J. Munro. 2013. Placebo effects in hearing-aid trials are reliable. *International Journal of Audiology* 52(7):472–477.

De Sousa, K. C., C. Smits, D. R. Moore, H. C. Myburgh, and W. Swanepoel. 2020a. Pure-tone audiometry without bone-conduction thresholds: Using the Digits-in-Noise test to detect conductive hearing loss. *International Journal of Audiology*59(10):801–808.

De Sousa, K. C., W. Swanepoel, D. R. Moore, H. C. Myburgh, and C. Smits. 2020b. Improving sensitivity of the Digits-in-Noise test using antiphasic stimuli. *Ear and Hearing* 41(2):442–450.

De Sousa, K. C., V. Manchaiah, D. R. Moore, M. A. Graham, and D. W. Swanepoel. 2023. Effectiveness of an over-the-counter self-fitting hearing aid compared with an audiologist-fitted hearing aid: A randomized clinical trial. *JAMA Otolaryngology - Head and Neck Surgery* 149(6):522–530.

de Vet, H. C., C. B. Terwee, R. W. Ostelo, H. Beckerman, D. L. Knol, and L. M. Bouter. 2006. Minimal changes in health status questionnaires: Distinction between minimally detectable change and minimally important change. *Health and Quality of Life Outcomes* 4:54.

de Vet, H. C. W., C. B. Terwee, L. B. Mokkink, and D. L. Knol. 2011. *Measurement in medicine: A practical guide, Practical guides to biostatistics and epidemiology*. Cambridge, UK: Cambridge University Press.

Dekker, J., M. de Boer, and R. Ostelo. 2024. Minimal important change and difference in health outcome: An overview of approaches, concepts, and methods. *Osteoarthritis and Cartilage* 32(1):8–17.

Demeester, K., V. Topsakal, J.-J. Hendrickx, E. Fransen, L. Van Laer, G. Van Camp, P. Van de Heyning, and A. Van Wieringen. 2012. Hearing disability measured by the Speech, Spatial, and Qualities of Hearing Scale in clinically normal-hearing and hearing-impaired middle-aged persons, and disability screening by means of a reduced SSQ (the SSQ5). *Ear and Hearing* 33(5):615–616.

Demorest, M. E., and S. A. Erdman. 1988. Retest stability of the communication profile for the hearing impaired. *Ear and Hearing* 9(5): 237–242.

Demorest, M. E., and B. E. Walden. 1984. Psychometric principles in the selection, interpretation, and evaluation of communication self-assessment inventories. *Journal of Speech and Hearing Disorders* 49(3):226–240.

Dillard, L. K., L. J. Matthews, and J. R. Dubno. 2024a. Change on the Revised Hearing Handicap Inventory and associated factors: Results from a longitudinal cohort study. *International Journal of Audiology*:1–11.

Dillard, L. K., L. J. Matthews, and J. R. Dubno. 2024b. The Revised Hearing Handicap Inventory and pure-tone average predict hearing aid use equally well. *American Journal of Audiology* 33(1):199–208.

Dillon, H., A. James, and J. Ginis. 1997. Client Oriented Scale of Improvement (COSI) and its relationship to several other measures of benefit and satisfaction provided by hearing aids. *Journal of the American Academy of Audiology* 8(1):27–43.

Dornhoffer, J. R., T. A. Meyer, J. R. Dubno, and T. R. McRackan. 2020. Assessment of hearing aid benefit using patient-reported outcomes and audiologic measures. *Audiology and Neurotology* 25(4):215–223.

Erdman, S. A. 2014. The biopsychosocial approach in patient- and relationship-centered care: Implications for audiologic counseling. In *Adult audiologic rehabilitation,* edited by J. J. Montano and J. B. Spitzer, 2nd ed. San Diego, CA: Plural Publishing Inc. Pp. 159–206.

Fitzgerald, M. B., S. P. Gianakas, Z. J. Qian, S. Losorelli, and A. C. Swanson. 2023. Preliminary guidelines for replacing word-recognition in quiet with speech in noise assessment in the routine audiologic test battery. *Ear and Hearing* 44(6):1548–1561.

Fitzgerald, M. B., K. M. Ward, S. P. Gianakas, M. L. Smith, N. H. Blevins, and A. P. Swanson. 2024. Speech-in-noise assessment in the routine audiologic test battery: Relationship to perceived auditory disability. *Ear and Hearing* 45(4):816–826.

Folmer, R. L., J. Vachhani, G. P. McMillan, C. Watson, G. R. Kidd, and M. P. Feeney. 2017. Validation of a computer-administered version of the Digits-in-Noise test for hearing screening in the United States. *Journal of the American Academy of Audiology* 28(2): 161–169.

Folmer, R. L., G. H. Saunders, J. J. Vachhani, R. H. Margolis, G. Saly, B. Yueh, R. A. McArdle, L. L. Feth, C. M. Roup, and M. P. Feeney. 2021. Hearing health care utilization following automated hearing screening. *Journal of the American Academy of Audiology* 32(4):235–245.

Fox, R. S., J. J. Manly, J. Slotkin, J. D. Peipert, and R. C. Gershon. 2021. Reliability and validity of the Spanish-language version of the NIH toolbox. *Assessment* 28(2):457–471.

Gatehouse, S. 2000. The impact of measurement goals on the design specification for outcome measures. *Ear and Hearing* 21(4 Suppl):100S–105S.

Gatehouse, S., and W. Noble. 2004. The Speech, Spatial and Qualities of Hearing Scale (SSQ). *International Journal of Audiology* 43(2):85–99.

Giolas, T. G., E. Owens, S. H. Lamb, and E. D. Schubert. 1979. Hearing performance inventory. *Journal of Speech and Hearing Disorders* 44(2):169–195.

Haley, S. M., and M. A. Fragala-Pinkham. 2006. Interpreting change scores of tests and measures used in physical therapy. *Physical Therapy* 86(5):735–743.

Hall, D. A., S. Zaragoza Domingo, L. Z. Hamdache, V. Manchaiah, S. Thammaiah, C. Evans, L. L. Wong, International Collegium of Rehabilitative Audiology and TINnitus Research NETwork. 2018. A good practice guide for translating and adapting hearing-related questionnaires for different languages and cultures. *International Journal of Audiology* 57(3):161–175.

Haskell, G. B., D. Noffsinger, V. D. Larson, D. W. Williams, R. A. Dobie, and J. L. Rogers. 2002. Subjective measures of hearing aid benefit in the NIDCD/VA clinical trial. *Ear and Hearing* 23(4):301–307.

Hays, R., and D. Hadorn. 1992. Responsiveness to change: An aspect of validity, not a separate dimension. *Quality of Life Research* 1:73–75.

Heffernan, E., B. E. Weinstein, and M. A. Ferguson. 2020. Application of Rasch analysis to the evaluation of the measurement properties of the Hearing Handicap Inventory for the Elderly. *Ear and Hearing* 41(5):1125–1134.

High, W. S., G. Fairbanks, and A. Glorig. 1964. Scale for self-assessment of hearing handicap. *Journal of Speech and Hearing Disorders* 29(3):215–230.

Holder, J. T., L. M. Levin, and R. H. Gifford. 2018. Speech recognition in noise for adults with normal hearing: Age-normative performance for AzBio, BKB-SIN, and QuickSIN. *Otology & Neurotology* 39(10):e972–e978.

Hoth, S. 2016. [The Freiburg speech intelligibility test: A pillar of speech audiometry in German-speaking countries]. *HNO* 64(8):540–548.

Humes, L. E. 1999. Dimensions of hearing aid outcome. *Journal of the American Academy of Audiology* 10(01):26–39.

Humes, L. E. 2003. Modeling and predicting hearing aid outcome. *Trends in Amplification* 7(2):41–75.

Humes, L. E. 2021. An approach to self-assessed auditory wellness in older adults. *Ear and Hearing* 42(4):745–761.

Humes, L. E., and V. Krull. 2012. Hearing aids for adults. *Evidence-Based Practice in Audiology* 61–92.

Humes, L. E., D. Halling, and M. Coughlin. 1996. Reliability and stability of various hearing-aid outcome measures in a group of elderly hearing-aid wearers. *Journal of Speech and Hearing Research* 39(5):923–935.

Humes, L. E., C. B. Garner, D. L. Wilson, and N. N. Barlow. 2001. Hearing-aid outcome measures following one month of hearing aid use by the elderly. *Journal of Speech, Language, and Hearing Research* 44(3):469–486.

Humes, L. E., D. L. Wilson, N. N. Barlow, and C. Garner. 2002. Changes in hearing-aid benefit following 1 or 2 years of hearing-aid use by older adults. *Journal of Speech, Language, and Hearing Research* 45(4):772–782.

Humes, L. E., D. L. Wilson, and A. C. Humes. 2003. Examination of differences between successful and unsuccessful elderly hearing aid candidates matched for age, hearing loss and gender. *International Journal of Audiology* 42(7):432–441.

Humes, L. E., G. R. Kidd, and J. J. Lentz. 2013. Auditory and cognitive factors underlying individual differences in aided speech-understanding among older adults. *Frontiers in Systems Neuroscience* 7:55.

Humes, L. E., S. E. Rogers, T. M. Quigley, A. K. Main, D. L. Kinney, and C. Herring. 2017. The effects of service-delivery model and purchase price on hearing-aid outcomes in older adults: A randomized double-blind placebo-controlled clinical trial. *American Journal of Audiology* 26(1):53–79.

Interacoustics. 2022. *Quick Speech in Noise (QuickSIN).* https://www.interacoustics.com/audiometers/ac40/support/quick-speech-in-noise-quicksin (accessed September 10, 2024).

Jaeschke, R., J. Singer, and G. H. Guyatt. 1989. Measurement of health status. Ascertaining the minimal clinically important difference. *Control Clin Trials* 10(4):407–415.

Jansen, S., H. Luts, K. C. Wagener, B. Kollmeier, M. Del Rio, R. Dauman, C. James, B. Fraysse, E. Vormès, B. Frachet, J. Wouters, and A. van Wieringen. 2012. Comparison of three types of French speech-in-noise tests: A multi-center study. *International Journal of Audiology* 51(3):164–173.

Jansen, S., H. Luts, P. Dejonckere, A. van Wieringen, and J. Wouters. 2013. Efficient hearing screening in noise-exposed listeners using the digit triplet test. *Ear and Hearing* 34(6):773–778.

Jerger, J., R. Chmiel, E. Florin, F. Pirozzolo, and N. Wilson. 1996. Comparison of conventional amplification and an assistive listening device in elderly persons. *Ear and Hearing* 17(6):490–504.

Johnson, J. A., R. M. Cox, and G. C. Alexander. 2010. Development of APHAB norms for WDRC hearing aids and comparisons with original norms. *Ear and Hearing* 31(1):47–55.

Johnson, J. A., J. Xu, and R. M. Cox. 2016. Impact of hearing aid technology on outcomes in daily life II: Speech understanding and listening effort. *Ear Hear* 37(5):529–540.

Johnson, J. A., J. Xu, and R. M. Cox. 2017. Impact of hearing aid technology on outcomes in daily life III: Localization. *Ear Hear* 38(6):746–759.

Kam, A. C., M. C. Tong, and A. van Hasselt. 2011. Cross-cultural adaptation and validation of the Chinese Abbreviated Profile of Hearing Aid Benefit. *International Journal of Audiology* 50(5):334–339.

Kamper, S. J., C. G. Maher, and G. Mackay. 2009. Global rating of change scales: A review of strengths and weaknesses and considerations for design. *Journal of Manual & Manipulative Therapy* 17(3):163–170.

Kiessling, J., M. Meis, and H. Meister. 2011. German translations of questionnaires SADL, ECHO and SSQ and their evaluation. *Audiological Acoustics* 50(1):6–16.

Kılıç, N., G. İ. Ş. Kamışlı, B. Gündüz, İ. Bayramoğlu, and Y. K. Kemaloğlu. 2021. Turkish validity and reliability study of the Speech, Spatial and Qualities of Hearing scale. *Turkish Archives of Otorhinolaryngology* 59(3):172.

Killion, M., and P. A. Niquette. 2000. What can the pure-tone audiogram tell us about a patient's SNR loss? *Hearing Journal* 53(3):46–48, 50, 52–53.

Killion, M. C., and E. Villchur. 1993. Kessler was right—partly: But SIN test shows some aids improve hearing in noise. *Hearing Journal* 46(9):31–35.

Killion, M. C., W. O. Olsen, C. L. Clifford, D. D. VanVliet, D. E. Rose, D. E. Bensen, M. W. Marion, P. A. Tillman, D. B. Hawkins, S. M. Dalzell, and D. A. Fabry. 1996. "Preliminary data on the SIN Test," presented at the annual convention of the American Academy of Audiology, Salt Lake City, UT.

Killion, M. C., P. A. Niquette, G. I. Gudmundsen, L. J. Revit, and S. Banerjee. 2004. Development of a Quick Speech-in-Noise test for measuring signal-to-noise ratio loss in normal-hearing and hearing-impaired listeners. *Journal of the Acoustical Society of America* 116(4 Pt 1):2395–2405.

Kochkin, S. 1997. Subjective measures of satisfaction and benefit: Establishing norms. *Seminars in Hearing* 18(1):37–48.

Koole, A., A. P. Nagtegaal, N. C. Homans, A. Hofman, R. J. Baatenburg de Jong, and A. Goedegebure. 2016. Using the Digits-in-Noise test to estimate age-related hearing loss. *Ear and Hearing* 37(5):508–513.

Kraus, E. M., J. A. Shohet, and P. J. Catalano. 2011. Envoy esteem totally implantable hearing system: Phase 2 trial, 1-year hearing results. *Otolaryngology—Head and Neck Surgery* 145(1):100–109.

Kwak, C., J. H. Seo, Y. Oh, and W. Han. 2022. Efficacy of the Digit-in-Noise test: A systematic review and meta-analysis. *Journal of Audiology & Otology* 26(1):10–21.

Lamb, S. H., E. Owens, and E. D. Schubert. 1983. The revised form of the hearing performance inventory. *Ear and Hearing* 4(3):152–157.

Larson, V. D., D. W. Williams, W. G. Henderson, L. E. Luethke, L. B. Beck, D. Noffsinger, R. H. Wilson, R. A. Dobie, G. B. Haskell, G. W. Bratt, J. E. Shanks, P. Stelmachowicz, G. A. Studebaker, A. E. Boysen, A. Donahue, R. Canalis, S. A. Fausti, B. Z. Rappaport, and f. t. P. o. t. N. V. H. A. C. T. Group. 2000. Efficacy of 3 commonly used hearing aid circuitsa crossover trial. *JAMA* 284(14):1806–1813.

Lichtenstein, M. J., F. H. Bess, and S. A. Logan. 1988. Validation of screening tools for identifying hearing-impaired elderly in primary care. *JAMA* 259(19):2875–2878.

Lin, F. R., J. R. Pike, M. S. Albert, M. Arnold, S. Burgard, T. Chisolm, D. Couper, J. A. Deal, A. M. Goman, N. W. Glynn, T. Gmelin, L. Gravens-Mueller, K. M. Hayden, A. R. Huang, D. Knopman, C. M. Mitchell, T. Mosley, J. S. Pankow, N. S. Reed, V. Sanchez, J. A. Schrack, B. G. Windham, and J. Coresh. 2023. Hearing intervention versus health education control to reduce cognitive decline in older adults with hearing loss in the USA (ACHIEVE): A multicentre, randomised controlled trial. *Lancet* 402(10404):786–797.

Löhler, J., F. Gräbner, B. Wollenberg, P. Schlattmann, and R. Schönweiler. 2017. Sensitivity and specificity of the Abbreviated Profile of Hearing Aid Benefit (APHAB). *European Archives of Oto-Rhino-Laryngology* 274(10):3593–3598.

Lotfi, Y., A. R. Nazeri, A. Asgari, A. Moosavi, and E. Bakhshi. 2016. Iranian version of Speech, Spatial, and Qualities of Hearing scale: A psychometric study. *Acta Medica Iranica* 756–764.

Lydick, E., and R. S. Epstein. 1993. Interpretation of quality of life changes. *Quality of Life Research* 2(3):221–226.

Lyzenga, J., and C. Smits. 2011. Effects of coarticulation, prosody, and noise freshness on the intelligibility of digit triplets in noise. *Journal of the American Academy of Audiology* 22(4):215–221.

Malinoff, R. L., and B. E. Weinstein. 1989. Measurement of hearing aid benefit in the elderly. *Ear and Hearing* 10(6):354–356.

McArdle, R. A., and R. H. Wilson. 2006. Homogeneity of the 18 QuickSIN lists. *Journal of the American Academy of Audiology* 17(3):157–167.

McArdle, R. A., R. H. Wilson, and C. A. Burks. 2005. Speech recognition in multitalker babble using digits, words, and sentences. *Journal of the American Academy of Audiology* 16(9):726–739.

McHorney, C. A., and A. Tarlov. 1995. Individual-patient monitoring in clinical practice: Are available health status surveys adequate? *Quality of Life Research* 4:293–307.

McLean, W. J., A. S. Hinton, J. T. J. Herby, A. N. Salt, J. J. Hartsock, S. Wilson, D. L. Lucchino, T. Lenarz, A. Warnecke, N. Prenzler, H. Schmitt, S. King, L. E. Jackson, J. Rosenbloom, G. Atiee, M. Bear, C. L. Runge, R. H. Gifford, S. D. Rauch, D. J. Lee, R. Langer, J. M. Karp, C. Loose, and C. LeBel. 2021. Improved speech intelligibility in subjects with stable sensorineural hearing loss following intratympanic dosing of FX-322 in a phase 1b study. *Otology & Neurotology* 42(7):e849–e857.

McShefferty, D., W. M. Whitmer, and M. A. Akeroyd. 2016. The just-meaningful difference in speech-to-noise ratio. *Trends in Hearing* 20:1–11.

Mehrkian, S., Z. Bayat, M. Javanbakht, H. Emamdjomeh, and E. Bakhshi. 2019. Effect of wireless remote microphone application on speech discrimination in noise in children with cochlear implants. *International Journal of Pediatric Otorhinolaryngology* 125:192–195.

Melo, I. M. M., A. R. X. Silva, R. Camargo, H. G. Cavalcanti, D. V. Ferrari, K. V. M. Taveira, and S. A. Balen. 2022. Accuracy of smartphone-based hearing screening tests: A systematic review. *CoDAS* 34(3):e20200380.

Mendel, L. L. 2007. Objective and subjective hearing aid assessment outcomes. *American Journal of Audiology* 16(2):118–129.

Meng, L., D. Hao, D. Li, J. Yue, Y. Wan, and L. Shi. 2024. Establishment of self-reported hearing cut-off value on the Chinese version of short form of Speech, Spatial and Qualities of Hearing scale (SSQ12). *International Journal of Audiology* 1–8.

Mokkink, L. B., C. B. Terwee, D. L. Patrick, J. Alonso, P. W. Stratford, D. L. Knol, L. M. Bouter, and H. C. W. de Vet. 2010. The COSMIN study reached international consensus on taxonomy, terminology, and definitions of measurement properties for health-related patient-reported outcomes. *Journal of Clinical Epidemiology* 63(7):737–745.

Motlagh Zadeh, L., N. H. Silbert, W. Swanepoel, and D. R. Moore. 2021. Improved sensitivity of Digits-in-Noise test to high-frequency hearing loss. *Ear and Hearing* 42(3):565–573.

Moulin, A., and C. Richard. 2016. Sources of variability of speech, spatial, and qualities of hearing scale (SSQ) scores in normal-hearing and hearing-impaired populations. *International Journal of Audiology* 55(2):101–109.

Moulin, A., A. Pauzie, and C. Richard. 2015. Validation of a French translation of the Speech, Spatial, and Qualities of Hearing Scale (SSQ) and comparison with other language versions. *International Journal of Audiology* 54(12):889–898.

Moulin, A., J. Vergne, S. Gallego, and C. Micheyl. 2019. A new Speech, Spatial, and Qualities of Hearing Scale short-form: Factor, cluster, and comparative analyses. *Ear and Hearing* 40(4):938–950.

Mueller, H. G. 2016. *Signia expert series: Speech-in-Noise testing for selection and fitting of hearing aids: Worth the effort?* https://www.audiologyonline.com/articles/signia-expert-series-speech-in-18336 (accessed January 12, 2025).

Mulrow, C. D., C. Aguilar, J. E. Endicott, M. R. Tuley, R. Velez, W. S. Charlip, M. C. Rhodes, J. A. Hill, and L. A. DeNino. 1990a. Quality-of-life changes and hearing impairment. A randomized trial. *Annals of Internal Medicine* 113(3):188–194.

Mulrow, C. D., M. R. Tuley, and C. Aguilar. 1990b. Discriminating and responsiveness abilities of two hearing handicap scales. *Ear and Hearing* 11(3):176–180.

Mulrow, C. D., M. R. Tuley, and C. Aguilar. 1992a. Correlates of successful hearing aid use in older adults. *Ear and Hearing* 13(2):108–113.

Mulrow, C. D., M. R. Tuley, and C. Aguilar. 1992b. Sustained benefits of hearing aids. *Journal of Speech and Hearing Research* 35(6):1402–1405.

Myhrum, M., M. G. Heldahl, A. K. Rødvik, O. E. Tvete, and G. E. Jablonski. 2024. Validation of the Norwegian version of the Speech, Spatial and Qualities of Hearing scale (SSQ). *Audiology and Neurotology* 29(2):124–135.

Neal, K., C. M. McMahon, S. E. Hughes, and I. Boisvert. 2022. Listening-based communication ability in adults with hearing loss: A scoping review of existing measures. *Front Psychol* 13:786347.

Newman, C. W., and B. E. Weinstein. 1988. The Hearing Handicap Inventory for the Elderly as a measure of hearing aid benefit. *Ear and Hearing* 9(2):81–85.

Newman, C. W., and B. E. Weinstein. 1989. Test-retest reliability of the Hearing Handicap Inventory for the Elderly using two administration approaches. *Ear and Hearing* 10(3):190–191.

Newman, C. W., B. E. Weinstein, G. P. Jacobson, and G. A. Hug. 1990. The Hearing Handicap Inventory for Adults: Psychometric adequacy and audiometric correlates. *Ear and Hearing* 11(6):430–433.

Newman, C. W., G. P. Jacobson, G. A. Hug, B. E. Weinstein, and R. L. Malinoff. 1991. Practical method for quantifying hearing aid benefit in older adults. *Journal of the American Academy of Audiology* 2(2):70–75.

Noble, W., G. Naylor, N. Bhullar, and M. A. Akeroyd. 2012. Self-assessed hearing abilities in middle-and older-age adults: A stratified sampling approach. *International Journal of Audiology* 51(3):174–180.

Noble, W., N. S. Jensen, G. Naylor, N. Bhullar, and M. A. Akeroyd. 2013. A short form of the Speech, Spatial, and Qualities of Hearing Scale suitable for clinical use: The SSQ12. *International Journal of Audiology* 52(6):409–412.

Öberg, M., T. Lunner, and G. Andersson. 2007. Psychometric evaluation of hearing specific self-report measures and their associations with psychosocial and demographic variables. *Audiological Medicine* 5(3):188–199.

Oremule, B., J. Abbas, G. Saunders, K. Kluk, R. Isba, S. Bate, and I. Bruce. 2024. Mobile audiometry for hearing threshold assessment: A systematic review and meta-analysis. *Clinical Otolaryngology* 49(1):74–86.

Ou, H., and M. Wetmore. 2020. Development of a revised performance-perceptual test using Quick Speech in Noise test material and its norms. *Journal of the American Academy of Audiology* 31(03):176–184.

Patro, A., A. C. Moberly, M. H. Freeman, E. L. Perkins, T. A. Jan, K. O. Tawfik, M. R. O'Malley, M. L. Bennett, R. H. Gifford, D. S. Haynes, and N. I. Chowdhury. 2024. Investigating the minimal clinically important difference for AzBIO and CNC speech recognition scores. *Otology & Neurotology* 45(9):e639–e643.

Pearsons, K. S., R. L. Bennett, and S. Fidell. 1977. *Speech levels in various noise environments (report no. EPA-600/1-77-025).* https://nepis.epa.gov/Exe/ZyPURL.cgi?Dockey=P100CWGS.TXT (accessed January 12, 2025).

Perron, M., B. Lau, and C. Alain. 2023. Interindividual variability in the benefits of personal sound amplification products on speech perception in noise: A randomized cross-over clinical trial. *PLoS One* 18(7):e0288434.

Phatak, S. A., B. M. Sheffield, D. S. Brungart, and K. W. Grant. 2018. Development of a test battery for evaluating speech perception in complex listening environments: Effects of sensorineural hearing loss. *Ear and Hearing* 39(3):449–456.

Potgieter, J. M., D. W. Swanepoel, H. C. Myburgh, T. C. Hopper, and C. Smits. 2015. Development and validation of a smartphone-based Digits-in-Noise hearing test in South African English. *International Journal of Audiology* 55(7):405–411.

Potgieter, J. M., W. Swanepoel, H. C. Myburgh, and C. Smits. 2018a. The South African English smartphone Digits-in-Noise hearing test: Effect of age, hearing loss, and speaking competence. *Ear and Hearing* 39(4):656–663.

Potgieter, J. M., W. Swanepoel, and C. Smits. 2018b. Evaluating a smartphone Digits-in-Noise test as part of the audiometric test battery. *South African Journal of Communication Disorders* 65(1):e1–e6.

Prinsen, C. A. C., S. Vohra, M. R. Rose, M. Boers, P. Tugwell, M. Clarke, P. R. Williamson, and C. B. Terwee. 2016. How to select outcome measurement instruments for outcomes included in a "core outcome set"—A practical guideline. *Trials* 17(1):449.

Radulescu, L., O. Astefanei, R. Serban, S. Cozma, C. Butnaru, and C. Martu. 2024. The validation of the Speech, Spatial and Qualities of Hearing scale SSQ12 for native Romanian speakers with and without hearing impairment. *Journal of Personalized Medicine* 14(1):90.

Reynard, P., J. Lagacé, C. A. Joly, L. Dodelé, E. Veuillet, and H. Thai-Van. 2022. Speech-in-noise audiometry in adults: A review of the available tests for French speakers. *Audiology and Neurotology* 27(3):185–199.

Roup, C. M., E. Post, and J. Lewis. 2018. Mild-gain hearing aids as a treatment for adults with self-reported hearing difficulties. *Journal of the American Academy of Audiology* 29(6):477–494.

Sabin, A. T., D. J. Van Tasell, B. Rabinowitz, and S. Dhar. 2020. Validation of a self-fitting method for over-the-counter hearing aids. *Trends in Hearing* 24:2331216519900589.

Samsa, G., D. Edelman, M. L. Rothman, G. R. Williams, J. Lipscomb, and D. Matchar. 1999. Determining clinically important differences in health status measures: A general approach with illustration to the Health Utilities Index Mark II. *Pharmacoeconomics* 15(2):141–155.

Sanchez, V. A., M. L. Arnold, E. E. Garcia Morales, N. S. Reed, S. Faucette, S. Burgard, H. N. Calloway, J. Coresh, J. A. Deal, and A. M. Goman. 2024. Effect of hearing intervention on communicative function: A secondary analysis of the ACHIEVE randomized controlled trial. *Journal of the American Geriatrics Society* 72(12):3784–3799.

Sanchez-Lopez, R., T. Dau, and W. M. Whitmer. 2022. Audiometric profiles and patterns of benefit: A data-driven analysis of subjective hearing difficulties and handicaps. *International Journal of Audiology* 61(4):301–310.

Saunders, G. H., and K. M. Cienkowski. 1997. Acclimatization to hearing aids. *Ear and Hearing* 18(2):129–139.

Saxena, U., S. K. Mishra, H. Rodrigo, and M. Choudhury. 2022. Functional consequences of extended high frequency hearing impairment: Evidence from the Speech, Spatial, and Qualities of Hearing scale. *Journal of the Acoustical Society of America* 152(5):2946–2952.

Schafer, E. C., J. Pogue, and T. Milrany. 2012. List equivalency of the AzBIO sentence test in noise for listeners with normal-hearing sensitivity or cochlear implants. *Journal of the American Academy of Audiology* 23(7):501–509.

Schimmel, C., V. Manchaiah, D. Swanepoel, and A. Sharma. 2024. Digits-in-Noise test as an assessment tool for hearing loss and hearing aids. *Audiology Research* 14:342–358.

Singh, G., and M. K. Pichora-Fuller. 2010. Older adults performance on the Speech, Spatial, and Qualities of Hearing Scale (SSQ): Test-retest reliability and a comparison of interview and self-administration methods. *International Journal of Audiology* 49(10):733–740.

Śliwińska-Kowalska, M. 2020. [Preventive hearing tests in workers exposed to noise and organic solvents]. *Medycyna Pracy* 71(4):493–505.

Smits, C., S. E. Kramer, and T. Houtgast. 2006. Speech reception thresholds in noise and self-reported hearing disability in a general adult population. *Ear and Hearing* 27(5): 538–549.

Smits, C., S. Theo Goverts, and J. M. Festen. 2013. The Digits-in-Noise test: Assessing auditory speech recognition abilities in noise. *Journal of the Acoustical Society of America* 133(3):1693–1706.

Spahr, A. J., M. F. Dorman, L. M. Litvak, S. Van Wie, R. H. Gifford, P. C. Loizou, L. M. Loiselle, T. Oakes, and S. Cook. 2012. Development and validation of the AzBIO sentence lists. *Ear and Hearing* 33(1):112–117.

Srinivasan, N., and S. O'Neill. 2023. Comparison of Speech, Spatial, and Qualities of Hearing scale (SSQ) and the Abbreviated Profile of Hearing Aid Benefit (APHAB) questionnaires in a large cohort of self-reported normal-hearing adult listeners. *Audiology Research* 13(1):143–150.

Stark, P., and L. Hickson. 2004. Outcomes of hearing aid fitting for older people with hearing impairment and their significant others. *International Journal of Audiology* 43(7):390–398.

Stenbäck, V., E. Marsja, R. Ellis, and J. Rönnberg. 2023. Relationships between behavioural and self-report measures in speech recognition in noise. *International Journal of Audiology* 62(2):101–109.

Streiner, D., G. Norman, and J. Cairney. 2015. *Health measurement scales: A practical guide to their development and use.* Oxford, UK: Oxford University Press.

Surr, R. K., M. T. Cord, and B. E. Walden. 1998. Long-term versus short-term hearing aid benefit. *Journal of the American Academy of Audiology* 9(3).

Taylor, K. S. 1993. Self-perceived and audiometric evaluations of hearing aid benefit in the elderly. *Ear and Hearing* 14(6):390–394.

Thorén, E. S., G. Andersson, and T. Lunner. 2012. The use of research questionnaires with hearing impaired adults: Online vs. paper-and-pencil administration. *BMC Ear, Nose and Throat Disorders* 12:1–6.

Tomioka, K., H. Ikeda, K. Hanaie, M. Morikawa, J. Iwamoto, N. Okamoto, K. Saeki, and N. Kurumatani. 2013. The Hearing Handicap Inventory for Elderly-Screening (HHIE-S) versus a single question: Reliability, validity, and relations with quality of life measures in the elderly community, Japan. *Quality of Life Research* 22(5):1151–1159.

Toolbox Assessments, Inc. 2024. *Words-in-Noise test.* https://nihtoolbox.org/test/words-in-noise-test (accessed January 12, 2025).

Toussaint, A., P. Hüsing, A. Gumz, K. Wingenfeld, M. Härter, E. Schramm, and B. Löwe. 2020. Sensitivity to change and minimal clinically important difference of the 7-item Generalized Anxiety Disorder Questionnaire (GAD-7). *Journal of Affective Disorders* 265:395–401.

Utoomprurkporn, N., J. Stott, S. G. Costafreda, and D. E. Bamiou. 2021. Lack of association between audiogram and hearing disability measures in mild cognitive impairment and dementia: What audiogram does not tell you. *Healthcare (Basel)* 9(6).

Van den Borre, E., S. Denys, A. van Wieringen, and J. Wouters. 2021. The digit triplet test: A scoping review. *International Journal of Audiology* 60(12):946–963.

Ventry, I. M., and B. E. Weinstein. 1982. The Hearing Handicap Inventory for the Elderly: A new tool. *Ear and Hearing* 3(3):128–134.

Ventry, I. M., and B. E. Weinstein. 1983. Identification of elderly people with hearing problems. *ASHA* 25(7):37–42.

Vermiglio, A. J., L. Leclerc, M. Thornton, H. Osborne, E. Bonilla, and X. Fang. 2021. Diagnostic accuracy of the AzBIO speech recognition in noise test. *Journal of Speech, Language, and Hearing Research* 64(8):3303–3316.

Walden, B. E. 1997. Toward a model clinical-trials protocol for substantiating hearing aid user-benefit claims. *American Journal of Audiology* 6(2):13–24.

Walden, T. C., and B. E. Walden. 2004. Predicting success with hearing aids in everyday living. *Journal of the American Academy of Audiology* 15(05):342–352.

Wang, S., and L. L. N. Wong. 2024. Development of the Mandarin Digit-in-Noise test and examination of the effect of the number of digits used in the test. *Ear and Hearing* 45(3):572–582.

Watson, C. S., G. R. Kidd, J. D. Miller, C. Smits, and L. E. Humes. 2012. Telephone screening tests for functionally impaired hearing: Current use in seven countries and development of a US version. *Journal of the American Academy of Audiology* 23(10):757–767.

Weinstein, B. E., and I. M. Ventry. 1983. Audiometric correlates of the Hearing Handicap Inventory for the Elderly. *Journal of Speech and Hearing Disorders* 48(4):379–384.

Weinstein, B. E., J. B. Spitzer, and I. M. Ventry. 1986. Test-retest reliability of the Hearing Handicap Inventory for the Elderly. *Ear and Hearing* 7(5):295–299.

Wilson, R. H. 2003. Development of a speech-in-multitalker-babble paradigm to assess word-recognition performance. *Journal of the American Academy of Audiology* 14(09):453–470.

Wilson, R. H. 2006. *Speech recognition and identification materials*, disc 4.0. https://chs.asu.edu/sites/default/files/2022-05/booklet-speech_recid_disc_4.0_0.pdf (accessed January 14, 2025).

Wilson, R. H. 2011. Clinical experience with the Words-in-Noise test on 3430 veterans: Comparisons with pure-tone thresholds and word recognition in quiet. *Journal of the American Academy of Audiology* 22(07):405–423.

Wilson, R. H., and A. Strouse. 2002. Northwestern University auditory test no. 6 in multi-talker babble: A preliminary report. *Journal of Rehabilitation Research and Development* 39(1).

Wilson, R. H., and D. G. Weakley. 2004. The use of digit triplets to evaluate word-recognition abilities in multitalker babble. *Seminars in Hearing* 25(1):93–111.

Wilson, R. H., and C. A. Burks. 2005. Use of 35 words for evaluation of hearing loss in signal-to-babble ratio: A clinic protocol. *Journal of Rehabilitation Research and Development* 42(6):839–852.

Wilson, R. H., and R. McArdle. 2007. Intra- and inter-session test, retest reliability of the Words-in-Noise (WIN) test. *Journal of the American Academy of Audiology* 18(10):813–825.

Wilson, R. H., and W. B. Cates. 2008. A comparison of two word-recognition tasks in multitalker babble: Speech Recognition in Noise Test (SPRINT) and Words-in-Noise test (WIN). *Journal of the American Academy of Audiology* 19(7):548–556.

Wilson, R. H., and K. L. Watts. 2012. The Words-in-Noise test (WIN), list 3: A practice list. *Journal of the American Academy of Audiology* 23(02):092–096.

Wilson, R. H., H. B. Abrams, and A. L. Pillion. 2003. A word-recognition task in multitalker babble using a descending presentation mode from 24 db to 0 db signal to babble. *Journal of Rehabilitation Research & Development* 40(4).

Wilson, R. H., C. A. Burks, and D. G. Weakley. 2005. Word recognition in multitalker babble measured with two psychophysical methods. *Journal of the American Academy of Audiology* 16(08):622–630.

Wilson, R. H., C. A. Burks, and D. G. Weakley. 2006. Word recognition of digit triplets and monosyllabic words in multitalker babble by listeners with sensorineural hearing loss. *Journal of the American Academy of Audiology* 17(06):385–397.

Wilson, R. H., C. S. Carnell, and A. L. Cleghorn. 2007a. The Words-in-Noise (WIN) test with multitalker babble and speech-spectrum noise maskers. *Journal of the American Academy of Audiology* 18(06):522–529.

Wilson, R. H., R. A. McArdle, and S. L. Smith. 2007b. An evaluation of the BKB-SIN, HINT, QuickSIN, AND WIN materials on listeners with normal hearing and listeners with hearing loss. *Journal of Speech, Language, and Hearing Research* 50(4):844–856.

Wilson, R. H., C. P. Trivette, D. A. Williams, and K. L. Watts. 2012. The effects of energetic and informational masking on the Words-in-Noise test (WIN). *Journal of the American Academy of Audiology* 23(07):522–533.

Wolinsky, F. D., G. Wan, and W. Tierney. 1998. Changes in the SF-36 in 12 months in a sample of disadvantaged older adults. *Medical Care* 36:1589–1598.

Wright, D., and J.-P. Gagné. 2021. Acclimatization to hearing aids by older adults. *Ear and Hearing* 42(1):193–205.

Wyrwich, K., W. M. Tierney, and F. D. Wolinsky. 1999. Further evidence supporting an SEM-based criterion for identifying meaningful intra-individual changes in health-related quality of life. *Journal of Clinical Epidemiology* 52:861–873.

Wyss, J., D. J. Mecklenburg, and P. L. Graham. 2020. Self-assessment of daily hearing function for implant recipients: A comparison of mean total scores for the Speech Spatial Qualities of Hearing Scale (SSQ49) with the SSQ12. *Cochlear Implants International* 21(3):167–178.

Zaar, J., P. Ihly, T. Nishiyama, S. Laugesen, S. Santurette, C. Tanaka, G. Jones, M. Vatti, D. Suzuki, and T. Kitama. 2023. Predicting speech-in-noise reception in hearing-impaired listeners with hearing aids using the Audible Contrast Threshold (ACT) test. [Preprint]. PsyArXiv Preprints. https://doi.org/10.31234/osf.io/m9khu.

Zaar, J., L. B. Simonsen, R. Sanchez-Lopez, and S. Laugesen. 2024. The Audible Contrast Threshold (ACT) test: A clinical spectro-temporal modulation detection test. *Hearing Research* 453:109103.

Zhang, Y., X. Xi, and Y. Huang. 2023. The anchor design of anchor-based method to determine the minimal clinically important difference: A systematic review. *Health and Quality of Life Outcomes* 21:74.

7

Dissemination and Implementation

As noted in Chapter 3, core outcome sets (COS) can enhance standardization and in turn help improve the usefulness of findings in health care research and clinical assessments to ultimately improve patient outcomes. However, these benefits are only realized if a COS is used. COS uptake in clinical research using randomized controlled trials varies substantially depending on the condition, and uptake has been found to be low in the development of practice guidelines (Hughes et al., 2021; Rhodes et al., 2024). While studies describing protocols used to develop, disseminate, and implement COSs are readily identified in the literature, analyses of the effectiveness of the dissemination and implementation protocols of those COSs are more limited (Bellucci et al., 2021; South et al., 2024). As noted in Chapter 3, one often cited strategy for increasing uptake of a COS is developing consensus during the process of creating the COS by engaging with those who will use it. An examination of the available literature related to barriers and facilitators for COS uptake, as well as dissemination and implementation in other areas such as evidence-based practice, can provide useful insights.

DISSEMINATION AND IMPLEMENTATION BASICS

Dissemination and implementation are often discussed collectively. However, dissemination and implementation are two separate but related areas. Dissemination refers to active efforts to spread information, typically research findings, to targeted audiences using planned strategies (Rabin et al., 2008).

Implementation refers to the process of translating that knowledge into action, typically in the form of adoption and integration of a given evidence-based practice, using planned strategies (Baumann et al., 2023; Rabin et al., 2008). Dissemination and implementation science is a growing field of research that investigates and develops approaches to increase uptake of research innovations and the resulting evidence-based interventions (Rabin et al., 2008; Yi et al., 2022). Both dissemination and implementation strategies seek to create a change in behavior that leads to uptake of a new practice, in this case use of the COS.

Dissemination strategies lay the foundation for, and contribute to, implementation strategies to support COS uptake. Therefore, dissemination and implementation processes are often guided by behavior science theory, such as the Capability, Opportunity, Motivation-Behavior (COM-B) model (see Figure 7-1) and the Behavior Change Wheel (see Figure 7-2) (Matvienko-Sikar et al., 2024; Michie et al., 2011).

The COM-B model posits that for a behavior to occur, an individual must have the capability, opportunity, and motivation to carry out that behavior (Matvienko-Sikar et al., 2024). Dissemination and implementation programs usually engage one or a combination of commonly used staged models, such as the reach, adoption, implementation, and maintenance (RE-AIM) framework to inform the selection of, and organize deployment of, strategies (Glasgow et al., 2019). A staged approach highlights the importance of dissemination and implementation activities beyond the point of initial uptake to support sustainable adoption (Proctor et al., 2013; Rabin et al., 2008).

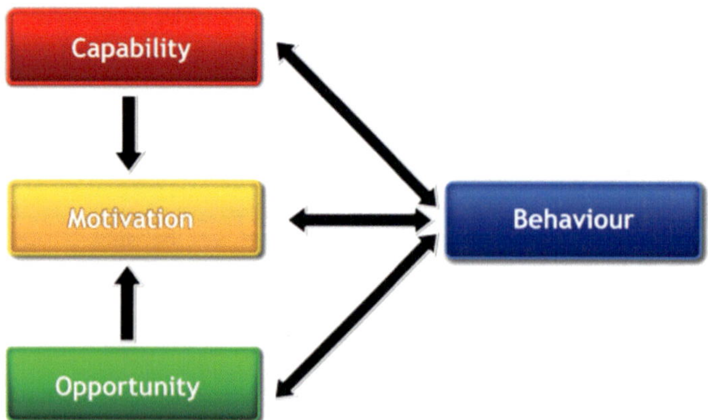

FIGURE 7-1 The COM-B system: A framework for understanding behavior.
NOTE: COM-B = Capability, Opportunity, Motivation-Behavior.
SOURCE: Michie et al., 2011. CC BY 2.0.

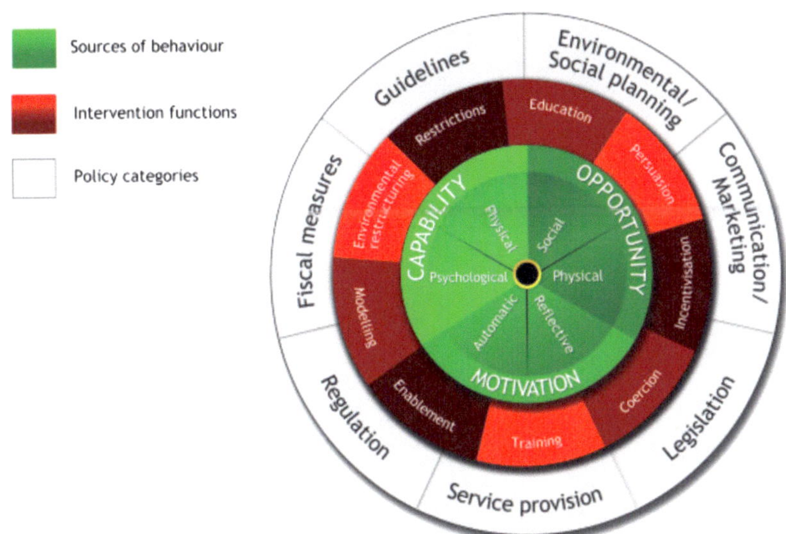

FIGURE 7-2 The behavior change wheel.
SOURCE: Michie et al., 2011. CC BY 2.0.

DISSEMINATION AND IMPLEMENTATION FOR CORE OUTCOME SET UPTAKE

Matvienko and colleagues (2024) applied the COM-B model and concepts from the Behavior Change Wheel to barriers and facilitators to the use of COSs commonly cited in studies, examining uptake by researchers to identify potential strategies for facilitating the uptake of COSs (Matvienko-Sikar et al., 2024). Table 7-1 highlights several facilitators and barriers specific to the uptake of a COS.

Improving Awareness of the COS

Several studies investigating the uptake of COSs have noted that researchers who were knowledgeable about COSs in general or for a specific condition were more likely to use a COS in their studies (Bellucci et al., 2021; Hughes et al., 2022). Additionally, those studies found that lack of awareness of the COS for a specific condition and lack of knowledge in general about COSs, as well as about the rigorous methodology involved in their development, were frequently cited as a reason for not using a COS (Bellucci et al., 2021; Hughes et al., 2021, 2022; Kirkham and Williamson, 2022; Saldanha et al., 2024). This highlights the importance

TABLE 7-1 Barriers and Facilitators to the Use of a COS Identified by Researchers or Clinical Trialists

Barriers	Facilitators
• Lack of awareness of COSs in general and for specific conditions	• Knowledge about COSs in general and for specific conditions
• Lack of knowledge about how to use a COS	• Understanding how to apply a COS
• Lack of knowledge about how to measure a COS	• Previous involvement developing a COS
• Unsure that COSs are current	• Easy to find and determine suitability of a COS
• Unsure which COS should be used when multiple options are available	• Understanding that COSs address inconsistencies in outcomes measured in trials
• Perception that a COS may not match scope and specificity for the planned trial	• Understanding that using a COS does not preclude inclusion of other outcomes
• Costs associated with measuring a COS	• Understanding that a COS helps identify outcomes for trials
• Challenges with measuring a COS related to availability and quality of existing and recommended measurements	• Understanding the robust examination of evidence and rigorous methodology used to develop a COS
• Too many COS outcomes to measure limits opportunity to use other outcomes	• Research community promotes and facilitates use of COSs
• Too many COS outcomes to measure overburdens participants and researchers	• Understanding that a COS improves research consistency and evidence synthesis as well as reduces waste
• Measurement approaches for the COS create additional burden for participants and researchers	• Perception that COS measurement will not overburden participants
• Research team is critical of methods used to develop and update the COS	
• Researcher prefers to use own outcomes or older COS	
• COSs are seen as limiting opportunity for innovation of new outcomes	
• Researchers want to control trial outcome	

NOTE: COS = Core Outcome Set.
SOURCE: Modified from Matvienko-Sikar et al., 2024. CC BY 4.0.

of first engaging in a robust dissemination strategy to ensure researchers, hearing health professionals, clinicians of first contact (e.g., primary care physicians, advanced practice registered nurses), and patients have the necessary knowledge of this COS for adult hearing health.

In 2013, a large systematic review by McCormack and colleagues (2013) sought to identify the most effective approaches to dissemination of research findings to inform evidence-based practice. That review, as well as a more recent large systematic review from South and colleagues (2024), found that multicomponent approaches that included some combination of strategies to improve the reach of information to multiple audiences and settings, strategies to increase motivation to use the information, or strategies to improve the ability to use the information were generally most effective (McCormack et al., 2013; South et al., 2024).

Systematic reviews have found that while the effect size was small, multicomponent approaches that include academic detailing (also referred to as educational outreach) were most often identified in the literature as having a positive effect on changing clinical practice (McCormack et al., 2013; O'Brien et al., 2007; South et al., 2024; Tomasone et al., 2020). Academic detailing is derived from the detailing approach used by pharmaceutical sales representatives in which they engaged in face-to-face engagement with physicians to promote prescription of certain drugs (Fischer, 2016). It uses principles of various models of behavior change in direct outreach and engagement with health care professionals to deliver evidence-based information to promote the adoption of a recommended change in clinical practice (Fischer, 2016; O'Brien et al., 2007). Key components of effective academic detailing (in general) include (Soumerai and Avorn, 1990):

- Conducting interviews with clinicians to determine their baseline knowledge and motivations for using their existing practice patterns (in this case outcome measurements);
- Defining specific educational and behavioral objectives for the academic detailing program;
- Focusing outreach efforts on specific categories of clinicians and relevant opinion leaders;
- Establishing credibility by referencing information from unbiased and authoritative sources, collaborating with respected organizations, and presenting diverse perspectives on any directly relevant controversial issues;
- Creating succinct educational materials that include graphics;
- Emphasizing and repeating the key messages during outreach interactions; and
- Using positive reinforcement during follow-up interactions.

Studies of academic detailing programs found the strategy effectively increased uptake of recommendations for changes in practice such as appropriate prescribing of opioids and naloxone, use of prescription monitoring programs, diabetes care in the primary care setting, managing behavioral symptoms of dementia, and others (Fischer, 2016; Kulbokas et al., 2021; Walaszek et al., 2023).

Conclusion 7-1: A robust multicomponent dissemination strategy that includes educational outreach can help ensure all key partners have the necessary knowledge of the COS (and corresponding measures).

Examples of Successful Strategies to Enhance Uptake of a COS

In terms of specific examples of successful dissemination and implementation strategies to enhance COS uptake in other fields, examinations of data from ClinicalTrials.gov and the World Health Organization International Clinical Trials Registry Platform found that the COS for rheumatoid arthritis has had particularly high uptake (Kirkham et al., 2017). Given the historically high uptake of the rheumatoid arthritis COS developed by the organization Outcome Measures in Rheumatoid Arthritis Clinical Trials, now referred to as Outcome Measures in Rheumatology (OMERACT), it is reasonable to consider their strategies for insight into applicable best practices.

The OMERACT organization itself is likely an important tool to support COS uptake. It serves as a central entity that has taken responsibility for developing and updating COSs, as well as their dissemination and implementation. Many of those strategies echo the components of effective academic detailing. The rheumatoid arthritis COS dissemination has been supported by key strategies to establish its credibility. One key strategy is the establishment of the OMERACT organization itself, which at its inception was affiliated with the International League of Associations of Rheumatology, a well-known and respected organization in the field (Tugwell et al., 2007). Additionally, the organization's first several conferences were hosted by the World Health Organization at its headquarters in Geneva, Switzerland (Tugwell et al., 2007). OMERACT's founders and current committees and working groups consist of highly regarded thought leaders and experts in rheumatology.

OMERACT uses a multicomponent education approach that supports dissemination of COSs. Working groups, which analyze evidence from research and conduct reviews that often lead to an updated or new COS, publish their work in respected professional journals well known to the professionals engaged in rheumatoid arthritis research and care. OMERACT maintains a website that includes a handbook that uses text and infographics to explain its COSs and the methodology used to develop them, a structured education program targeted at COS users, and information about past and upcoming events (OMERACT, 2024). In addition to OMERACT's biannual conferences, committee leaders present at professional meetings for experts in related fields, such as neurology and radiology (Tugwell et al., 2007).

Because of the vast nature of implementation and dissemination science surrounding COSs, there is a need for continued research to further identify additional key facilitators and barriers to increasing the uptake of COSs in research and practice (Bellucci et al., 2021; South et al., 2024). A strong understanding of what makes an implementation framework successful allows for reproducible research and a clearer understanding of the findings and lends itself to recommendations for practice and guideline development (Smith et al., 2020). Further research in this area will continue to guide researchers and practitioners in effective dissemination and implementation practices, which is necessary for the uptake of COSs.

Conclusion 7-2: More research is needed to better understand the key facilitators, barriers, and approaches to the uptake of a COS (and corresponding measures) in research and practice, both for uptake of COSs in general as well as specific strategies in hearing health.

Conclusion 7-3: Having a centralized entity take responsibility for developing and updating the core outcome set is a highly effective strategy to encourage uptake.

STRATEGIES TO INCREASING THE UPTAKE OF A CORE OUTCOME SET FOR HEARING HEALTH OUTCOMES

Several strategies based on dissemination and implementation science, findings from research into barriers and facilitators to COS uptake, and examples from other successful endeavors can be applied to support the uptake of a hearing health COS.

The committee hosted a public webinar to hear directly from representatives of professional organizations including the American Academy of Audiology (AAA), the Academy of Doctors of Audiology (ADA), the American Speech-Language Hearing Society (ASHA), and the International Hearing Society (IHS).[1] The webinar focused on these organizations' experiences with disseminating new information to their constituencies to learn about which approaches have worked best to improve awareness and encourage the implementation of new practices as well as to learn about the challenges that these organizations face, particularly as they relate to outcome measurement (see Box 7-1).

Education

Dissemination and implementation strategies that target training and education are important for addressing many of the barriers to using COSs that have been identified in the literature. As previously noted, a multicomponent approach that includes academic detailing has been found beneficial. One-on-one outreach is inefficient and not cost-effective. Alternatively, group educational events such as conferences and workshops have been

---

[1] The webinar recording can be accessed at https://www.nationalacademies.org/event/43762_10-2024_meaningful-outcome-measures-in-adult-hearing-health-care-webinar-3.

BOX 7-1
Approaches to Dissemination and Implementation
of New Information in Hearing Health

"We're instructing on [outcome measurement] in both our entry level and our advanced education that's available to our membership and to our customers at large [. . .] We produce what's called our distance learning course for hearing health care professionals, which is the book work that an apprenticeship will do in conjunction with their hands-on training. It guides their trainer as to what they should be teaching them and trying to help make sure that the trainer and the trainee are both up to date on best practices. What we have found is that given that the vast majority of new hearing aid specialists are using the IHS materials, we have a huge opportunity there to be disseminating information."

—Sierra Sharpe, IHS

"We try to focus very heavily on making sure our members can have both some form of written material that they can reference at any time, day or night . . . but we also know that having that interaction with live webinars and live presentations can be helpful as well."

—Alicia Spoor, ADA

"The implementation piece . . . is hard to know. It's hard to measure, so we do ask our membership to give us some information when we do surveys about the practices that they use. If we ask something about how many of you use real-ear verification, we're depending on them to tell us that back. And we're also depending upon the sampling, and so depending on what that sample is and depending on who answers it. It's hard to know about the implementation piece, to really have a good grasp on how many of our members are implementing a practice that the community feels is evidence-based and needs to be happening."

—Donna Smiley, ASHA

"So how do we get that in front of people's faces? Presentations at conferences, particularly our annual conference, has been a big point, especially in some of the more highlighted, featured session talks where they have a large attendance, and people can pick up those new concepts or new guidelines. Other things like publications, whether it's our journal or our magazine, *Audiology Today*, helping to get it in front of people. Also targeting specific stakeholders. [. . .] as well as working with other audiology organizations, particularly state organizations to help keep them involved and keep them aware of what's going on at the national level."

—Patricia Gaffney, AAA

These quotes were collected from the committee's webinars.

identified as a beneficial approach (Forsetlund et al., 2021). These convenings may be led by the institution responsible for developing a COS measurement instrument, such as the PROMIS Health Organization, which holds events to train health care professionals in use of its Patient-Reported Outcome Measurement Information System (PROMIS) for measurement of person-centered outcomes (PROMIS Health Organization, 2024).

As noted in Chapter 3, patient-reported outcome measures (PROMs) gather data directly from patients about their health status and outcomes. These measures seek feedback on general outcomes, meaning "examine aspects that fit a variety of different conditions and allow comparison across these various medical conditions," or disease-specific outcomes, meaning measures that are "designed to identify specific symptoms and their impact on the function of those specific conditions" (Weldring and Smith, 2013, p. 63). PROMs have not only helped shape clinical decision making and contributed to patient-centered care, but they also offer valuable insight into symptoms and functioning that may have been missed by traditional clinical measures, allowing for a more holistic view (Adeghe et al., 2024). Presentations and workshops can also be embedded in relevant professional organizations' scientific meetings.

Webinars and other virtual learning options can be used to deliver education about COSs and their use in a convenient manner. OMERACT has an educational initiative referred to as OMER-ED that includes courses about the different rheumatoid arthritis COSs, the development process for its COS, and how to select the correct rheumatoid arthritis COS instrument (OMERACT, 2025). A similar virtual educational platform could be developed for the hearing health COS, with modules tailored to relevant audiences and accessibility needs.

Conclusion 7-4: Conferences, workshops, and webinars (and other virtual learning options) are effective strategies for enhancing education about COSs (and corresponding measures).

Regulation and Incentives

Institutions engaged in funding and regulating research can support the uptake of COSs. The International Standard Randomized Controlled Trial Number Registry website, which includes studies beyond randomized controlled trials (RCTs), advises researchers to identify outcome measures in their applications and refers them to the Core Outcome Measures in Effectiveness Trials (COMET) Initiative (BMC, 2025). *Standard Protocol Items: Recommendations for Interventional Trials* (SPIRIT) guidelines encourage researchers to identify relevant COSs by consulting COMET (Chan et al., 2013). Cochrane's author guidelines encourage review authors to use

OMERACT COSs (Tugwell et al., 2007). The Health Research Authority of the UK's National Health Service (NHS) includes information about the use of COSs in the best practices section of their website and provides a link to the COMET Initiative for additional education and support (NHS, 2019).

Research funding sources may create an incentive to use COSs. A study of OMERACT COS uptake in clinical trials registered on ClinicalTrials.gov and the World Health Organization-International Clinical Trials Registry Platform found that industry-funded trials were more likely to use a COS (Kirkham et al., 2019). This also suggests commercial research funders are an important group to include in educational outreach efforts to increase uptake of COSs. Notably, that study also found that registered clinical trials that were not commercially funded were less likely to plan to measure those COSs. OMERACT is currently seeking to increase collaboration with regulatory bodies, such as the Food and Drug Administration (FDA) to ensure its methodologies are consistent with FDA regulations (OMERACT, 2023). Academic detailing efforts that extend to regulators and funding agencies can increase awareness of the hearing health COS, which is an important first step toward a regulatory or funding requirement. There is precedent for agencies requiring the use of COSs in studies they support. The National Institutes of Health Helping to End Addiction Long-term (HEAL) Initiative developed a set of patient-reported core outcomes related to pain and requires clinical trials that are part of that initiative to use those COSs.[2]

One additional driver for increasing uptake of COSs in the clinical setting could be the growing interest in value-based care. Value-based care emphasizes measuring patient-reported outcomes, which share similarities with COSs (Kearney et al., 2023). Because of the overlap in patient-centered outcome measures (the measures developed and used for value-based health care) and COSs, requiring the use of COSs for value-based health care practices could be an avenue for consistent use of COSs.

Also, the implementation of COSs into patient portals integrated with electronic health records (EHR) systems could allow for a streamlined approach to incorporate the Abbreviated Profile of Hearing Aid Benefit (APHAB) and the Revised Hearing Handicap Inventory (RHHI) into the health record system. Integrating COSs into EHR systems could allow for COSs to become routine data collection and in turn inform future research and guideline development (Dodd et al., 2020). EHR systems have been widely implemented into the health care system to increase the ease of

---

[2] For more information, see https://rethinkingclinicaltrials.org/chapters/conduct/real-world-evidence-patient-reported-outcomes-pros/nih-heal-fda-and-other-core-outcome-sets (accessed October 9, 2024).

patient data collection and transfer (CMS, 2024). Using the systems already in practice could lead to the uptake of COSs.

Conclusion 7-5: Required use of COSs (and corresponding measures) by funders of research and insurers (when measures are required), as well as integration of the COSs into EHRs, can create effective incentives for the use of the COSs.

Data Repositories

At the 2024 Midwinter Meeting of the Association for Research in Otolaryngology, the topic of "big data" was discussed in an organized symposium. "Good Data in, Big Data out" presentations included:

- *Standardization of Threshold and Supra-Threshold Measures in Clinical Trials Assessing Investigational Inner Ear Medicines* (Le Prell, 2024).
- *The Role of Consistent Clinical Practice Approaches for Data-Informed Hearing Care* (Poling, 2024).
- *Here Hear Share* (Hertzano, 2024).
- *From Club Good to Pure Public Good: Some Barriers and Solutions to Sharing Health-Related Data* (Cummings, 2024).
- *Big Data, Big Possibilities* (Reavis, 2024).

Of particular relevance to the topic of databases, Poling noted that standardizing data collection and integration practices can improve clinical processes and improve patient care delivery. In addition, she highlighted the need for consistency in clinical practices to allow for data harmonization and the ability to use the full potential of big data from clinical audiology. Hertzano followed, noting that audiology has yet to establish a unified approach for harmonizing, sharing, analyzing, and visualizing data, with no large audiometric databases. To address this unmet need, Hertzano presented her team's efforts to develop a secure cloud-based platform, built upon the Probing Outcomes Data with Visual Analytics (POD-Vis) software, that can host hearing data. As noted in her meeting abstract, the development of this tool is led by the HearShare consortium, which includes Duke University, the National Institute on Deafness and Other Communication Disorders (NIDCD), Massachusetts Eye and Ear Infirmary, Mayo Clinic, Medical University of South Carolina, University of Maryland College Park, and the University of Maryland Baltimore. Collectively, these institutions have amassed a vast dataset that includes hearing thresholds, tympanometry, acoustic reflex thresholds, and speech audiometry (recognition scores in quiet and noise) from over 500,000 unique adult patients aged 18 years and above.

The National Institutes of Health (NIH) broadly supports the sharing of data in an appropriate repository.[3] NIDCD is highly supportive of data repositories (Tucci, 2023) and maintains a list of publicly available databases that NIDCD-funded scientists can access.[4] Of note, NIH currently hosts a pediatric hearing database.[5] Also worth noting is the NIH-supported gene Expression Analysis Resource (gEAR)[6] database, which provides an example of a data repository that supports not only data submission but also display, analysis, and interrogation, with users able to customize their own data displays and compare their data to other uploaded datasets (Orvis et al., 2021). The gEAR database is highly relevant to hearing loss (Hertzano and Mahurkar, 2022; Taiber et al., 2022). Tools within gEAR have been used to investigate genes associated with adult onset hearing loss (Lewis et al., 2023) and age-related hearing loss (Schubert et al., 2022). There are a host of issues related to database development and data sharing (Eckert et al., 2023). Thus, centralized support from government and other organizations is essential to the success of data harmonization and data-sharing repositories

Conclusion 7-6: Centralized data repositories can help researchers and clinicians benchmark their use of the COS and corresponding measures, compare results, and allow for pooling of data.

FINDINGS

Finding 7-1: Dissemination refers to the active efforts taken to spread information; implementation refers to translating that information into action.

Finding 7-2: A combination of strategies is typically needed to encourage the uptake and use of new information.

Finding 7-3: Multicomponent approaches that include some combination of strategies to improve the reach of information to multiple audiences and settings, strategies to increase motivation to use the information, or strategies to improve the ability to use the information are generally most effective.

---

[3] For more information see https://sharing.nih.gov/data-management-and-sharing-policy/sharing-scientific-data/repositories-for-sharing-scientific-data (accessed January 13, 2025).

[4] For more information see https://www.nidcd.nih.gov/research/population-clinical-database-resources-nidcd-mission-areas#hearing (accessed January 13, 2025).

[5] For more information see https://audgendb.github.io/ (accessed January 13, 2025).

[6] For more information see https://umgear.org/ (accessed January 13, 2025).

Finding 7-4: Known facilitators to uptake of COSs include:

- Knowledge of the COS (including its purpose),
- Understanding how to use the COS and recognizing that its use does not preclude the use of other outcomes,
- Understanding that the COS addresses inconsistencies in outcomes measured in trials, and
- Understanding the rigor of the development of the COS.

Finding 7-5: Known barriers for uptake of COSs include:

- Lack of awareness,
- Costs,
- Measurement burden,
- Perception that the COS may not match the scope and specificity for planned trials,
- Perception that the COS limits opportunities for innovation of new outcomes, and
- Preference for continuing current practices.

Finding 7-6: Researchers who know about COSs are more likely to use them in their studies.

Finding 7-7: Successful mechanisms to encourage the uptake of a COS include having a central entity responsible for developing and updating the COS and hosting conferences on the topic. Key dissemination and implementation strategies include education, typically through educational outreach; conferences and training events; and regulation and funding incentives, such as required use by research funders or registries

RECOMMENDATIONS

The first step in encouraging adoption of the COS and corresponding measures includes engaging in a robust dissemination strategy to ensure that researchers, health care professionals, and adults with hearing difficulties have the necessary knowledge of the COS and its measures.

Recommendation 7-1: Health academic organizations and programs, professional organizations, researchers, and consumer groups should disseminate information about the importance of the core outcome set to clinicians of first contact (e.g., primary care clinicians), hearing health clinicians (e.g., students, audiologists, otolaryngologists), and adults with hearing difficulties.

Strategies for dissemination include providing information and training on the COS and corresponding measures through formal educational, clinical, and research-focused training programs, websites, meetings, continuing education, and webinars. The committee notes that disseminating this information to different partners will likely require a multipronged approach. The committee purposefully includes primary care and other clinicians of first contact among the targets of dissemination because these partners will often be the first to evaluate the concerns of patients reporting hearing difficulty and patients may ask questions regarding the COS. Furthermore, adults with hearing difficulties themselves need to be included in the dissemination efforts to encourage a whole health approach to care.

Dissemination of information alone, however, is insufficient to ensure the uptake of a COS. It will be important to develop strategies for creating incentives to use the COS and corresponding measures as well as strategies for alleviating burdens to its use. Such strategies can come from a variety of sources, including requirements for use in research, incorporation of the outcome measures into electronic health records, and use in value-based care.

> **Recommendation 7-2: To create incentives for the use of the core outcome set and corresponding measures the following should occur:**
> a. Sponsors of research on hearing health interventions should require the use of the core outcome set and corresponding measures (at a minimum), unless scientifically justified for exclusion.
> b. Electronic health record (EHR) vendors should incorporate the Abbreviated Profile of Hearing Aid Benefit and Revised Hearing Handicap Inventory into EHRs.
> c. Insurers who require outcome measures should require the use of the recommended measures.

In particular, the committee notes that the recommended Words-in-Noise test (WIN) (see Chapter 6) is conducted through an audiometer and its results can be recorded in the EHR. The committee recommends the inclusion of the recommended self-report questionnaires (APHAB-Global and the RHHI) in the EHR both to allow for ease of use by the clinician and to enable patients to answer these questionnaires in advance of a clinical visit.

One of the main purposes of developing and using a COS and corresponding measures is to allow for the pooling of data, in part to compare the effectiveness of interventions, as well as develop a more robust evidence base that helps improve clinical care. The committee recognizes that NIH already has existing platforms for the centralized sharing of data.

> **Recommendation 7-3: To facilitate big data meta-analyses, the National Institutes of Health should develop a national database to allow**

clinicians and researchers to benchmark the use of the core outcome set and corresponding measures, as well as their results.

One highly effective strategy for encouraging the uptake of COSs in other fields is having a central entity take responsibility for developing and updating the COS. The committee recognizes the importance of ensuring the consistency of what is measured and how it is measured over time. However, as new evidence emerges, the COS will need to be revisited. The purpose will not be to just add more core outcomes, but to consider which ones should remain part of the core, or which ones should be considered for supplemental measurement as appropriate. As noted in Chapters 4 and 5, several outcomes (e.g., quality of life, cognition, listening fatigue) are widely meaningful, but the evidence bases for the ability of hearing interventions to affect the outcomes are mixed and evolving. The committee notes that several federal agencies provide substantial funding and work in hearing health research and hearing health care delivery and therefore are well positioned to collaborate to support ongoing evaluation and support for a COS.

> **Recommendation 7-4: After an adequate level of new research has been gathered, the National Institutes of Health, the Department of Defense, and the Veterans Administration should collaborate to revisit the core outcome set.**

Finally, while following the recommendations for dissemination and implementation of the COS and corresponding measures can help encourage uptake, there will still likely be gaps in understanding for which approaches work best for specific target audiences in the hearing health field. For example, tailoring the dissemination of information to various audiences will likely require research on specific strategies for each target population.

> **Recommendation 7-5: Sponsors of hearing health research should fund research on comprehensive implementation science approaches to identify additional key facilitators for and barriers to the uptake and use of the core outcome set and corresponding measures.**

REFERENCES

Adeghe, E. P., C. A. Okolo, and O. T. Ojeyinka. 2024. The influence of patient-reported outcome measures on healthcare delivery: A review of methodologies and applications. *OARJ of Biology and Pharmacy* 10(02):013–021.

Baumann, A. A., R. C. Shelton, S. Kumanyika, and D. Haire-Joshu. 2023. Advancing health-care equity through dissemination and implementation science. *Health Services Research* 58(Suppl 3):327–344.

Bellucci, C., K. Hughes, E. Toomey, P. R. Williamson, and K. Matvienko-Sikar. 2021. A survey of knowledge, perceptions and use of core outcome sets among clinical trialists. *Trials* 22(1):937.

BMC (BioMedCentral). 2025. *ISRCTN Registry - The UK's clinical study registry.* https://www.isrctn.com/page/definitions#primaryOutcomeMeasures (accessed January 7, 2025).

Chan, A. W., J. M. Tetzlaff, P. C. Gøtzsche, D. G. Altman, H. Mann, J. A. Berlin, K. Dickersin, A. Hróbjartsson, K. F. Schulz, W. R. Parulekar, K. Krleza-Jeric, A. Laupacis, and D. Moher. 2013. Spirit 2013 explanation and elaboration: Guidance for protocols of clinical trials. *British Medical Journal* 346:e7586.

CMS (Centers for Medicare & Medicaid Services). 2024. *Electronic health records.* https://www.cms.gov/priorities/key-initiatives/e-health/records (accessed December 19, 2024).

Cummings, M. 2024. *From club good to pure public good: Some barriers and solutions to sharing health-related data.* Paper presented at the 2024 Association for Research in Otolaryngology MidWinter Meeting, Orlando, FL.

Dodd, S., N. Harman, N. Taske, M. Minchin, T. Tan, and P. R. Williamson. 2020. Core outcome sets through the healthcare ecosystem: The case of type 2 diabetes mellitus. *Trials* 21(1): 570.

Eckert, M. A., F. T. Husain, D. M. P. Jayakody, W. Schlee, and C. R. Cederroth. 2023. An opportunity for constructing the future of data sharing in otolaryngology. *Journal of the Association for Research in Otolaryngology* 24(4):397–399.

Fischer, M. A. 2016. Academic detailing in diabetes: Using outreach education to improve the quality of care. *Current Diabetes Reports* 16(10):98.

Forsetlund, L., M. A. O'Brien, L. Forsén, L. M. Reinar, M. P. Okwen, T. Horsley, and C. J. Rose. 2021. Continuing education meetings and workshops: Effects on professional practice and healthcare outcomes. *Cochrane Database of Systematic Reviews* 9(9):Cd003030.

Glasgow, R. E., S. M. Harden, B. Gaglio, B. Rabin, M. L. Smith, G. C. Porter, M. G. Ory, and P. A. Estabrooks. 2019. RE-AIM planning and evaluation framework: Adapting to new science and practice with a 20-year review. *Frontiers in Public Health* 7(64). https://doi.org/10.2289/fpubh.

Hertzano, R. 2024. *Here Hear Share!* Paper presented at the 2024 Association for Research in Otolaryngology MidWinter Meeting, Orlando, FL.

Hertzano, R., and A. Mahurkar. 2022. Advancing discovery in hearing research via biologist-friendly access to multi-omic data. *Human Genetics* 141(3):319–322.

Hughes, K. L., M. Clarke, and P. R. Williamson. 2021. A systematic review finds core outcome set uptake varies widely across different areas of health. *Journal of Clinical Epidemiology* 129:114–123.

Hughes, K. L., P. R. Williamson, and B. Young. 2022. In-depth qualitative interviews identified barriers and facilitators that influenced chief investigators' use of core outcome sets in randomised controlled trials. *Journal of Clinical Epidemiology* 144:111–120.

Kearney, A., E. Gargon, J. W. Mitchell, S. Callaghan, F. Yameen, P. R. Williamson, and S. Dodd. 2023. A systematic review of studies reporting the development of core outcome sets for use in routine care. *Journal of Clinical Epidemiology* 158:34–43.

Kirkham, J. J., and P. Williamson. 2022. Core outcome sets in medical research. *BMJ Medicine* 1(1):e000284.

Kirkham, J. J., M. Clarke, and P. R. Williamson. 2017. A methodological approach for assessing the uptake of core outcome sets using ClinicalTrials.gov: Findings from a review of randomised controlled trials of rheumatoid arthritis. *BMJ.* https://doi.org/10.1136/bmj.j2262.

Kirkham, J. J., M. Bracken, L. Hind, K. Pennington, M. Clarke, and P. R. Williamson. 2019. Industry funding was associated with increased use of core outcome sets. *Journal of Clinical Epidemiology* 115:90–97.

Kulbokas, V., K. A. Hanson, M. H. Smart, M. R. Mandava, T. A. Lee, and A. S. Pickard. 2021. Academic detailing interventions for opioid-related outcomes: A scoping review. *Drugs Context* 10:2021-7-7.

Le Prell, C. 2024. *Standardization of threshold and supra-threshold measures in clinical trials assessing investigational inner ear medicines.* Paper presented at the 2024 Association for Research in Otolaryngology MidWinter Meeting, Orlando, FL.

Lewis, M. A., J. Schulte, L. Matthews, K. I. Vaden Jr., C. J. Steves, F. M. Williams, B. A. Schulte, J. R. Dubno, and K. P. Steel. 2023. Accurate phenotypic classification and exome sequencing allow identification of novel genes and variants associated with adult-onset hearing loss. *PLoS Genetics* 19(11):e1011058.

Matvienko-Sikar, K., S. Hussey, K. Mellor, M. Byrne, M. Clarke, J. J. Kirkham, J. Kottner, F. Quirke, I. J. Saldanha, V. Smith, E. Toomey, and P. R. Williamson. 2024. Using behavioral science to increase core outcome set use in trials. *Journal of Clinical Epidemiology* 168:111285.

McCormack, L., S. Sheridan, M. Lewis, V. Boudewyns, C. L. Melvin, C. Kistler, L. J. Lux, K. Cullen, and K. N. Lohr. 2013. Communication and dissemination strategies to facilitate the use of health-related evidence. *Evidence Report Technology Assessment* 213:1–520.

Michie, S., M. M. van Stralen, and R. West. 2011. The behaviour change wheel: A new method for characterising and designing behaviour change interventions. *Implementation Science* 6(52). https://doi.org/10.1186/1748-5908-6-42.

NHS (National Health Service). 2019. *Outcome measures.* https://www.hra.nhs.uk/planning-and-improving-research/best-practice/outcome-measures/ (accessed October 9, 2024).

O'Brien, M. A., S. Rogers, G. Jamtvedt, A. D. Oxman, J. Odgaard-Jensen, D. T. Kristoffersen, L. Forsetlund, D. Bainbridge, N. Freemantle, D. A. Davis, R. B. Haynes, and E. L. Harvey. 2007. Educational outreach visits: Effects on professional practice and health care outcomes. *Cochrane Database of Systematic Reviews* 2007(4):Cd000409.

OMERACT (Outcome Measures in Rheumatology). 2023. *2023 year end report.* Ottawa, Canada: OMERACT.

OMERACT. 2024. *OMERACT: Outcome measures in rheumatology.* https://omeract.org (accessed June 25, 2024).

OMERACT. 2025. *OMER-ED.* https://omeract.org/elearning/ (accessed January 7, 2025).

Orvis, J., B. Gottfried, J. Kancherla, R. S. Adkins, Y. Song, A. A. Dror, D. Olley, K. Rose, E. Chrysostomou, and M. C. Kelly. 2021. gEAR: gene Expression Analysis Resource portal for community-driven, multi-omic data exploration. *Nature Methods* 18(8):843–844.

Poling, G. 2024. *The role of consistent clinical practice approaches for data-informed hearing care.* Paper presented at the 2024 Association for Research in Otolaryngology MidWinter Meeting, Orlando, FL.

Proctor, E. K., B. J. Powell, and J. C. McMillen. 2013. Implementation strategies: Recommendations for specifying and reporting. *Implementation Science* 8(139). https://doi.org/10.1186/1748-5908-8-139.

PROMIS (Patient-Reported Outcomes Measurement Information System) Health Organization. 2024. *What is PROMIS.* https://www.promishealth.org/57461-2 (accessed September 30, 2024).

Rabin, B. A., R. C. Brownson, D. Haire-Joshu, M. W. Kreuter, and N. L. Weaver. 2008. A glossary for dissemination and implementation research in health. *Journal of Public Health Management and Practice* 14(2):117–123.

Reavis, K. 2024. *Big data, big possibilities.* Paper presented at the 2024 Association for Research in Otolaryngology MidWinter Meeting, Orlando, FL.

Rhodes, S., S. Dodd, S. Deckert, L. Vasanthan, R. Qiu, J. F. Rohde, I. D. Florez, J. Schmitt, R. Nieuwlaat, J. Kirkham, and P. R. Williamson. 2024. Representation of published core outcome sets in practice guidelines. *Journal of Clinical Epidemiology* 169:111311.

Saldanha, I. J., K. L. Hughes, S. Dodd, T. Lasserson, J. J. Kirkham, Y. Wu, S. W. Lucas, and P. R. Williamson. 2024. Study found increasing use of core outcome sets in Cochrane Systematic Reviews and identified facilitators and barriers. *Journal of Clinical Epidemiology* 169:111277.

Schubert, N. M., M. van Tuinen, and S. J. Pyott. 2022. Transcriptome-guided identification of drugs for repurposing to treat age-related hearing loss. *Biomolecules* 12(4):498.

Smith, J. D., D. H. Li, and M. R. Rafferty. 2020. The implementation research logic model: A method for planning, executing, reporting, and synthesizing implementation projects. *Implementation Science* 15(1):84.

Soumerai, S. B., and J. Avorn. 1990. Principles of educational outreach ('academic detailing') to improve clinical decision making. *Journal of the American Medical Association* 263(4):549–556.

South, A., J. V. Bailey, M. K. B. Parmar, and C. L. Vale. 2024. The effectiveness of interventions to disseminate the results of non-commercial randomised clinical trials to healthcare professionals: A systematic review. *Implementation Science* 19(1):8.

Taiber, S., K. Gwilliam, R. Hertzano, and K. B. Avraham. 2022. The genomics of auditory function and disease. *Annual Review of Genomics and Human Genetics* 23(1):275–299.

Tomasone, J. R., K. D. Kauffeldt, R. Chaudhary, and M. C. Brouwers. 2020. Effectiveness of guideline dissemination and implementation strategies on health care professionals' behaviour and patient outcomes in the cancer care context: A systematic review. *Implementation Science* 15(1):41.

Tucci, D. L. 2023. NIDCD's 5-year strategic plan describes scientific priorities and commitment to basic science. *Journal of the Association for Research in Otolaryngology* 24(3):265–268.

Tugwell, P., M. Boers, P. Brooks, L. Simon, V. Strand, and L. Idzerda. 2007. OMERACT: An international initiative to improve outcome measurement in rheumatology. *Trials* 8:38.

Walaszek, A., T. Albrecht, M. Schroeder, T. J. LeCaire, S. Houston, M. Recinos, and C. M. Carlsson. 2023. Using academic detailing to enhance the knowledge, skills, and attitudes of clinicians caring for persons with behavioral and psychological symptoms of dementia. *Journal of the American Medical Directors Association* 24(12):1981–1983.

Weldring, T., and S. M. S. Smith. 2013. Patient-reported outcomes (PROs) and patient-reported outcome measures (PROMs). *Health Services Insights* 6:61–68.

Yi, J. A., A. Hakimi, and A. K. Vavra. 2022. Application of dissemination and implementation science frameworks to surgical research. *Seminars in Vascular Surgery* 35(4):456–463.

Appendix A

Glossary

The committee presents a glossary of select terms that are defined in the context in which they are used in the report. This list of terms is not exhaustive, and some terms are discussed more fully in Chapters 1 and 6.

GLOSSARY

Acquired hearing loss A hearing loss that appears after birth, at any time in one's life, perhaps as a result of a disease, a condition, aging, or an injury.

Adult-onset hearing loss Hearing loss that develops during adulthood.

Audibility Detection of sound.

Clinical significance Assessment of whether findings contribute to medical care resulting in the improvement of individual physical function and ability to engage in social life.

Clinicians of first contact The first health care provider an individual may encounter who could support an intervention pathway for a problem. In the case of hearing health care, this may be a primary care clinician or in some cases, patients may be able to directly access hearing health care from an audiologist.

Cognitive health Refers to the ability to clearly think, learn, and remember.

Communication The exchange of ideas and thoughts among two or more individuals.

Community partners A person with an interest or concern in a topic of interest.

Complex listening situation Any listening situation that requires listening effort because of interfering signals (e.g., noise or other competing sound, accented speech, unfamiliar language).

Core set of outcomes An agreed-upon standardized minimum set of outcomes that are measured and reported across settings and interventions.

Detection The ability to identify that a sound (e.g., beeps, tones, speech, or other sound output) is present.

Distal outcomes Outcomes that are downstream from an intervention and that take time to actualize.

Effectiveness The performance of an intervention under real-world circumstances.

Efficacy The performance of an intervention under ideal and controlled circumstances.

Health outcome The effect of a health care service or intervention (or a lack of a health care service or intervention).

Health-related quality of life The physical and mental health aspects of quality of life.

Hearing The mental and physical ability to perceive sounds.

Hearing health care Care for the assessment and treatment of hearing-related conditions.

Hearing-related quality of life The hearing health aspects of quality of life.

Implementation science The scientific study of methods and strategies that facilitate the uptake of evidence-based practice and research into regular use by practitioners and policy makers.

Listening effort The resources or energy necessary or used by a listener in real time to meet the cognitive demand needed to understand when people are speaking.

Listening fatigue Cognitive exhaustion caused by increased efforts to listen and comprehend others when they are speaking that accumulate over time.

Localization The ability to identify the placement of a sound source in a sound field.

Loneliness The perception of social isolation or the subjective feeling of being lonely.

Meaningful outcome A result from treatment that is important to the adult with hearing difficulties and the clinician.

Measurement bias Nonrandom difference from a true measurement.

Measurement error The difference between the observed value (the result of measurement) and the actual value of what is being measured (contains random and nonrandom error).

Noise Any unwanted signal that interferes with the signal of interest. Wanted sound, such as loud music at a concert venue, may also interfere with communication, but is not included in the definition of noise.

Outcome domain A grouping category that encompasses a family of related outcomes.

Outcome measure A tool that assesses or captures the impact of an intervention on an outcome.

Participation Involvement in a life situation.

Participation restriction Limitation of involvement in a life situation.

Patient-reported outcome measures (PROM) An assessment of an outcome that is directly reported by the patient who experienced it or their proxy.

Physical function The ability to perform basic and complex activities of daily living.

Proximal outcome An immediate outcome of a treatment. For hearing health interventions, the proximal outcome is verification of audibility.

Psychological health Encompasses emotional, psychological, and social well-being, influencing cognition, perception, and behavior.

Quality of life An individual's subjective well-being and ability to lead a fulfilling life. Common facets of quality of life include such things as physical and mental health, relationships, work environment, social status, wealth, a sense of security and safety, freedom, social belonging, and physical surroundings.

Reliability The degree to which the content of a measurement instrument is an adequate reflection of the construct to be measured.

Sensitivity to change The ability of a measurement instrument to detect change over time in the construct to be measured. Also known as responsiveness.

Social connection An umbrella term that encompasses the structural, functional, and quality aspects of how individuals connect to each other.

Social isolation The objective state of having few social relationships or infrequent social contact with others.

Speech communication The use of the oral medium of passing information, whether formally or informally, by a speaker to an audience.

Speech in noise The ability to detect and understand speech in complex listening environments (e.g., background speech, music, accents, unfamiliar words, reverberation).

Validity The extent to which the results of a measurement actually reflect what they are intended to measure; how accurate is the measure.

Verification Confirmation that the treatment at the most basic level is doing what it was intended to do (e.g., a hearing aid is making sound audible).

Appendix B

Measure Inventory

This appendix includes the measures by outcome domain as cataloged by the committee early in its evidence-gathering phase. These measures were identified through a review of which measures are typically used in the published literature, as well as committee judgment. This list is not comprehensive; instead, it is intended to give a sense of the large range of measures available and exemplifies the need for standardization in the field. Some of these measures are used primarily for diagnostic purposes. The committee did not perform an in-depth analysis of all of these measures, but it did review the overall availability and make a high-level overview of the quality of measures by outcome or domain.

Cognition
- Alzheimer's Disease Assessment Scale-Cognitive (ADAS-COG)
- Auditory Verbal Learning Test (AVLT)
- Behavioral Dyscontrol Scale II (BDS-2)
- Digit Symbol Substitution Test (DSST)
- General Practitioner Assessment of Cognition (GP-COG)
- Mini COG
- Mini Mental State Examination (MMSE)
- Montreal Cognitive Assessment (MoCA)
- Reading Span Test (RST)
- Symbol Digits Modalities Test (SDMT)
- Trail Making Test (TMT)
- Verbal Fluency Test (VFT)

Hearing-Related Psychosocial Health (also see Quality of Life measures below)
* Communication Profile for Hearing Impaired (CPHI)
* Hearing Handicap Inventory for Adults - Screening Version (HHIA-S)
* Hearing Handicap Inventory for Adults (HHIA)
* Hearing Handicap Inventory for the Elderly - Screening Version (HHIE-S)
* Hearing Handicap Inventory for the Elderly (HHIE)
* Revised Hearing Handicap Inventory - Screening Version (RHHI-S)
* Revised Hearing Handicap Inventory (RHHI)

Listening Effort and Fatigue
* Behavioral
  o Cognitive spare capacity
  o False alarm rate
  o Hit rate
  o Lapse of attention
  o Listening span
  o Reaction times
  o Running memory
  o Word recall
* Physiological
  o Electrophysiological
    * Biventricular pacing (BVP)
    * Electroencephalogram (EEG)
    * Facial electromyography (fEMG)
    * Heart rate variability (HRV)
    * Peripheral vasoconstriction
    * Pupillometry
    * Skin conductance
  o Functional imaging
    * Functional magnetic resonance imaging (fMRI)
    * Functional near-infrared spectroscopy (fNIRS)
  o Hormonal
    * Alpha amylase
    * Chromogranin A
    * Cortisol
* Self-report
  o Amsterdam Checklist
  o Checklist Individual Strength (CIS) questionnaire
  o Effort Assessment Scale
  o Fatigue Assessment Scale
  o Fatigue Scale

  o   LE Scale
  o   NASA Task Load Index (modified and various forms)
  o   Need for Recovery
  o   Perceived Listening Effort
  o   Profile of Mood States (POMS)
  o   SSQ qualities subscale
  o   Subjective Mental Effort
  o   Visual Analog Scale – Effort
  o   Visual Analog Scale – Fatigue

Mental/Behavioral Health
- Center for Epidemiologic Studies Depression Scale 5 (CESD-5)
- General Anxiety Disorder (GAD-7)
- Geriatric Depression Scale (GDS)
- Hamilton Depression Rating Scale (HDRS)
- Hospital Anxiety and Depression Scale (HADS)
- Neuropsychiatric Inventory Questionnaire (NPIQ)
- Patient Health Questionnaire (PHQ-9)
- Positive and Negative Affect Schedule (PANAS)
- Psychosis Screening Questionnaire (PSQ)
- State Trait Anxiety Index (STAI)

Participation Restrictions
- Committee elected not to inventory measures based on elimination of outcome domain from consideration for core outcome set and paucity of specific measures.

Physical Health
- Committee elected not to inventory measures based on elimination of outcome domain from consideration for core outcome set and paucity of specific measures.

Physiological Response to Sound
- Acoustic Reflex
- Auditory Brainstem Response (ABR)
- Measures of Central Auditory Function (MLR, P300, P600)
- Otoacoustic Emissions (DPOAE, TEOAE)
- Tympanometry

Social Connection
- Berkman-Syme Social Network Index
- Campaign to End Loneliness Measurement Scale

- Cornwell Perceived Isolation Scale
- De Jong Gierveld Loneliness Scale
- Duke Social Support Index
- Lubben Social Network Scale
- Social Disconnectedness and Perceived Isolation Scales
- Social Participation Restrictions Questionnaire (SPaRQ)
- Steptoe Social Isolation Index
- UCLA Loneliness Scale

Social-Economic Impacts
- Committee elected not to inventory measures based on elimination of outcome domain from consideration for core outcome set and paucity of specific measures.

Sound Localization
- Everyday Sounds Localization Test
- Spatial Hearing Questionnaire (SHQ)
- Speech and Spatial Qualities of Hearing (SSQ49)
- Speech and Spatial Qualities of Hearing 12-items (SSQ12)
- Speech and Spatial Qualities of Hearing 15-items (SSQ15)
- Speech and Spatial Qualities of Hearing 17-items (SSQ17)
- Speech and Spatial Qualities of Hearing 5-item Screener (SSQ5)
- York Binaural Hearing-Related Quality of Life (YBHRQL) Questionnaire

Speech Communication
- Abbreviated Profile of Hearing Aid Benefit (APHAB)/Abbreviated Profile of Hearing Aid Profile (APHAP)
- Acceptable Noise Level (ANL)
- Articulation Index (AI)
- Audible Contrast Threshold (ACT)
- AzBio Sentence Test
- Bamford-Kowal-Bench Speech-in-Noise (BKB-SIN)
- Central Institute for the Deaf Word List (CID W-22)
- Client-Oriented Scale of Improvement (COSI)
- Connected Speech Test (CST)
- Coordinate Response Measure (CRM)
- Digits-in-Noise (DIN)
- Extended Speech Intelligibility Index (ESII)
- Glasgow Hearing Aid Benefit Profile (GHABP)
- Hearing in Noise Test (HINT)
- International Outcome Inventory-Hearing Aids (IOI-HA)

- Maryland Consonant-Nucleus-Consonant (CNC) Test
- Modified Speech Transmission Index (mSTI)
- Northwestern University Auditory No. 6 (NU-6) Test
- Phonetically Balanced 50-Word List (PB-50)
- Phonetically Balanced Word List for Kindergarten Children (PBK)
- Profile of Hearing Aid Benefit (PHAB)/Profile of Hearing Aid Performance (PHAP)
- Quick Sentences-in-Noise (QuickSIN)
- Revised Speech Perception in Noise (R-SPIN)
- Speech and Spatial Qualities of Hearing (SSQ49)
- Speech and Spatial Qualities of Hearing 12-items (SSQ12)
- Speech and Spatial Qualities of Hearing 15-items (SSQ15)
- Speech and Spatial Qualities of Hearing 17-items (SSQ17)
- Speech and Spatial Qualities of Hearing 5-item Screener (SSQ5)
- Speech Intelligibility Index (SII)
- Speech Intelligibility Rating (SIR)
- Speech Perception in Noise (SPIN)
- Speech Recognition in Noise Test (SPRINT)
- Speech Recognition Sensitivity Model
- Speech Recognition Threshold (SRT)
- Speech Transmission Index (STI)
- Words-in-Noise (WIN) Test

Quality of Life
- 12-Item Short Form Survey (SF-12)
- European Quality of Life 5-Dimension (EQ-5D)
- Health and Activities Limitation Index (HALex)
- Health Utilities Index 2 and 3 (HUI2, HUI3)
- Health Utility Index (HUI)
- Impact of Hearing Loss Inventory Tool (IHEAR-IT)
- Medical Outcomes Study SF-36
- Patient-Reported Outcomes Measurement Information System 29 (PROMIS-29)
- PROMIS 29+2
- PROMIS Overall Life Satisfaction Short Form
- Scale of the Subjective Well-Being of Older Adults With Hearing Loss (SWB-HL)
- Short Form 36 Health Survey Questionnaire (SF-36)
- Short Form 36 Health Survey Questionnaire for Veterans (SF-36 V)
- Short Form 6-Dimension (SF-6D)
- WHO Disability Assessment Scale (WHODAS)

Appendix C

223

Measure Evaluation Worksheet

The criteria and rating system presented in Table C-1 was adopted from Terwee and colleagues (2007) and modified to fit the committee's process for evaluating measures of interest. For many of the considered measures, the level of evidence needed to evaluate each criterion was not available and therefore not every component was applicable. However, the committee used the existing evidence to assess each candidate measure based on as many of these criteria as possible to select the best outcome for each measure.

TABLE C-1 Committee Criteria and Rating System for Outcome Measure Evaluation

Measurement Property	Rating*	Criteria
Content validity	+	All items refer to relevant aspects of the construct to be measured AND are relevant for the target population AND are relevant for the context of use AND together comprehensively reflect the construct to be measured
(including face validity)	?	Not all information for '+' reported
	–	Criteria for '+' not met
Structural validity	+	**Classical Test Theory (CTT):**
		Unidimensionality: Exploratory factor analysis: First factor accounts for at least 20% of the variability AND ratio of the variance explained by the first to the second factor greater than 4 OR Bi-factor model: Standardized loadings on a common factor > 0.30 AND correlation between individual scores under a bi-factor and unidimensional model > 0.90
		Structural validity: Comparative fit index (CFI) or Tucker-Lewis Index (TLI) comparable measure > 0.95 AND root mean square error of approximation (RMSEA) < 0.06 OR standardized root mean residuals (SRMR) < 0.08
		Rasch/Item Response Theory (IRT):
		At least limited evidence for unidimensionality or positive structural validity AND no evidence for violation of local independence: Rasch: standardized item-person fit residuals between –2.5 and 2.5; OR IRT: residual correlations among the items after controlling for the dominant factor < 0.20 OR Q3s < 0.37 AND no evidence for violation of monotonicity: adequate looking graphs OR item scalability > 0.30 AND adequate model fit: Rasch: infit and outfit mean squares $\geq$ 0.5 and $\leq$ 1.5 OR Z-standardized values > –2 and < 2; OR IRT: G2 > 0.01;
		Optional additional evidence:
		Adequate targeting; Rasch: adequate person-item threshold distribution; IRT: adequate threshold range
		No important differential item functioning for relevant subject characteristics (such as age, gender, education), McFadden's R2 < 0.02
	?	CTT: Not all information for '+' reported
		IRT: Model fit not reported
	–	Criteria for '+' not met
	No data available	If the element hasn't been tested/reported, leave the cell blank (this is different from having a negative finding).

TABLE C-1 Continued

Measurement Property	Rating*	Criteria
Internal consistency	+	At least limited evidence for unidimensionality or positive structural validity AND Cronbach's alpha(s) ≥ 0.70 and ≤ 0.95
	?	Not all information for '+' reported OR conflicting evidence for unidimensionality or structural validity OR evidence for lack of unidimensionality or negative structural validity
	–	Criteria for '+' not met
Reliability	+	Intraclass correlation coefficient (ICC) or weighted Kappa ≥ 0.70
	?	ICC or weighted Kappa not reported
	–	Criteria for '+' not met
Measurement error	+	Smallest detectable change (SDC) or limits of agreement (LOA) < minimal important change (MIC)
	?	MIC not defined
	–	Criteria for '+' not met
Hypotheses testing	+	At least 75% of the results are in accordance with the hypotheses
	?	No correlations with instrument(s) measuring related construct(s) AND no differences between relevant groups reported
	–	Criteria for '+' not met
Criterion validity	+	Convincing arguments that gold standard is "gold" AND correlation with gold standard ≥ 0.70
	?	Not all information for '+' reported
	–	Criteria for '+' not met
Responsiveness	+	At least 75% of the results are in accordance with the hypotheses
	?	No correlations with changes in instrument(s) measuring related construct(s) AND no differences between changes in relevant groups reported
	–	Criteria for '+' not met

NOTE: * "+" = positive rating, "?" = indeterminate rating, "–" = negative rating.
SOURCE: Modified from Terwee et al., 2007. Reprinted with permission from Elsevier.

REFERENCE

Terwee, C. B., S. D. Bot, M. R. de Boer, D. A. van der Windt, D. L. Knol, J. Dekker, L. M. Bouter, and H. C. de Vet. 2007. Quality criteria were proposed for measurement properties of health status questionnaires. *Journal of Clinical Epidemiology* 60(1):34–42.

Appendix D

WIN vs. QuickSIN Table

The following table provides a side-by-side comparison of the evidence from studies of the psychometric quality of the Words-in-Noise (WIN) test versus the Quick Speech-in-Noise (QuickSIN) test.

TABLE D-1 Comparison of the Psychometric Evidence for WIN vs QuickSIN

	WIN: Maintains the level of the babble (60 dB HL), varies background speech level (60–84 dB HL) in 4 dB steps (0–24 dB SNR range); uses NU-6 words as basis	QuickSIN: Maintains the speech level (70 dB HL), varies the babble level (70–95 dB HL) in 5 dB steps (0–25 dB SNR range); uses IEEE sentences as basis
Normative data (young adult listeners/ normal hearing listeners[1])	N = 24 (Wilson and Strouse, 2002) (Wilson *et al.*, 2003) N = 24 (Wilson *et al.*, 2003) N = 96, across four experiments (Wilson, 2003) N = 36 (McArdle *et al.*, 2005) N = 24 (Wilson *et al.*, 2007a) N = 24 (Wilson *et al.*, 2007b) N = 24 (Wilson and Cates, 2008) N = 80, across 3 experiments (Wilson *et al.*, 2012) N = 24 (Wilson and Watts, 2012	N = 3 (Killion and Villchur, 1993) N = 20 (Bentler, 2000)[2] N = 73, across four experiments (Killion *et al.*, 2004) N = 36 (McArdle *et al.*, 2005) N = 24 (McArdle and Wilson, 2006)
Normative data (older adult listeners/ listeners with hearing loss[3])	N = 50 (Wilson and Strouse, 2002) N = 24 (Wilson *et al.*, 2003) N = 96, across four experiments (Wilson, 2003) N = 72 (McArdle *et al.*, 2005) N = 120 (Wilson and Burks, 2005) N = 40 (Wilson *et al.*, 2005) N = 48 (Wilson *et al.*, 2007a) N = 72 (Wilson *et al.*, 2007b) N = 411 across two experiments (Wilson and McArdle, 2007) N = 48 (Wilson and Cates, 2008) N = 64, across 3 experiments (Wilson *et al.*, 2012) N = 24 (Wilson and Watts, 2012	N = 3 (Killion and Villchur, 1993) N = 20 (Bentler, 2000) N = 26, across four experiments (Killion *et al.*, 2004) N = 72 (McArdle *et al.*, 2005) N = 72 (McArdle and Wilson, 2006)
Effects of age and hearing loss	N = 15 participants per decade, from 20–79 yrs (Wilson and Strouse, 2002) N = 3430: Ages 20–89, new patient examinations in the Audiology Clinic at the VA Medical Center, Mountain Home, Tennessee (Wilson, 2011) N = 10 young normal hearing, N = 10 old normal hearing, N = 10 old hearing loss (Billings *et al.*, 2023)	N = 6; three adults in their 20's and three adults in their 60's (Killion and Villchur, 1993) N = 5808: Ages 18–101 with a range of wide range of auditory pathologies; patients examined at the Stanford Ear Institute (Fitzgerald *et al.*, 2023) N = 10 young normal hearing, N = 10 old normal hearing, N = 10 old hearing loss (Billings *et al.*, 2023)

[1] See individual studies for definitions of "young" and "normal hearing."

[2] This study included but was not limited to sentences incorporated in the QuickSIN.

[3] See individual studies for definitions of "old" and "hearing loss."

TABLE D-1 Continued

	WIN: Maintains the level of the babble (60 dB HL), varies background speech level (60–84 dB HL) in 4 dB steps (0–24 dB SNR range); uses NU-6 words as basis	QuickSIN: Maintains the speech level (70 dB HL), varies the babble level (70–95 dB HL) in 5 dB steps (0–25 dB SNR range); uses IEEE sentences as basis
Psychometric development of test	NU 6 lists 3, 4 divided into 70-word lists, SNRs –10 to 20 in 5-dB steps (Wilson and Strouse, 2002) NU 6 lists 2, 3, 4 divided into 25-word lists; SNRs –4 to 16 or 4 to 24 in 4 dB steps; multiple babble levels compared; monaural vs binaural conditions compared (Wilson, 2003) NU 6 lists 2, 3, 4 divided into 70-word lists, SNRs 0 to 24 in 4 dB steps –10 and –5 dB SNRs omitted; step size decreased from 5 dB to 4 dB; words time locked to specific babble section; multiple randomizations assessed (Wilson *et al.*, 2003) Two 35-word lists assessed for equivalence (Wilson and Burks, 2005) Reanalyzed data from 573 listeners with hearing loss to establish lists of equivalent difficulty (Wilson and Burks, 2005) Words presented with either descending level or random level order (Wilson *et al.*, 2005) Background manipulated with multi-talker babble versus speech-spectrum noise (Wilson *et al.*, 2007a) Test-retest reliability assessed (Wilson and McArdle, 2007) Standard (forward) babble compared with reversed babble (Wilson *et al.*, 2012) Lists 1, 2, and 3 assessed for equivalence (Wilson and Watts, 2012)	List equivalency assessed across 12 IEEE sentence lists (Bentler, 2000) IEEE sentences narrowed to 18 lists of six sentences each, plus three practice lists, across a series of four experiments (Killion *et al.*, 2004) List equivalency assessed across 18 IEEE sentence lists (McArdle and Wilson, 2006) Alternative conditions including time-compressed, reverberant speech and a condition with an in-phase noise masker and out of phase speech targets were assessed (Phatak *et al.*, 2018)

continued

TABLE D-1 Continued

	WIN: Maintains the level of the babble (60 dB HL), varies background speech level (60–84 dB HL) in 4 dB steps (0–24 dB SNR range); uses NU-6 words as basis	QuickSIN: Maintains the speech level (70 dB HL), varies the babble level (70–95 dB HL) in 5 dB steps (0–25 dB SNR range); uses IEEE sentences as basis
Test-retest reliability assessed	No learning effect for run 2 versus run 1; test-retest < 1 dB (McArdle *et al.*, 2005) Small (0.4 dB) learning effect across 4 trials, not statistically significant (Wilson and Burks, 2005) 0.3 dB difference from test 1 (12.5 dB S/B) to test 2 (12.8 dB S/B) was statistically significant for two tests 12 months apart (Wilson and McArdle, 2007); intra-class correlation coefficient = 0.88 No significant intra-session differences for two tests 40 days apart (Wilson and McArdle, 2007); the intra-class correlation for the test retest data were 0.89 for the mild hearing loss group and 0.91 for the moderate hearing loss group No significant inter-session differences for two tests within same test session (Wilson and McArdle, 2007)	Test-retest assessed for three IEEE lists; correlation coefficient was 0.92 for normal hearing listeners and 0.97 for listeners with hearing loss (p's <0.01) (Bentler, 2000) Averaging results of several lists improved reliability; one list; 95% confidence level = ±2.7 dB, two lists: 95% confidence level = ±1.9 dB, three lists: 95% confidence level = ±1.6 dB (Killion *et al.*, 2004) Learning effect inferred from more participants having better performance on run 2 than run 1; test retest < 1 dB (McArdle *et al.*, 2005)
Sound level for the fixed element (WIN background noise, QuickSIN speech targets), as reported by authors[4]	50 dB HL (70 dB SPL) (Wilson and Strouse, 2002) 70 dB SPL (Experiments 1 and 2, Wilson, 2003) 70, 80, and 90 dB SPL (Experiment 3, Wilson, 2003) 70 and 90 dB SPL (Experiment 4, Wilson, 2003) 60 dB HL (Wilson *et al.*, 2003) 80 dB SPL (McArdle *et al.*, 2005) 80 dB SPL (Wilson and Burks, 2005) 80 dB SPL (Wilson *et al.*, 2005) 70 dB SPL (Wilson *et al.*, 2007a) 80 dB SPL (Wilson *et al.*, 2007b)	80 dB SPL (65 dB HL) and 50 dB SPL (35 dB HL) (Killion and Villchur, 1993) 83 dB SPL and 53 dB SPL (Bentler, 2000) 70 dB HL (Killion *et al.*, 2004) 90 dB SPL (McArdle *et al.*, 2005) 70 dB HL (Walden and Walden, 2004) 90 dB SPL (McArdle *et al.*, 2005) 70 dB HL (McArdle and Wilson, 2006) 100 dB SPL (Wilson *et al.*, 2007b) 70 dB HL (Billings *et al.*, 2023) 70 dB HL, unless levels were required to be increased due to audibility concerns (Fitzgerald *et al.*, 2023)

---

[4] Individual studies report levels in either dB SPL or dB HL; this table uses data reported in each manuscript. If authors provided a conversion factor, those are listed here.

TABLE D-1 Continued

	WIN: Maintains the level of the babble (60 dB HL), varies background speech level (60–84 dB HL) in 4 dB steps (0–24 dB SNR range); uses NU-6 words as basis	QuickSIN: Maintains the speech level (70 dB HL), varies the babble level (70–95 dB HL) in 5 dB steps (0–25 dB SNR range); uses IEEE sentences as basis
	60 dB HL (Experiment 1); 60 dB HL (mild to severe HL) and 70 dB HL (moderate to severe HL) (Wilson and McArdle, 2007) 60 dB HL (Wilson and Cates, 2008) 80 dB SPL (Experiments 1 and 2) (Wilson *et al.*, 2012) 70 dB SPL (Experiment 3) (Wilson *et al.*, 2012) 80 dB SPL (Wilson and Watts, 2012) 60 dB HL (Billings *et al.*, 2023)	
Sound level for the roving element (WIN speech targets, QuickSIN background noise) and SNRs, as reported by authors[5]	40 to 70 dB HL (–10 to 20 dB SNR) (Wilson and Strouse, 2002) 66 to 86 dB SPL (–4 to 16 dB SNR for normal hearing listeners) or 74 to 84 dB SPL (4 to 24 dB SNR for hearing impaired listeners) (Experiments 1 and 2, Wilson, 2003) 70 to 94 dB SPL; 80 to 104 dB SPL, and 90 to 114 dB SPL (0 to 24 dB SNR for all three babble levels) (Experiment 3, Wilson, 2003) 70 to 94 dB SPL or 90 to 114 dB SPL (0 to 24 dB SNR for both babble levels) (Experiment 4, Wilson, 2003) 60 to 84 dB HL (0 to 24 dB SNR) (Wilson *et al.*, 2003) 80 to 104 dB SPL (0 to 24 dB SNR) (McArdle *et al.*, 2005) 80 to 104 dB SPL(0 to 24 dB SNR) (Wilson and Burks, 2005) 80 to 104 dB SPL(0 to 24 dB SNR) (Wilson *et al.*, 2005) 70 to 94 dB SPL(0 to 24 dB SNR) (Wilson *et al.*, 2007a) 80 to 104 dB SPL (0 to 24 dB SNR) (Wilson *et al.*, 2007b)	65 to 80 dB SPL or 35 to 50 dB SPL (0 to 15 dB SNR) (Killion and Villchur, 1993) 68 to 83 dB SPL or 38 to 53 dB SPL (0 to 15 dB SNR) (Bentler, 2000) 45 to 70 dB HL (0 to 25 dB SNR) (Killion *et al.*, 2004) 45 to 70 dB HL (0 to 25 dB SNR) (Walden & Walden, 2004) 65 to 90 dB SPL (0 to 25 dB SNR) (McArdle *et al.*, 2005) 45 to 70 dB HL (0 to 25 dB SNR) (McArdle and Wilson, 2006) 75 to 100 dB SPL (0 to 25 dB SNR) (Wilson *et al.*, 2007b) 45 to 70 dB HL (0 to 25 dB SNR) (Billings, 2023)

continued

---

[5] Individual studies report levels in either dB SPL or dB HL; this table uses data reported in each manuscript. If authors provided a conversion factor, those are listed here.

TABLE D-1 Continued

	WIN: Maintains the level of the babble (60 dB HL), varies background speech level (60–84 dB HL) in 4 dB steps (0–24 dB SNR range); uses NU-6 words as basis	QuickSIN: Maintains the speech level (70 dB HL), varies the babble level (70–95 dB HL) in 5 dB steps (0–25 dB SNR range); uses IEEE sentences as basis
	60 to 84 dB HL (Experiment 1); 60 to 84 dB HL (mild to severe HL) and 70 to 94 dB HL (moderate to severe HL) (0 to 24 dB SNR) (Wilson and McArdle, 2007) 60 to 84 dB HL (0 to 24 dB SNR) (Wilson and Cates, 2008) 80 to 104 dB SPL (0 to 24 dB SNR) (Experiments 1 and 2) (Wilson et al., 2012) 70 to 78 dB SPL (0 and 4 dB SNR) (Experiment 3) (Wilson et al., 2012) 80 to 104 dB SPL (0 to 24 dB SNR) (Wilson and Watts, 2012) 60 to 84 dB HL (0 to 24 dB SNR) (Billings, 2023)	
Monaural vs binaural presentation[6]	Monaural (Wilson and Strouse, 2002) Binaural (Experiments 1–3) or both binaural and monaural with masking (Experiment 4); Binaural thresholds lower (better) than monaural thresholds (~1 dB) (Wilson, 2003) Binaural (Wilson et al., 2003) Monaural (McArdle et al., 2005) Monaural (Wilson and Burks, 2005) Monaural (Wilson et al., 2005) Monaural (Wilson et al., 2007a) Monaural (Wilson et al., 2007b) Monaural (Wilson and McArdle, 2007) Binaural (Wilson and Cates, 2008) Monaural (Wilson et al., 2012)	Binaural (Killion and Villchur, 1993) Binaural (N = 37) and Monaural (N = 3) (Bentler, 2000) Binaural (N = 41) and Monaural (N = 5) (Killion et al., 2004) Monaural (McArdle et al., 2005) Monaural (McArdle and Wilson, 2006) Monaural (Wilson et al., 2007b)

---

[6] If authors did not explicitly state testing was monaural or binaural, testing mode is not reported. Binaural testing typically provides a statistically significant advantage over monaural testing when outcomes are directly compared.

TABLE D-1 Continued

	WIN: Maintains the level of the babble (60 dB HL), varies background speech level (60–84 dB HL) in 4 dB steps (0–24 dB SNR range); uses NU-6 words as basis	QuickSIN: Maintains the speech level (70 dB HL), varies the babble level (70–95 dB HL) in 5 dB steps (0–25 dB SNR range); uses IEEE sentences as basis
Benchmark test comparisons (Benchmark tests are listed)	QuickSIN (McArdle *et al.*, 2005); mean 50% point on QuickSIN and WIN were not significantly different QuickSIN, BKB-SIN, and HINT (Wilson *et al.*, 2007b); QuickSIN and WIN were more difficult than BKB-SIN and HINT (more semantic content in the latter tests) QuickSIN, Listening in Spatialized Noise-Sentences (LiSN-S), and Coordinate Response Measure (CRM) (Billings *et al.*, 2023); WIN was the most difficult, followed by QuickSIN; LiSN-S and SRM scores were better than WIN and QuickSIN SPRINT (Wilson and Cates, 2008); SPRINT and WIN were significantly correlated (r = –0.81, p < 0.01) Digits in Noise (McArdle *et al.*, 2005); approx. 16–17 dB difference in SNR (closed set vs open set) Digits in Noise (Wilson *et al.*, 2006); approx. 15–19 dB difference in SNR (closed set vs open set)	WIN (McArdle *et al.*, 2005); mean 50% point on QuickSIN and WIN were not significantly different WIN, BKB-SIN, and HINT (Wilson *et al.*, 2007b); QuickSIN and WIN were more difficult than BKB-SIN and HINT (more semantic content in the latter tests) WIN, Listening in Spatialized Noise-Sentences (LiSN-S), and Coordinate Response Measure (CRM) (Billings *et al.*, 2023); WIN was the most difficult, followed by QuickSIN; LiSN-S and SRM scores were better than WIN and QuickSIN
Correlation with subjective rating of listening difficulty	Statistically significant relationship with difficulty rating (rho = 0.673; p<0.001) (McArdle *et al.*, 2005) No significant relationships detected with difficulty rating (Wilson *et al.*, 2005) No significant relationships with difficulty rating (Wilson *et al.*, 2006)	Statistically significant relationship with difficulty rating (rho = 0.571; p<0.001) (McArdle *et al.*, 2005) QuickSIN SNR loss accounted for a significant amount of variance in SSQ12-Speech5 score (Fitzgerald *et al.*, 2024)
Test duration	Average test time was 3:33 (Wilson *et al.*, 2005) Less than 2 min per list (McArdle *et al.*, 2005) Typically less than 2.5 min per list (Wilson and Burks, 2005)	A QuickSIN score obtained in 1 min from a single list is accurate to ±2.7 dB at the 95% confidence level (Killion *et al.*, 2004) ~55 sec per list (McArdle and Wilson, 2006)

continued

TABLE D-1 Continued

	WIN: Maintains the level of the babble (60 dB HL), varies background speech level (60–84 dB HL) in 4 dB steps (0–24 dB SNR range); uses NU-6 words as basis	QuickSIN: Maintains the speech level (70 dB HL), varies the babble level (70–95 dB HL) in 5 dB steps (0–25 dB SNR range); uses IEEE sentences as basis
Critical Difference	3.1–3.5 dB (Wilson and McArdle, 2007)	Critical differences varied with List and hearing status (Bentler, 2000) 1.96 dB (Killion *et al.*, 2004, summary of unpublished data presented at a conference) 3.9 dB with one list per condition; 1.9 dB with four lists per condition; 1.4 dB with eight lists per condition (Killion *et al.*, 2004)
Use Assessing Evidence of Benefit	Statistically significant improvement (1.3 dB) in WIN threshold for group treated with FX322 but not placebo group (McLean *et al.*, 2021) Statistically significant improvement on WIN with remote microphone use in children with cochlear implants (34% vs 65%) (Mehrkian *et al.*, 2019)	Amplification improved aided performance in some test conditions (Killion and Villchur, 1993) Amplification improved aided performance for some participants (Killion and Niquette, 2000, based on unpublished data shared by Bentler and Duve) SNR loss was statistically significantly smaller (4.6 dB vs 6.3 dB) during testing of the aided QuickSIN versus testing of the unaided QuickSIN (p<0.01) (Walden and Walden, 2004) SNR loss was statistically significantly smaller (5.75 dB vs 7.9 dB) during testing of the aided QuickSIN versus testing of the unaided QuickSIN (p = 0.03) (Mendel, 2007) Contrast between aided QuickSIN score actual performance) and patient perception of performance is the basis of the Revised Performance-Perceptual Test (revised-PPT) (Ou and Wetmore, 2020) No significant benefits shown on QuickSIN after implant with Envoy Esteem device (Kraus *et al.*, 2011)

NOTES: IEEE = Institute of Electrical and Electronics Engineers; NU-6 = Northwestern University Auditory Test No. 6.

REFERENCES

Bentler, R. A. 2000. List equivalency and test-retest reliability of the speech in noise test. *American Journal of Audiology* 9(2):84–100.

Billings, C. J., T. M. Olsen, L. Charney, B. M. Madsen, and C. E. Holmes. 2023. Speech-in-noise testing: An introduction for audiologists. Paper read at Seminars in Hearing.

Fitzgerald, M. B., S. P. Gianakas, Z. J. Qian, S. Losorelli, and A. C. Swanson. 2023. Preliminary guidelines for replacing word-recognition in quiet with speech in noise assessment in the routine audiologic test battery. *Ear and Hearing* 44(6):1548–1561.

Fitzgerald, M. B., K. M. Ward, S. P. Gianakas, M. L. Smith, N. H. Blevins, and A. P. Swanson. 2024. Speech-in-noise assessment in the routine audiologic test battery: Relationship to perceived auditory disability. *Ear and Hearing* 45(4):816–826.

Killion, M. C., and E. Villchur. 1993. Kessler was right - partly: But SIN test shows some aids improve hearing in noise. *The Hearing Journal* 46(9):31–35.

Killion, M. C., and P. A. Niquette. 2000. What can the pure-tone audiogram tell us about a patient's SNR loss? *The Hearing Journal* 53(3):46–48.

Killion, M. C., P. A. Niquette, G. I. Gudmundsen, L. J. Revit, and S. Banerjee. 2004. Development of a quick speech-in-noise test for measuring signal-to-noise ratio loss in normal-hearing and hearing-impaired listeners. *Journal of the Acoustical Society of America* 116(4 Pt 1):2395–2405.

Kraus, E. M., J. A. Shohet, and P. J. Catalano. 2011. Envoy esteem totally implantable hearing system: Phase 2 trial, 1-year hearing results. *Otolaryngology—Head and Neck Surgery* 145(1):100–109.

McArdle, R. A., and R. H. Wilson. 2006. Homogeneity of the 18 QuickSIN lists. *Journal of the American Academy of Audiology* 17(3):157–167.

McArdle, R. A., R. H. Wilson, and C. A. Burks. 2005. Speech recognition in multitalker babble using digits, words, and sentences. *Journal of the American Academy of Audiology* 16(9):726–739; quiz 763–764.

McLean, W. J., A. S. Hinton, J. T. J. Herby, A. N. Salt, J. J. Hartsock, S. Wilson, D. L. Lucchino, T. Lenarz, A. Warnecke, N. Prenzler, H. Schmitt, S. King, L. E. Jackson, J. Rosenbloom, G. Atiee, M. Bear, C. L. Runge, R. H. Gifford, S. D. Rauch, D. J. Lee, R. Langer, J. M. Karp, C. Loose, and C. LeBel. 2021. Improved speech intelligibility in subjects with stable sensorineural hearing loss following intratympanic dosing of FX-322 in a phase 1b study. *Otology & Neurotology: Official Publication of the American Otological Society, American Neurotology Society [and] European Academy of Otology and Neurotology* 42(7):e849–e857.

Mehrkian, S., Z. Bayat, M. Javanbakht, H. Emamdjomeh, and E. Bakhshi. 2019. Effect of wireless remote microphone application on speech discrimination in noise in children with cochlear implants. *International Journal of Pediatric Otorhinolaryngology* 125:192–195.

Mendel, L. L. 2007. Objective and subjective hearing aid assessment outcomes. *American Journal of Audiology* 16(2):118–129.

Ou, H., and M. Wetmore. 2020. Development of a revised performance-perceptual test using quick speech in noise test material and its norms. *Journal of the American Academy of Audiology* 31(03):176–184.

Phatak, S. A., B. M. Sheffield, D. S. Brungart, and K. W. Grant. 2018. Development of a test battery for evaluating speech perception in complex listening environments: Effects of sensorineural hearing loss. *Ear and Hearing* 39(3):449–456.

Walden, T. C., and B. E. Walden. 2004. Predicting success with hearing aids in everyday living. *Journal of the American Academy of Audiology* 15(05):342–352.

Wilson, R. H. 2003. Development of a speech-in-multitalker-babble paradigm to assess word-recognition performance. *Journal of the American Academy of Audiology* 14(09):453–470.

Wilson, R. H. 2011. Clinical experience with the Words-in-Noise test on 3430 veterans: Comparisons with pure-tone thresholds and word recognition in quiet. *Journal of the American Academy of Audiology* 22(7):405–423.

Wilson, R. H., and A. Strouse. 2002. Northwestern University auditory test no. 6 in multi-talker babble: A preliminary report. *Journal of Rehabilitation Research & Development* 39(1).

Wilson, R. H., and C. A. Burks. 2005. Use of 35 words for evaluation of hearing loss in signal-to-babble ratio: A clinic protocol. *Journal of Rehabilitation Research & Development* 42(6):839–852.

Wilson, R. H., and R. McArdle. 2007. Intra- and inter-session test, retest reliability of the Words-in-Noise (WIN) test. *Journal of the American Academy of Audiology* 18(10): 813–825.

Wilson, R. H., and W. B. Cates. 2008. A comparison of two word-recognition tasks in multitalker babble: Speech Recognition in Noise Test (SPRINT) and Words-in-Noise test (WIN). *Journal of the American Academy of Audiology* 19(7):548–556.

Wilson, R. H., and K. L. Watts. 2012. The Words-in-Noise test (WIN), list 3: A practice list. *Journal of the American Academy of Audiology* 23(02):092–096.

Wilson, R. H., H. B. Abrams, and A. L. Pillion. 2003. A word-recognition task in multitalker babble using a descending presentation mode from 24 db to 0 db signal to babble. *Journal of Rehabilitation Research & Development* 40(4).

Wilson, R. H., C. A. Burks, and D. G. Weakley. 2005. Word recognition in multitalker babble measured with two psychophysical methods. *Journal of the American Academy of Audiology* 16(08):622–630.

Wilson, R. H., C. A. Burks, and D. G. Weakley. 2006. Word recognition of digit triplets and monosyllabic words in multitalker babble by listeners with sensorineural hearing loss. *Journal of the American Academy of Audiology* 17(06):385–397.

Wilson, R. H., C. S. Carnell, and A. L. Cleghorn. 2007a. The Words-in-Noise (WIN) test with multitalker babble and speech-spectrum noise maskers. *Journal of the American Academy of Audiology* 18(6):522–529.

Wilson, R. H., R. A. McArdle, and S. L. Smith. 2007b. An evaluation of the BKB-SIN, HINT, QuickSIN, and WIN materials on listeners with normal hearing and listeners with hearing loss. *Journal of Speech, Language, and Hearing Research* 50(4):844–856.

Wilson, R. H., C. P. Trivette, D. A. Williams, and K. L. Watts. 2012. The effects of energetic and informational masking on the Words-in-Noise test (WIN). *Journal of the American Academy of Audiology* 23(07):522–533.

Appendix E

Biographical Sketches of Committee Members and Staff

COMMITTEE MEMBERS

Theodore G. Ganiats, M.D. (*Chair*), is professor emeritus of family medicine at the University of California, San Diego (UCSD). Dr. Ganiats is a member of many professional associations, including the Society for Medical Decision Making, Academy Health, the American Public Health Association, and the International Society for Quality of Life Research. He was the founder and first executive director of the UCSD Health Services Research Program. He has served as a member or chair of more than 50 national guideline, quality, and performance panels spanning multiple disciplines. He served as the first director of the National Center for Excellence in Primary Care Research at the Agency for Healthcare Research and Quality. In 2017–2018, he participated in a project with the American Academy of Otolaryngology-Head and Neck Surgery related to the development of measures of quality of care for age-related hearing loss. Dr. Ganiats has an M.D. from UCSD. He is an elected member of the National Academy of Medicine.

Kendall M. Campbell, M.D., is professor and chair of the Department of Family Medicine at the University of Texas Medical Branch in Galveston, Texas. He is the Sealy Hutchings and Lucille Wright Hutchings Chair in Family Medicine. Dr. Campbell is nationally recognized for his research affecting underrepresented groups in medicine. He has published over 100 peer-reviewed manuscripts, several book chapters, and has contributed to National Academy of Medicine publications. He has received honors and awards for his service including the Martin Luther King, Jr., Distinguished Service Award, the Exemplary Teacher Award, and the 2021 Society of Teachers in Family Medicine President's Award. Dr. Campbell is a founding director of the Society of Teachers in Family Medicine Leadership through Scholarship Fellowship through which he mentors and provides faculty and leadership development to early career family medicine faculty all over the country. He has received funding through the Health Resources and Services Administration to expand this work to faculty beyond family medicine. Dr. Campbell was elected to the National Academy of Medicine as part of the class of 2021. He completed his medical training at the University of Florida College of Medicine and residency at Tallahassee Memorial Healthcare.

Tamala David, Ph.D., M.P.A., M.S., FNP, is a native resident of Rochester, New York; an area with a large deaf population. She grew up in a household with a deaf grandmother (a sign language user) and is passionate about issues related to the health and well-being of deaf and older adults who are hard of hearing. Dr. David received her bachelor's degree in nursing and master's degree in public administration (with an emphasis in health care and a certificate in nonprofit management) from the State University of New York College at Brockport. She received her master's degree in nursing, with a specialty as a family nurse practitioner, and a Ph.D. in health practice research from the University of Rochester. In general, her projects have addressed population health issues at local, national, and international levels. She has more than a decade of experience providing education related to community health nursing and deaf health to nurses and physicians at all levels locally, nationally, and internationally. At the State University of New York College at Brockport, Dr. David teaches courses related to community health nursing, locally and internationally. She has received compensation as a member of the Rochester Prevention Research Center: National Center for Deaf Health Research at the University of Rochester since 2004 and has been a member of other research/health project teams at the University of Rochester since 2015. She has served in uncompensated roles on advisory committees and the board for the Rochester Chapter of the Hearing Loss Association of America since 2017.

Larry E. Humes, Ph.D., is a distinguished professor emeritus at Indiana University. He has served as associate editor, editor, and editorial board member for several audiology journals. Dr. Humes has received the Honors of the Association and the Alfred Kawana Award for Lifetime Achievement in Publications from the American Speech-Language-Hearing Association and the James Jerger Career Award for Research in Audiology and a Presidential Award from the American Academy of Audiology. He is a fellow of the Acoustical Society of America and of the International Collegium on Rehabilitative Audiology. His most recent research activities have focused on age-related changes in auditory perception, including speech-understanding ability, and on outcome measures for hearing aids. He is currently a co-principal investigator on a research contract from the Patient-Centered Outcomes Research Institute evaluating hearing aid fitting methods. Dr. Humes received his Ph.D. in audiology from Northwestern University, where he now holds an appointment as an adjunct professor.

Alan M. Jette, Ph.D., is emeritus professor and dean at Boston University's Sargent College of Health and Rehabilitation Sciences and served as Professor of Health Policy and Management at the Boston University School of Public Health from 2005 to 2017. He also served as Professor of Rehabilitation Sciences at the Massachusetts General Hospital Institute of Health Professions from 2012 to 2021. Dr. Jette is an international expert on rehabilitation and a leader in developing patient-centered rehabilitation outcome measures in a range of challenging clinical areas such as work disability, post-acute care, spinal cord injury, and neurological, orthopedic, and geriatric conditions. He has authored more than 250 publications in the rehabilitation sciences field and served as a principal investigator for numerous studies funded by the National Institutes for Health, the National Institute on Disability, Independent Living, and Rehabilitation Research, the Agency for Healthcare Quality and Research, and several foundations. Dr. Jette has served as a member of more than a dozen boards and committees at the National Academies of Sciences, Engineering, and Medicine. He chaired the Institute of Medicine (IOM) committee that authored the 2007 report, *The Future of Disability in America*. In addition to cochairing the IOM Forum on Aging, Disability, and Independence he was chair of the IOM Committee on the Use of Selected Assistive Products and Technologies in Eliminating or Reducing the Effects of Impairments. Dr. Jette was elected to the National Academy of Medicine in 2013. He earned a bachelor's degree in physical therapy from the State University of New York at Buffalo and a master's degree and Ph.D. in public health from the University of Michigan.

Colleen G. Le Prell, Ph.D., is the head of the Department of Speech, Language, and Hearing and the director of the recently launched Clinical and Translational Research Center at the University of Texas at Dallas, where she holds the Emilie and Phil Schepps Professorship in Hearing Science. Dr. Le Prell has received funding from government, industry, and philanthropic sources for research that programmatically advances the understanding and prevention of noise-induced hearing loss. Her research activities are currently funded by the National Institutes of Health (NIH) and the

Department of Defense. She has previously led clinical trials evaluating possible prevention of noise-induced hearing loss and recently published two comprehensive review papers discussing hearing loss endpoints. Dr. Le Prell previously served as president and in other leadership roles for the National Hearing Conservation Association, and from 2017 to 2025 she served as an invited member of the Centers for Disease Control and Prevention's National Institute for Occupational Safety and Health National Occupational Research Agenda Hearing Loss Prevention Cross Sector Council. She is an invited participant in the World Health Organization "Make Listening Safe" campaign. Since October 2024, she has served as chair of the Auditory System Study Section for the NIH Center for Scientific Review. She is an associate editor for the *Journal of Acoustical Society of America* and the *International Journal of Audiology*, and she serves on the editorial board for *Hearing Research*. In 2020, she was compensated for participation in the Technical Advisory Board Annual Meeting for Hearing Lab Technology. Since 2021, she has received compensation for leading the Scientific Advisory Board for Bellucci Translational Hearing Center Creighton University. From 2021 to 2023, she was a coeditor for a journal supplement on behalf of the Defense Hearing Center of Excellence Pharmaceutical Interventions for Hearing Loss committee: working group on patient outcomes. From 2019 to 2022, Dr. Le Prell was a Board Member for the American Academy of Audiology Foundation and on a leadership advisory team for the National Hearing Conservation Association. From 2018 to 2019 she was a member of the American Academy of Audiology Task Force on the Role of Audiologists in the Provision of Pharmaceutical Agents for the Prevention or Treatment of Hearing loss. From 2018 to 2019 she was a member of the American Academy of Audiology Musician Task Force for Best Practices for Working with Musicians. She completed a Ph.D. in psychology and a postdoctoral fellowship in auditory pharmacology at the University of Michigan in laboratories located at the Kresge Hearing Research Institute.

Uchechukwu Megwalu, M.D., M.P.H., is a professor in the Department of Otolaryngology-Head & Neck Surgery and division chief of comprehensive otolaryngology at Stanford University School of Medicine. He received his undergraduate degree from McMaster University in Hamilton, Ontario, Canada. Dr. Megwalu received his medical degree from Washington University School of Medicine, completed his residency at New York Eye and Ear Infirmary, and received his M.P.H. degree from Icahn School of Medicine at Mount Sinai. After residency, Dr. Megwalu joined the faculty at Icahn School of Medicine at Mount Sinai, where he served as director of otolaryngology at Queens Hospital Center, and assistant regional director of otolaryngology for Queens Health Network from 2011 to 2015. Dr. Megwalu joined the Division of Comprehensive Otolaryngology at Stanford in 2016.

His clinical interests include thyroid and parathyroid disorders, head and neck tumors, sinusitis, and chronic ear disorders. Dr. Megwalu conducts outcomes/health services research, with a focus on health literacy, health disparities, and comparative effectiveness research.

Catherine V. Palmer, Ph.D., is a professor in the Departments of Communication Science and Disorders and Otolaryngology at the University of Pittsburgh and serves as the director of audiology for the University of Pittsburgh Medical Center Integrated Health System. Dr. Palmer conducts funded research in the areas of auditory learning post hearing aid fitting, the relationship between hearing and health outcomes, and matching technology to individual needs. She is currently in the process of developing a hearing screening product, but it is not on the market. She has published over 150 articles and book chapters in these topic areas as well as provided over 200 national and international presentations. Dr. Palmer teaches graduate level amplification courses at the University of Pittsburgh and serves as editor-in-chief of *Seminars in Hearing*. She is a licensed audiologist in the state of Pennsylvania. Dr. Palmer is a past president of the American Academy of Audiology and received the Honors of the Academy in 2023. She received her Ph.D. from Northwestern University prior to joining the faculty at the University of Pittsburgh.

Carla Perissinotto, M.D., M.H.S., served as the first associate chief for geriatrics clinical programs at the University of California, San Francisco, from 2017 to 2021. In that role, she managed both inpatient and outpatient clinical programs. Dr. Perissinotto is a professor in the Division of Geriatrics, Department of Medicine. She is board certified in internal medicine, geriatrics, and palliative medicine. Her main work has been in home-based medical care where she provides medical care to homebound older adults. Dr. Perissinotto is passionate about working with diverse communities and improving the training of internal medicine residents and all learners in the care of older adults. She is also a recipient of the highly competitive Health Resources and Services Administration Geriatric Academic Career Award 2010-2015, with which she developed curricula to teach a wide range of learners on the care of elderly patients in diverse settings. Dr. Perissinotto has also gained national and international recognition for her research on the effects of loneliness on the health of older adults. She is frequently invited to discuss her research and discuss the clinical and policy implications of the health effects of loneliness.

Thomas A. Powers, Ph.D., is the founder/managing member of Powers Consulting, LLC, providing management consulting to the hearing health industry. He serves as an expert audiology consultant and strategic advisor for the Hearing Industries Association, and a limited partner in Amplifi, LLC. Dr. Powers received his B.S. from the State University of New York at Geneseo, and his M.A. and Ph.D. in Audiology from Ohio University. He began his career as a partner in an audiology private practice and has over 35 years of experience in the hearing health care industry. Prior to his current role, he was vice-president, government services and professional relations, for Sivantos, Inc. During his tenure at Siemens/Sivantos he was the compliance officer for 7 years. Dr. Powers is a member of American Academy of Audiology, Academy of Dispensing Audiologists, American Speech, Language and Hearing Association, International Society of Audiology, is a Distinguished Policy Fellow in the National Academies of Practice, and is a member of the American Auditory Society and served as president from 2004 to 2006. Dr. Powers currently holds an appointment as assistant professor in the Graduate Faculty in Biomedicine at Salus University and as adjunct research professor at Ohio University. In addition to his professional experience, Dr. Powers is also a hearing aid user.

Nicholas Reed, Au.D., Ph.D., is an associate professor in the Optimal Aging Institute with appointments in the Departments of Otolaryngology-Head and Neck Surgery and Population at the New York University Grossman School of Medicine. He is the director of an audiology core, where he oversees the integration and management of hearing measures into multiple large epidemiologic cohort studies and clinical trials. His research focuses on the association of hearing loss among older adults and healthy aging outcomes including cognitive decline and health resource utilization, the effect of hearing intervention on health outcomes, and novel models of hearing care delivery. He was awarded the Early Career Research Award in 2021 from the American Auditory Society. He is currently compensated as an editor for the *American Journal of Audiology* and previously served in uncompensated roles on scientific advisory boards for Shoebox Audiometry from 2018 to 2021 and Neosensory from 2021 to 2023. In 2022, Dr. Reed coauthored an editorial on the use of the pure-tone average as a universal metric of hearing to improve public awareness and understanding of hearing. Dr. Reed completed his clinical doctorate at Towson University, an audiology clinical fellowship at Georgetown University Hospital, and his research doctorate at Johns Hopkins University. He previously served on the National Academies committees *Evaluating Hearing Loss for Individuals with Cochlear Implants* and *Review of Relevant Literature Regarding Adverse Events Associated with Vaccines.*

Sherri L. Smith, Au.D., Ph.D., is an associate professor in the Department of Head and Neck Surgery & Communication Sciences and is the chief of audiology across the Duke University Health System. She holds a faculty appointment in the Department of Population Health Sciences and is a senior fellow in the Center for Aging. Prior to joining Duke in 2018, she spent 15 years at the Mountain Home Tennessee Veterans Affairs Medical Center and was an associate professor at East Tennessee State University. Dr. Smith's clinical, research, and teaching experience focuses on hearing rehabilitation in older adults, with an emphasis on hearing aids, cochlear implants, and patient-centered audiologic rehabilitation. She has a background in patient-reported outcome measure (PROM) development, and the use of several PROMs in the assessment of self-perceived hearing difficulty and hearing rehabilitation outcomes in clinic and in research studies. Dr. Smith is a member of the American Auditory Society, Academy of Rehabilitative Audiology, and the American Speech-Language-Hearing Association. She was recently elected Fellow of the American Speech-Language-Hearing Association. Dr. Smith's training includes her Au.D. and Ph.D. from the University of Florida (2001/2003), followed by completion of the Veterans Administration Research Career Development program (2005–2013).

Fan-Gang Zeng, Ph.D., is a professor of otolaryngology in the School of Medicine, professor of biomedical engineering in the Samueli School of Engineering, and the founder and director of the Hearing and Speech Laboratory at the University of California, Irvine. Dr. Zeng has expertise in engineering better treatments for hearing loss and tinnitus. He is a member of the Collegium Oto-Rhino-Larygologicum Amicitiae Sacrum and a fellow of the American Institute for Medical and Biological Engineering, the Acoustical Society of America, and the Institute of Electrical and Electronics Engineers. Dr. Zeng works closely with industry; he holds several patents as well as stock in several companies, but none directly in the space of outcome measures for adult hearing loss. He was elected to the National Academy of Engineering in 2023.

NATIONAL ACADEMY OF MEDICINE FELLOWS

Cameron Gettel, M.D., M.H.S., is an assistant professor in the Department of Emergency Medicine and a clinical investigator at the Yale Center for Outcomes Research and Evaluation. He also serves as the codirector of the Yale Emergency Scholars Fellowship. Dr. Gettel's research aims to advance the understanding of emergency department care transitions in the growing geriatric population through the identification and development of patient- and caregiver-reported outcome measures and then to design, implement, and validate innovative care transition strategies and interventions to improve clinical outcome. At the Yale Center for Outcomes Research and Evaluation, he works to develop the next generation of performance measures across multiple care settings. Dr. Gettel has led work with the Society for Academic Emergency Medicine and the American College of Emergency Physicians, respectively addressing fundamental emergency workforce topics and developing innovative models to improve quality measure reporting within the specialty. Dr. Gettel received a B.S. from Elizabethtown College and an M.D. from Pennsylvania State College of Medicine. He completed a residency in emergency medicine at Brown University followed by a health services research and policy fellowship in the National Clinician Scholars Program at Yale University.

Paule Joseph, CRNP, Ph.D., is an early-career Afro-Latina nurse scientist, educator, and philanthropist who was born and raised in Venezuela, South America. As an international expert in chemosensation and metabolic diseases, she bridges the intersections of nursing, science, nutrition, public health, policy, and health disparities. She is a 2019 NIH Lasker Scholar and Distinguished Scholar. She is chief of the Section of Sensory Science and Metabolism in the Division of Intramural Clinical and Biological Research at the National Institute on Alcohol Abuse and Alcoholism with a dual appointment at the National Institute of Nursing Research. Dr. Joseph leads a multidimensional translational research program combining research and clinical practice focused on chemosensation (taste and smell), obesity, and substance abuse. Her interdisciplinary laboratory team conducts research focused on understanding neurological and molecular mechanisms underlying chemosensation and motivational pathways of eating behaviors and how they might differ among individuals with obesity, alcohol, and substance use disorders. Dr. Joseph is a leader of national and global nonprofit organizations dedicated to decreasing health disparities and increasing minority health promotion and access. When individuals reported taste and smell loss during the COVID-19 pandemic, Dr. Joseph and her team began investigating the effects of the SARS-CoV-2 virus on the chemical senses.

NATIONAL ACADEMIES STAFF

Tracy A. Lustig, D.P.M., M.P.H. (*Study Director*), is a senior program officer with the Health and Medicine Division of the National Academies of Sciences, Engineering, and Medicine (the National Academies). Dr. Lustig was trained in podiatric medicine and surgery and spent several years in private practice. In 1999 she was awarded a congressional fellowship with the American Association for the Advancement of Science and spent 1 year working in the office of Ron Wyden of the U.S. Senate. Dr. Lustig joined the National Academies in 2004. She has directed consensus studies on the geriatrics workforce, oral health, ovarian cancer research, social isolation and loneliness, and the pediatric subspecialty workforce, and served as the codirector for a 2022 study on nursing home quality. She has also directed workshops on hearing loss and healthy aging, the allied health workforce, the use of telehealth to serve rural populations, assistive technologies, and biomarkers of disability. In 2009 Dr. Lustig staffed an Academies-wide initiative on the "Grand Challenges of an Aging Society" and subsequently helped to launch the Forum on Aging, Disability, and Independence. She is the study director for the Committee on Meaningful Outcome Measures in Adult Hearing Health Care. Dr. Lustig has a doctor of podiatric medicine degree from Temple University and an M.P.H. with a concentration in health policy from the George Washington University.

Ella Morse, M.P.H., is a research associate with the Health and Medicine Division of the National Academies of Sciences, Engineering, and Medicine (the National Academies). Before working at the National Academies, she directed the Arlington Public Schools COVID-19 Response Team as lead pandemic coordinator. In this role, she served 42 schools, 28,000 students, and 7,000 staff members by managing weekly in-school testing and case investigations, implementing mitigation strategies, and safeguarding isolation guidelines and procedures. Previously, Ms. Morse completed internships focusing on COVID-19 surveillance for the New Hampshire Department of Health and Human Services and women's health research for the New Hampshire Women's Foundation. She holds a B.S. in public health with a minor in sustainability and an M.P.H. concentrating in epidemiology, both from the George Washington University.

Abian Hailu, B.S., is a senior program assistant with the Health and Medicine Division of the National Academies of Sciences, Engineering, and Medicine (the National Academies). Prior to joining the National Academies, he worked as an intern for two maternal health organizations focusing on policy research and reproductive justice. In this role, Mr. Hailu helped implement a new program aimed at supporting fathers alongside mothers during the postpartum period. Additionally, he created and helped distribute a comprehensive nutrition database specifically tailored to promote perinatal health in underserved areas. Mr. Hailu holds a B.S. from Virginia Commonwealth University in health sciences with a minor in psychology.

Sharyl J. Nass, Ph.D., serves as senior board director of the Board on Health Care Services and co-director of the National Cancer Policy Forum at the National Academies of Sciences, Engineering, and Medicine (the National Academies). The National Academies provide independent, objective analysis and advice to the nation to solve complex problems and inform public policy decisions related to science, technology, and medicine. To enable the best possible care for all patients, the board undertakes scholarly analysis of the organization, financing, effectiveness, workforce, and delivery of health care, with emphasis on quality, cost, and accessibility. The forum examines policy issues pertaining to the entire continuum of cancer research and care. For more than two decades, Dr. Nass has worked on a broad range of health and science policy topics that includes the quality and safety of health care and clinical trials, developing technologies for precision medicine, and strategies to support clinician well-being. She has a Ph.D. from Georgetown University and undertook postdoctoral training at the Johns Hopkins University School of Medicine, as well as a research fellowship at the Max Planck Institute in Germany. She also holds a B.S. and an M.S. from the University of Wisconsin–Madison. She has been the recipient of the Cecil Medal for Excellence in Health Policy Research, a Distinguished Service Award from the National Academies, and the Institute of Medicine staff team achievement award (as team leader).